THE ANTHROPOLOGY OF MEDICINE

D0060960

THE ANTHROPOLOGY OF MEDICINE

_____ From Culture to Method

Third Edition

Edited by
Lola Romanucci-Ross
Daniel E. Moerman
Laurence R. Tancredi

BERGIN & GARVEY
Westport, Connecticut • London

Library of Congress Cataloging-in-Publication Data

The anthropology of medicine : from culture to method / edited by Lola
    Romanucci-Ross, Daniel E. Moerman, and Laurence R. Tancredi.—3rd
    ed.
        p. cm.
    Includes bibliographical references and index.
    ISBN 0–89789–490–1 (alk. paper).—ISBN 0–89789–516–9 (pbk. :
alk. paper)
        1. Medical anthropology. 2. Traditional medicine. 3. Materia
    medica, Vegetable. 4. Mental illness—Social aspects.
    5. Psychiatry, Transcultural. I. Romanucci-Ross, Lola.
    II. Moerman, Daniel E. III. Tancredi, Laurence R.
    GN296.A63   1997
    306.4'61—DC21   96–53993

British Library Cataloguing in Publication Data is available.

Library of Congress Catalog Card Number: 96–53993
ISBN: 0–89789–490–1
        0–89789–516–9 (pbk.)

First published in 1997

Bergin & Garvey, 88 Post Road West, Westport, CT 06881
An imprint of Greenwood Publishing Group, Inc.

Printed in the United States of America

The paper used in this book complies with the
Permanent Paper Standard issued by the National
Information Standards Organization (Z39.48–1984).

10 9 8 7 6 5 4 3 2 1

Copyright Acknowledgment

CONTENTS

PREFACE: THE CULTURAL CONTEXT OF MEDICINE AND THE BIOHUMAN PARADIGM

Medical systems emerge from attempts to survive disease and surmount death, and from social and cultural responses to illness and the sick role. Descriptions and analyses of this process in world cultures define a field known as medical anthropology. Although this process is an ancient one—perhaps 60,000 years old—with roots in the middle Paleolithic, the field of study is a relatively new one that began with systematic inquiries by anthropologists into health practices and explanations of disease in technologically primitive and peasant cultures.

This volume represents various aspects of the state of the art of medical anthropology, emphasizing what we have called the anthropology of medicine: a study of medical thought and problem solving, the acculturation process of the healer and physician in diverse cultural settings, and the social and cultural context of medicine. Our approach is from the perspective of cultural and medical anthropologists who have taught and worked with Western-educated physicians immersed in clinical and research medicine, as well as those who have worked with other healers and patients outside the bounds of modern biomedicine and surgery. One of us provides, in addition, the perspective of a physician.

Anthropological field research is an experience in abstraction; it is an exercise in putting particulars in brackets as we search for universals in elements and the relations among them. In this sense we have chosen to fuse the particulars of Western medicine with those from other cultures for conceptual analysis in what we have called the anthropology of medicine. Beyond the surface differences, we try to expose similarities of deep structure, to demonstrate that there is a path beyond culture and that one may focus on method.

We believe that medicine, in a very real sense, stands astride both the cultural and the biological dimensions of humankind, and we elaborate on this in particular in one chapter of Part IV. We believe that medicine is a kind of applied anthropology in the broadest sense of the term: action for human beings. As anthropologists who have learned a great deal from physicians and surgeons, we hope that the perspective we can bring to this complex cultural and biological exchange will be of value to those who, so much closer to the action, are in the very trenches we learn so much by observing.

This book, then, is designed for physicians and medical students, public health administrators and workers, and students in related health-science fields, as well as students and professionals in anthropology and social science who are interested in the practice of theory of health and healing. It is, in brief, a text for both the health sciences and anthropology.

For a century in the West, there have been two literatures regarding the health sciences. They have represented two different canons, or paradigms: the approaches of biomedical science and of behavioral science. To simplify somewhat, the biomedical paradigm tells that, for example, tuberculosis is "caused" by *Mycobacterium tuberculosis*, whereas the behavioral-science paradigm tells us that tuberculosis is "caused" by poverty and malnutrition. It is our contention that these two approaches can be integrated into one bio-human paradigm; further, we contend that the unifying factor is the concept of culture. By culture we mean the system of meaning—belief, knowledge, and action—by which people organize their lives. Such organization structures the diseases to which people are subject. As a simple case, schistosomiasis is a disease of irrigation agriculture; as a less simple case, the *windigo* psychosis of Algonquian Indians is a disease (characterized by homicidal behavior and cannibalistic fears) of a hunting people subject to great environmental fluctuations.

Diseases, however, are never experienced directly; illnesses, cultural constructs of "dis-ease," are what people experience. Illnesses are constructed of belief and knowledge, which vary with both space and time. A contemporary example might be hyperactivity, an illness with associated treatment(s) that did not exist before the 1970s. People debate whether it is a new "disease," a response, perhaps, to new environmental toxins (i.e., food additives), or whether it was "always there" but not recognized. *Either case* provides an example (slightly different ones, to be sure) of the role of the cultural process in sickness and health. If it was always there but not recognized, then we have a case of an invented illness. If it is a new disease, we have a case of cultural concerns (for "altered" foods) that have created a novel physiological disorder.

The theoretical value of such an approach seems evident. Human beings are simultaneously cultural and biological creatures, and these two dimensions necessarily interact. The study of human health and healing, in which people *attempt to influence directly the relationship between biology and culture*, is one rich with potential for learning fundamental things about what it means to be human.

The anthropologist takes a broad view of the world, and sees pre-modern Europe as a very unusual and special case—one of the least healthy societies in human history—subject to dozens of new and terrifying diseases as a consequence, essentially, of the great growth of the population of both humans and domesticated animals. This "one-two punch" of domestication and urbanization created conditions for the evolution and communication of infectious disease organisms on a scale unprecedented in human history, well beyond the abilities of the best-intentioned physician to control or prevent.

Consider, as an ideal comparison, the health status of Europeans and Native Americans in the year 1480. Paleopathological evidence indicates that the Native Americans were extremely healthy: they had a life expectancy longer than that of Europeans of the time. Life was difficult, and they suffered from accidents, fractures, rheumatic conditions, and, perhaps, trichinosis contracted from animals that they hunted. Scholarly debate rages regarding the origins of syphilis; some argue that it was introduced into Europe from America by members of Columbus's crew, while others state that it was an Old World disease. It is, however, the *only* ambiguous case; all the other diseases transmitted from one continent to the other went westward: smallpox, measles, typhoid, tuberculosis, cholera, diphtheria, plague—the list seems endless. These diseases had ravaged Europe for generations. They were also the single most important cause of the cataclysmic drop in the Native American population. The most recent available estimates suggest that between 1490 and 1890, the native population of the 48 contiguous United States dropped 90 percent, from 1.9 million to 200,000 (Thornton and Marsh-Thornton 1981). Similarly, it is estimated that the Australian aboriginal population dropped by 80 percent between 1788 and 1933 (White 1977). The poor health status of native peoples in colonial times was a consequence of colonialism, not a measure of indigenous health.

That Native Americans or aboriginal Australians had little medical wherewithal when confronted with cancer or influenza seems a misplaced criticism. What is most striking about non-Western medicine is how much people did with what they had. That many of the herbal remedies of the past have been supplanted by synthetic ones—many of which are, after all, modified natural products (for example, aspirin)—should not detract from the perspicacity of the original discoverers; and, as chapters attest, there may be much more of value that we can learn from non-Western medicine to enhance the biochemical basis of modern medicine.

But, perhaps because of the relative lack of powerful specific drugs in the non-Western pharmacopoeia, it is clear that many of these peoples were far more sophisticated and far more inventive than we in manipulating the social and human dimensions of medicine. This aspect of non-Western medicine may ultimately have the most to teach us about healing. Once one recognizes that the *form* of medical treatment affects the *outcome* of treatment, one can hardly leave it to chance, any more than one can prescribe drugs (however effective) by chance. The chapters in this book demonstrate that this *is* the case, and they show some of the forms that medical treatment can take; they show as well how deeply medical systems are embedded in culture.

Human beings are simultaneously biological and cultural organisms. For physicians to achieve their goal—to optimize human health—they must be intensely aware of this human duality. Our purpose is not to undercut the grounding of medicine in biology (tuberculosis *is* caused by a bacillus) but to assert that "medicine" is also grounded in culture (tuberculosis is *also* caused by poverty and malnutrition); moreover, and most importantly, these two dimensions are interconnected in many and complex ways.

As a very specific example, consider the character of medical diagnosis. Physicians, during the long years of training in which they gain their expertise, increasingly become members of the medical subculture—with a language, a system of values, and a conceptual framework for decision making—and, at least for a time, are separated from the arena in which they are later to be effective. Moreover, physicians must learn how to cope with the inevitable internal duality of medicine as both scientific and clinical. Whereas scientific medicine involves public research on aggregates, clinical medicine involves private treatment of individuals; the former is statistical, the latter is idiosyncratic; the former is concerned with the course of a disease, the latter with the history of an illness. As clinicians confront patients they have to mold them into categories, transforming unique constellations of experience, notions, beliefs, symptoms, and disease into types, a "case of the measles" or "lyme disease." For the clinician this is almost a necessity, but for patients it is simultaneously clarifying and dehumanizing. Whatever they "have" rules out other possibilities, but they are no longer discrete sufferers but members of a class.

And likewise for the physician: To diagnose is to classify and to predict a course and a treatment based on the vagaries of statistics and experience; it is to take what can always be a very serious risk. This risk has both structural and statistical dimensions. It is a structural risk in that validation is essentially derived from the response to treatment, which is temporally remote. It is a statistical risk in that "classic cases" are rare, in that medical theory must be manipulated to fit the unique characteristics of infinitely varying patients. To do this at all is to *ignore* much of what patients present and to select as *meaningful* a segment of their existence that is particularly diagnostic, that is, to ignore things that patients think are important, to dismiss some (perhaps much) of their lives as *unimportant*. Here we see a mutual commitment of patient and physician to an intrinsically categorical process—an intrinsically dehumanizing and distancing process—and this must occur regardless of the cultural distance between physician and patient. Indeed, the experience of many physicians is that among the most difficult patients are other physicians; perhaps it is only here that the physician can more easily translate the patient's discontent—and, perhaps, less easily ignore it. This dehumanization can only be exacerbated by additional cultural differences in general education, class, ethnic origins, and the like.

Whatever else diagnosis may be, it is first a social process based on interpersonal communication between the scientifically knowledgeable physician and the concerned patient. The physician should understand why and when a person seeks medical attention, how the patient views his or her own sickness, how the patient reports his or her symptoms and interprets his or her feelings, and what changes occur in the patient's life because of the illness or treatment. These factors are always influenced by the cultural backgrounds of patient and physician. Wide variation in patients' backgrounds and the cultural differences between doctor and patient may profoundly influence the diagnostic process and therapeutic course (Romanucci-Ross and Tancredi 1987).

Yet if the patient cannot act in concert with the physician, how is the physician to control the course of the patient's disease? As the patient gives up uniqueness for a diagnosis, he or she also gives up independence. And the new dependence is on the physician. Dependence can take many forms. The skill with which the physician projects an appropriate, empathetic concern and strikes a responsive chord in the patient will affect the richness and utility of the interchange. If the process is to be dehumanizing, it may as well be as useful as possible. The therapeutic exchange can be so structured that the patient can develop a sense of trust and security while the physician can develop a sense of responsibility and confidence, which will facilitate healing.

The physician must remember that when a diagnosis is pronounced, there should be no assumption that the patient understands it. The patient may never have heard the word before; if he or she has, it is inconceivable that he or she understands the term as the physician does. And it is the patient's *understanding* that will influence the response to treatment.

Furthermore, there is increasing evidence that a significant group of patients, even those among the highly educated lay public, are unable to comprehend the nature of the medical information provided in order to obtain an informed consent (Tancredi 1982). The physician has to be sensitive to the many medical and emotional factors affecting the patient.

The technique of patient interviewing can be a highly honed skill—focused but not rigidly structured; it should be flexible to adjust to the patient's perhaps abnormal attitudes and behavior (the patient is, after all, at least by his or her own definition, sick) but organized to elicit sufficient pertinent information in the available time to allow the physician room to take the diagnostic risk; and it should be so organized that the patient has an *appropriate understanding* of the diagnosis.

This third edition comprises chapters on research in medical anthropology; some are new, and a number have been thoroughly revised, since the nature of the data in some chapters necessitated updating. We believe they provide a foundation for a biohuman medical paradigm by demonstrating how culture—human belief, knowledge, and action—structures the human experience of disease, affects the ways in which *both physicians and patients* perceive and define illness, and influences the matrices of decision making in the subcultures attempting to communicate about problems of health care and medical research.

REFERENCES

Romanucci-Ross, L., and L. R. Tancredi. 1987. "The Anthropology of Healing." In *In Search of the Modern Hippocrates*. Roger J. Bulger, ed. Iowa City: University of Iowa Press, 127–46.

Tancredi, L. R. 1982. "Competency for Informed Consent: Conceptual Limits of Empirical Data." *International Journal of Law and Psychiatry* 5:51–63.

Thornton, R., and J. Marsh-Thornton. 1981. "Estimating Prehistoric American Indian Population Size for United States Area: Implications of the Nineteenth Century Population Decline and Nadir." *American Journal of Physical Anthropology* 55:47–54.

White, I. M. 1977. "Pitfalls to Avoid: The Australian Experience." In I. M. White, *Health and Disease in Tribal Society*. Amsterdam: Elsevier.

PART I

MEDICAL SYSTEMS AND THE USES OF CHOICE

The exchange of ideas between cultures concerning health and illness is no simple matter, and the interacting of medical systems provides a rich context for understanding the relationships between biology and the culture of medicine. In any particular case, how and which specific disease and disease concepts and specific medicines and ideas about their use and effectiveness are exchanged is an empirical question. But models for the nature of the exchange and the historicocultural context for the exchange provide an important focus for analyses that can (and often do) make prediction, and therefore health planning, possible.

The common conceit of the West—that the benefits of scientific medicine are obvious, as are the truths on which those benefits are based—is a conceit held by all people regarding their own medical systems. It was as true for the bleeding and purging physicians of the nineteenth century as it is for the neurosurgeons and cardiologists of the twentieth. These ideas, associated with fundamental principles of belief about the major cosmological issues of life and death, generally are very deeply held. In the United States in recent years, major political and social conflicts have raged over what can be narrowly conceived as medical issues. Abortion, the definition of death (or medical death), and the notion of "death with dignity" are examples of such issues where broad, deeply held beliefs influence medical matters.

Medical systems are, of course, part of the larger cultural system of any group. Ideas about sickness, health, and curing constitute a system—that is, one can consider the parts and analyze the relations among the parts. Such beliefs within cultural systems in contact are either reinforced or become diminished or distorted; the reason for this is that the system must, and does, include those persons whose perception and cognition conceptualize the system. A dramatic example of this involves the enormous social and ecological changes undergone by the northeastern subarctic Algonquian Indians in response to the introduction of European diseases (Martin 1978). Martin, in what is nominally a history of the fur trade, argues that the commercial involvement of Indians in the fur trade was more apparent than real. For a people whose essential notion of all illness was that it represented retaliation by the spirits of mistreated prey animals, the vast epidemics of European diseases (often occurring long before the Indians actually encountered Europeans) presented a serious enigma. They had not mistreated the animals; why, then, were the animals killing them? Martin's argument is, in effect, that the Indians decided that, for unknown reasons, the animals had declared war on them. Adopting, when available, the providential armaments of the newly appearing Europeans (guns and steel traps), they fought back. The result was the Indian involvement in the fur trade and, not incidentally, the extermination of much of the animal life of North America.

The most extraordinary aspect of this case appears in ethnographic accounts of the descendants of these fur traders (Tanner 1979). They are today returning to a pattern very similar to the one they pursued four centuries ago, carefully harvesting animals with appropriate reverence and ceremony. The great epidemics of the past are, of course, gone, and (vaccinated) hunters may be as healthy as their ancestors were. The war, it seems, is over; and, after four centuries of incomprehensible social change, at least some essential notions of health for these people are unchanged.

The chapters in this section all focus on the ways in which the conceptual portions of medical systems change (or do not change) as a result of culture contact.

Romanucci-Ross's discussion of medicine in Italy describes the medicalization of folk medicine by Western medicine—the active attempt by official providers of health care to impose a standard structure on diagnostic and curing practices. Despite massive propaganda, and even apparent complicity—seen in repeated visits to state insurance doctors—traditional ideas of body image and dysfunction prevail. Here a population is engaged in creating a grammar and rhetoric of a health culture and life-style that begins to link its traditions to what it learns of medical scientific method, both in practice and from the media. Conjoining these modalities, the people explore therapeutic choices and evolve new ethnotherapies.

In Kidwell's account of the relationship between Aztec and Spanish medicine, we find that these systems exchanged a broad range of items that facilitated the identification and cure of a variety of diseases. Indigenous plants were used by the conquerors for the diseases they found in the New World; more problematic for the host populations were the diseases brought to them. Analysis of the Spanish and Aztec sources from the period can isolate features of the crosscultural transactions in cognition. Upon what bases could the exchange of information occur? In this case, herbal medicine became a primary focus of exchange. Even though the Spanish used the Galenic binary structure of hot and cold, whereas the Aztecs classified plants by their uses, both groups found plants useful as food, medicine, and ornament. Aztec epidemiology and pharmacology fused with Greek and Galenic views; in time, the Mexican folk-medicine system emerged, perhaps the most fully syncretic medical system known.

In contrast, in the Admiralty Islands (Manus) of New Guinea during the 1960s, curative practices appeared to involve a critical usage of Western medical resources that fell into patterns of acculturative and counteracculturative sequences (see Romanucci-Ross 1977). For the more traditional Manus, Western medicine excelled in lower-level descriptions of disease; it was, however, incomplete and did not admit to multiple etiology in a bio-social-moral frame. One could predict which cures would be selected by knowing where the family or individual stood on the acculturation gradient. There was also a general attempt to match "whiteman's medicine" with "whiteman's diseases."

Crandon-Malamud gives us an illustration of illness and medicine as a trope to make statements about social relations. Medical dialogue occurring in a pluralistic and stratified society may often provide a context for the construction and negotiation of ethnic identity among Aymara Indians and *mestizos* in a rural Bolivian village on the altiplano. Diagnostic opinions are simultaneously statements about a condition, the sick person, the person delivering the opinion, and nosological and etiological categories deriving from the various medical traditions in the culture (Indian, folk, and Western).

These cases represent a range of medical interactions. The Mexican case represents a fully syncretic system; the Italian case represents a stable, unshakable one; and the Bolivian case demonstrates that medical choices are often driven by narratives that affirm or create ethnic identity. Exactly what determines the ultimate outcome of the interaction of medical systems is not yet clear. However, it *is* clear that this interaction is a complex and difficult one, not susceptible to facile prediction.

REFERENCES

Martin, C. 1978. *Keepers of the Game: Indian-Animal Relationships and the Fur Trade.* Berkeley: University of California Press.

Romanucci-Ross, Lola. 1977. "The Hierarchy of Resort in Curative Practices: The Admiralty Islands, Melanesia." In *Culture, Disease, and Healing.* David Landy, ed. New York: Macmillan, 481–86.

Tanner, Adrian. 1979. *Bringing Home Animals: Religious Ideology and Mode of Production among Mistassini Cree Hunters.* New York: St. Martin's Press.

1

CREATIVITY IN ILLNESS: METHODOLOGICAL LINKAGES TO THE LOGIC AND LANGUAGE OF SCIENCE IN FOLK PURSUIT OF HEALTH IN CENTRAL ITALY

LOLA ROMANUCCI-ROSS

For primitive societies and for folk or peasant cultures in the Europeanized world, including the United States, we have access to a considerable body of literature on health-seeking behavior and the contexts in which thera-peutic decisions are made (Landy 1977; Logan and Hunt 1978). Investigators of illness and healing in different cultures have tended to agree on the universality of some aspects of health-seeking behavior regardless of other manifest differences in those cultures: One of the areas of agreement con-cerns client management of alternative systems of curative practices. Strat-egies employed by patients, or by their families on their behalf, range from serial exclusion of one system in preference of another to making decisions that combine elements of several systems. Such combinations appear to the patient to maximize medical effectiveness.

The serial exclusion principle was well exemplified in the search for cures in a primitive group in the Admiralty Islands of Melanesia, where I was able to observe and record traditional medicine and the very beginnings of West-ern medicalization. What was occurring here could be described as shifting game strategies in curing events when the choices were multiple and the choosers were persons whose behavior ranged from traditional to "decultur-ated" to somewhat well adapted to living between two cultural models. Depending on the locus of the person on the acculturation continuum, the progression of resort to curing practices in health-seeking behavior was pre-dictable. Among the somewhat acculturated, Western medicine was chosen

Reprinted from *Social Science and Medicine* 23(1), Lola Romanucci-Ross, "Creativity in Illness: Methodological Linkages to the Logic and Language of Science in Folk Pursuit of Health in Central Italy," copyright 1986, Pergamon Press PLC, with kind permission from Elsevier Sci-ence Ltd, The Boulevard, Langford Lane, Kidlington OX5 1GB, UK.

first; when this failed, traditional medicine was sought. The reverse was true for the traditional individual. The patterning became more complex in response to external political events, but the choices remained serial and temporally mutually exclusive (Schwartz 1969).

Such a process in a society based on kinship relationships provides a sharp contrast to a society that functions primarily through political and economic institutions. In the United States, groups pressuring public opinion regarding proper professional help in regaining health were instrumental in institutionalizing the historical defeat, so to speak, of many alternative systems of health care so that allopathic medicine won the field. It did so, shortly after the turn of the century, by marshaling all the strategic resources at its command: the political, the judicial, the scientific (including technological advances), and the growing public confidence in the idea of progress and expertise (Cohen 1983).

The culture under discussion in this chapter includes some elements and some combinatorial rules similar to those in both the above-mentioned groups. Aspects of a process of what might appear to be an eclectic approach to health-seeking behavior will be examined. We will consider similarities and differences between the country folk and the urban dwellers in assumptions about the body and body image and in uses of ecological resources such as plants, animals, other persons, and "natural laws." We will explore the roles of healer and client and indicate borrowed models for behavior from other spheres and arenas in the culture. In particular, we emphasize that in this culture we find a manner of creating a grammar from sectors of experience, a grammar that poses no difficulty in combining mythology, religion, "natural law," and the logic and language of modern science.

We focus on a rural area of small villages (with a large town, Ascoli Piceno, included as a reference point) in the eastern-central portion of Italy (Romanucci-Ross 1983). Ascoli Piceno, the town, is the province of Ascoli Piceno and in the region of the Marches, which is surrounded by Tuscany, Umbria, Lazio, Abruzzi, and the Adriatic Sea. Ascoli Piceno, the province, contains both rural and urban communes *(comuni)* further divided into *frazioni*, or smaller units, of which the urban *comune* of Ascoli has fifteen. Less than one-fourth of the communal populations are now engaged in agriculture, with the rest in small businesses or service and other industries that include power plants, metallurgy, engine repairs, textiles, paper, and chemical products. Agricultural activities include the raising of grain and grapes, and animal husbandry. Among the rural population, less than half own their own farmlands; the others are part of the *mezzadria*, a sharecropping system, and about 6 percent are hired laborers (see *Monografia Regionale* 1977). Many of the people living in the town have migrated from the countryside or have relatives there. Although there is a slow but continuous flow of rural people into the town, the past several years have witnessed a slow but steady flow of town people moving into country houses (sometimes within the villages);

they drive to work each day. Not only do rural areas maintain their own dialects in an energetic bilingualism that small children can negotiate, but the town has its own dialect, Ascolano.

Ascoli had its own identity prior to commercial and political exchanges with Rome. There is early archaeological evidence that the Sabines from the north and the Illyrians from the coast came and settled among early Neolithic inhabitants (Balena 1979). Ascoli was dominated and culturally influenced by the French under both Charlemagne and Napoleon. The period from 300 to 800 has been called by some "the abortive Germanization of Italy" (Pulgram 1958). Early German dialects left some traces, particularly in this area, and the patron saint of Ascoli is Saint Emidio, one of its early bishops of German provenience. Except for a brief period as a republic, Ascoli was a papal possession for hundreds of years (Berselli 1961).

At the present time, ethnomedicine in the region appears eclectic, and we will examine the process leading to such an end point. As for the basic features of what might be called folk medicine (see below), these are more akin to Sebald's description of its rural German counterparts (Sebald 1980) than they are to the system described by De Martino (1961) for a region of southern Italy. In the south, De Martino found the rich symbolism of the bite of the tarantula, aesthetic uses of color and music in cures, and possession, all within a cultural-historical context of early Greek versions of Christianity. We do not intend to describe in detail the folk medicine of Ascoli and its *frazioni*, for this has, in part, been done elsewhere (Romanucci-Ross 1982, 1983), and a description of folk medical practices for a nearby region in the Abruzzi is also available (Moss and Cappannari 1960). As indicated earlier, we will focus on continuity and change in health care.

Many features of the folk medical model in this area, it should be noted, are shared by both urban and rural populations. In the countryside one can still see red ribbons on oxen, strands of garlic on some entry doors, sprigs of rue on windows, a branch of pine in a child's bedroom. The sprigs and branches can be found in some urban houses also, just as the red or gold horns worn as amulets are found everywhere, for fear of the evil eye is not just a rural phenomenon. If in the country one fears the destruction of crops or animals by the evil eye, in the town one fears that the *mal occhio* will cause a son to fail an examination at a professional school or ruin a daughter's chances for a good marriage. In both rural and urban groups one finds healing and curing attended to through the uses of the rituals of religion (Catholicism), fear of witches, use of healers, uses of herbals,[1] foods as medicinals, and cures at spas and other watering places.

The folk medical model makes the following assumptions about illness and curing: Illness can occur through indifference to the "natural law" of the need for psychosomatic system balance; that is, all things should be done or consumed in moderation. One must not exert oneself physically or emotionally, for too much passion can be ruinous. (Common targets for excesses of emotion are the liver, and the gastrointestinal tract.) One must avoid extremes of temperature or sudden temperature change. Too much air is harmful, especially for small children. The image of the body in good health is one that has a sufficient mass and density that it cannot "waste away" easily, hence being somewhat overweight is considered a sign of good health. The blood can become "impure," of course, through the lack of attention to system balance.

An individual does have control over illness caused by this lack of attention, and the remedies are to be found in nature itself through foods as medicinals, plants, mountain air, sulfurous waters, sunshine, ocean and shore, and mineral waters. Privileged natural states can be used to bring relief from pain: A man with rheumatism can be stepped over many times by a pregnant woman who recites a formula. Honored moral states are curative: A man afflicted with a mental or "nervous" illness can regain his normal mental state by giving a shirt of his to a "man of virtue" to wear and to return to him, then wearing that shirt. A privileged genealogy can heal: One can go to the town of Amatrice to a family that, having in the distant past hosted St. Peter, has had, and still has, the power to heal (with oil and salt) the effects of the bite of a viper both in sheep and in humans. There is healing to be found in a town with deep mythico-historical roots: Offida, named after *ophis*, which means "snake" in Greek, has a long tradition of venerating serpents and has long had a sanctuary for cures.

But there are illnesses for which one is not expected to assume responsibility, and over these one has little control. Being victimized by ghostly or spiritual phenomena is considered an external cause, as is a soured social relationship. If one is dealing with a witch, these two causes can coalesce. Persons who possess the "evil eye" are often not to blame for the strong gaze that harms others, but one must try to avoid them. One also can try not to be too successful or talk too much about one's success, for that will attract envy and the evil eye. The witch *(strega)* appears to be an ordinary person going about her business, but she can be causing harm to you or your animals. A bewitched horse, ill, sweating, and with braided mane, has been ridden (and braided) by a witch who just keeps working at the washing fountain as though it had nothing to do with her. Against such incursions one has only the "horn" or medals or prayers, the touching of iron, and the knowledge instilled in every child that to be overtly and conspicuously successful is to invite disaster through illness or loss. Animal spirits can bring illness or bad luck, but this seems to be a function of the happenstance of being at the wrong place at the wrong time.

Remedies for the above are the use of the healers (women) and the *mago* (a male herbalist and magic-worker who can counter the wickedness of female witches and restore good health or good fortune), for healer and witch are never the same person. Preventive medicine in the folk medical model exhorts one to obey "natural laws" of avoiding excess, and the rules of social relationships exhort one to avoid envy, although it is acknowledged to be almost impossible.

The folk model is an ideology shared by healer and patient. Nevertheless, the Western allopathic physicians in the city seek to restructure the interpretation of health and illness through use of their professional model, which is in constant transformation because of scientific innovations (Romanucci-Ross 1982). These physicians are consulted from time to time and, at first glance, there appears to be an affinity in behavior among the village people in this area and what others do elsewhere concerning health-seeking behavior. Such behavior does follow the pattern of a hierarchy of resort in curative practices (Schwartz 1969), but the combinatorial aspects of the process in this region of Italy were unlike those I had observed in other cultures.

Through the local pathologist and general practitioner in the large town, I began to find a number of healers and diagnosticians who were active in the referral group that linked folk and Western medicine; that is, their patients were (and often correctly) sent to a specialist in Ascoli Piceno. This referral pattern tends to foster meaningful information exchanges among the strata of healers. The patient never feels he or she is abandoning an ideological system because it is the healer or diagnostician who refers the patient to the allopathic physician; and the physician does not belittle the gifts of the healer who sent him the patient. These healers were referred to (by clients) as "the one who can be trusted" or "the one who knows."[2]

Clients of folk practitioners and healers represent a diversity of socioeconomic backgrounds. Among those who spoke freely and at great length to me of their hierarchies of resort in curative practices were middle-class housewives and wives of professionals, entrepreneurs, or other businessmen. Some of the clients were men; among them were a judge, a lawyer, a businessman, and a schoolteacher. In short, the sometime clients of folk healers are by no means characterized as rural and/or poor.

The three individuals named below, in particular, were frequented by a large number of persons in the urban and rural area.

Pasqualina, a diagnostician and healer, was called a *paragnostica* ("she who knows what is adjacent or peripheral"); she diagnosed by auscultation and by almost—but not quite—touching soft body parts, with trance behavior signaling the end of the physical examination. Her calling is considered scientifically validated because psychologists from the University of Bologna and other parapsychologists presumably had studied her. Her waiting room is usually overflowing with patients, who busily diagnose each other's presenting symptoms as they wait.

Another healer is called Maria La Santa. She seemed to me to be a living example of the syntactic structuring of folk symbols uniting religious passion, illness, and healing. She was described to me by some physicians as a "true hysteric"; her stigmata, covered by bandages or gloves, are said to bleed on certain Fridays preceding religious holidays.

The latest fad in healers is Olga, a pranotherapist; she has strong "electrical forces" in her hands and heals by touching. Patients bring her bottles of mineral water that she tosses into a vat. After washing her hands with baking soda, she runs her hands through the water and pours it back into bottles. This water has restored appetites and "cured malignant tumors." Through her thoughts, she resurrected her aunt in Philadelphia and cured a child in New York City by sending a packet in the mail. Laws of time and space do not exist for magic, anywhere. Olga has printed a book at her own expense, *Io ti segno, dio ti cura* (I mark you, God cures you), which her clients feel privileged to purchase. This story of her life and healing contains photographs of her curing practices, including one of her aunt rising from the casket. The iconography is religious but the language is "scientific"; she speaks of forces, vectors, and gravity. "Before" and "after" X-ray pictures of Olga's cures are included, yet she wants patients to be religious believers.

These three healers represent others who are referred to as mystic or *sensitiva*. Some, but not all, of the following qualifications need to be present in such a healer: stigmata on the palms of the hands, visions, revelations, clairvoyant episodes, out-of-body experiences, hyperesthesia, and a profoundly altered sense of time. Any or all of these validate divine power, and they usually appear after a long and painful illness. Often the voice of a dead father provides the final incentive to use the power. But the power is not always welcome. The provocation in an unprepared person of the sudden emergence of paranormal faculties is thought to cause mental illness. Hence, dealing with psychic healers is not without risk. One woman was told by her summoned mother's spirit, "Maria, stop this nonsense and learn to live *in the world!*" Efficacy and power of healers are a function of distance from the patient; the further the distance to be traveled, the greater the belief in curative powers. Maria La Santa was highly touted by those who came from Abruzzi to be healed; and reaching Olga and Pasqualina required a drive of some eighty kilometers. Some patients go to the Black Madonna, which requires several hours' driving. Her miracles are particular for certain illness and infertility (Moss and Cappannari 1953).

Such healers function in a culture in which there is a great interest in emotional states and, as for Wilhelm Reich, the language of emotions is the language of the body (Reich 1969). Ecstatic, hysterical, or dream states, hypnotic states, meditative states, and trances are not considered irrelevant to the business of life in the world, but are viewed as central to meaning in the teleological unraveling of one's destiny. These states are grounded in the religious experience. In addition, and in the present time, however, we find a configuration also deeply embedded in Italian culture, the language and logic of science, from which those who create new epistemes in health can borrow in abundance. Both in verbal communication and in journalistic writings, individuals and groups adopt the language of science to describe healing techniques. For example, emotional states create "bioenergetics" that allow the healer to absorb energy from the universe that can be transmitted to others. "Bioenergetics" can also be absorbed from archaeological sites; it provides power to cure rheumatics and arthritics in a process known as bioradiant, or biomagnetic, therapy. Such healers allow themselves to be studied "so that science might learn" about the natural laws expressed in their persons. These studies provide a scientific testimonial to these powers.

Folk healers, then, have been affected by the media and have joined a syncretic movement to link proofs of treatment efficacy from religion, medicine, and technology. Although there have been many cultural exchanges between nation-state and peasant enclaves, the nature of the exchange has been transformed radically. In the past it was occasioned mainly through migratory movements or administrative contact. In recent times the media-mediated information has blitzed the countryside as well as urban centers, engendering a syncretism of rational and metaphorical thought in reconstructing the path from illness to health.

Pharmacists in the region have joined the syncretic revolution and sell not only pharmaceuticals from commercial laboratories but also herbals and plant medicinals. With the client (patient) they discuss the virtues, the drawbacks, and the side effects of natural and of synthetic compounds from the pharmaceutical firms. Many pharmacists and some others interested in medical care are part of a *farmacognosia* movement whose members hold congresses and publish materials on all aspects of the study of drugs of plant origin. Gathered and classified are any materials dealing with the morphology and physiology of medicinal plants, pharmacological properties of botanicals and their active ingredients, or the gathering, conserving, or preparing of medicinals from botanicals. Old folk remedies once scoffed at are believed if read about in the newspaper. It is thought quaint and authenticating to read that "animals go for certain plants when sick" or a biblical tale about curing an ulcer with a poultice of figs. But such deference to ingenuity will not be shown to one's own folk predecessors. Through the young, the folk are once again learning to use words such as *decotto* (decoction) and *infuso* (infusion), and there are small lexicons of the most used medicinal terms. They are read to from dictionaries of infirmities with corresponding herbal remedies, and once more become believers. This goes beyond the reinforcement of traditional culture. In reversing the path of learning by going from younger to older, and by learning from print and other media, the tradition changes, yet elements that might have dropped out are preserved.

In the conscious models of thought about natural healing, some plants are considered to be only medicinal, but some are used both as food and as medicinals simultaneously (see Table 1.1). For example, onions, garlic, almonds, chestnuts, lettuce, rice, and many other everyday foods are consciously included in meals for their medicinal properties. One or more family members may need temporary relief from distressing symptoms or a minor affliction. A continuum exists from nutrient to medicinal usage, depending

Table 1.1
Conscious Models of Plants Used Both as Foods and as Medicinals

Name		Scientific Name	Local Usage	Parts Used
Almond	mandorlo	Prunus amygdalus Batsch	constipation, digestion, burns	fruit
Anise	anice	Pimpinella anisum L.	indigestion, stomach, spasms, cough, toothache	seeds
Apple	melo	Malus communis Poir	convalesence, constipation, diarrhea, stomach, hypertension	fruit
Asparagus	asparago	Asparagus officinalis L.	liver, intestinal cleaning, lungs, anemia	plant
Barberry	crespino (uva de la Madonna)	Berberis vulgaris L.	constipation, appetite, menstruation, as scorbutic	fruit, leaves
Basil	basilico	Ocinum basilicum L.	nervousness, cough, cold, spasm	plant
Beet	bietola	Beta vulgaris L.	anemia, cystitis, kidney, constipation	fruit, leaves
Carob	carrubo	Ceratonia siliqua L.	diarrhea, weight reduction	seeds, fruit
Chestnut	castagno	Castanea sativa Mill	diarrhea, cough	fruit, young leaves
Chicory	cicoria	Cichorum intybus L.	appetite, anemia, liver, skin, constipation, spring tonic	leaves, roots
Chili pepper	peperoncino	Capiscum annum L.	rheumatism, diarrhea, lungs	fruit
Coriander	coriandolo	Coriandrum sativum L.	digestion, spasm, dizziness	leaves
Cucumber	cetriolo	Cucumis sativus L.	colic, pruritis, skin problems	fruit

Elder tree	sambuco	Sambucus nigra L.	hemorrhoids, nervousness, constipation, colds	flowers, leaves fruit
Fennel	finocchio	Foeniculum vulgare (Mill) Gaertn	bronchitis, diarrhea, impotence, cough, nursing mothers	fresh leaves, roots
Fig	fico	Ficus carica L.	constipation, cough, pregnancy	fruit
Garlic	aglio	Allium sativum L.	parasites, thought to have antibiotic qualities, prevents respiratory illnesses	bulb
Hazelnut	nocciolo	Corylus avellana L.	fever, circulatory problems	leaves, seeds, fruit
Lemon	limone	Citrus limon L.	cleansing, skin, hair, teeth; digestion, diarrhea	fruit
Lettuce	lattuga	Lactuca sativa L.	skin problems, nervousness	leaves
Licorice	liquirizia	Glycyrrhiza glabra L.	stomach, spasm, cough	roots, rhizome
Mallow	malva	Malva silvestris L.	constipation, appetite, menstruation, as scorbutic	roots, leaves, flowers
Marjoram	maggiorana	Origanum majorana L.	nervousness, stomach problems, dizziness	plant
Medlar tree	nespolo	Mespilus germanica L.	stomach, skin, diarrhea	fruit, nuts, leaves
Mint	mente	Mentha rotundifolia L.	appetite, digestion, mouth cleanser, cough, hiccups, convulsions	leaves, flowerets

13

Table 1.1 (Continued)

Name		Scientific Name	Local Usage	Parts Used
Mustard	senape	Brassica nigra L.	bronchitis, respiratory illness	seeds
Oats	avena	Avena sativa L.	diabetes, skin disorders	seeds
Olive	olivo	Olea europea L.	hypertension, rheumatism, burns, hair care, liver, constipation	fruit
Onion	cipolla	Allium cepa L.	cleansing of respiratory system	bulb
Orange	arancio	Citrus simensis Osbeck	appetite, digestion, nervousness	fruit
Parsley	prezzemolo	Petroselinum sativum Hoffm.	anemia, digestion, rheumatism	plant
Rice	riso	Oryza sativa L.	diarrhea and other gastro-intestinal problems	grain
Rosemary	rosmarino	Rosmarinus officinalis L.	heart, liver, nervousness	flowering plant, leaves
Sage	salvia	Salvia officinalis L.	depression, impotence, frigidity, menstruation, gums, emphysema	leaves, flowerets
Strawberry	fragola	Fragaria vesca L.	angina, diarrhea, kidneys	fruit, young leaves
Sunflower	girasole	Helianthus annus L.	fever, hypertension, nervousness	leaves, flowers, seeds
Wheat	frumento	Triticum vulgare vill.	pregnancy, impotence	grain

on the framing and context. A nutrient in one meal may be a medicinal in another. Table 1.1 indicates that most disturbances are gastrointestinal. These somatic expressions relate to a loss of control over interpersonal relations (Romanucci-Ross 1983).

Since the mid-1980s an interest in psychotherapy and psychoanalysis has existed in this region. A psychoanalyst from Rome came to give classes in analysis to a group of five or six people in the city. Psychoanalytic percepts have filtered into the reports of workers in the child welfare center. Wayward children are often described in Freudian terms, and so are their performances on the Rorschach, Thematic Apperception, or other projective tests. Several rural people have begun to send problem children to a young psychoanalyst at his residence in the country. In his opinion, these people probably would not go to his office in the city.[3]

The incipient practice of psychoanalysis has had the curious effect of providing more clients to healers like Pasqualina, Maria La Santa, and Olga. Their therapies inform bored and disaffected middle-class, middle-aged housewives of former lives they have lived in Egypt or India, or the Himalayas. "Pasts" are described in great detail, with the appropriate psychological terminology for the reasons and the meanings of their experiential transformations through time. The clients I have interviewed seemed very pleased with healers in this respect. Why are they pleased? First of all, what does classic or neoclassic Freudian analysis purport to do for the patient? It rephrases the problem (the neurosis, the psychosis, the malaise, the malfunctioning) experientially and existentially. You are not who you think you are, precisely, nor have you understood the nature of the bonding to those who have caused or are causing your grief. You are told that some of these present relationships are transferences of an earlier unconscious or subconscious life. (Since you are not aware of them, they might just as well have been in another life, in another epoch.) So, not unlike the psychoanalyst, this type of healer provides the fantasy framework within which these women can formulate and try to resolve their problems.

This method of the *sensitiva* provides her patient with an extraordinary advantage, for this cultural group, of not calling into question the virtues of the constellations of bondings known as the family. Here the patient is not an oppressed individual seeking liberation from the constraints of the nuclear family at a certain stage of development. The problem pinpointed is that a dyad or constellation of characters from former times must patiently work out a solution. No one here and now is at fault. Regardless of the etiology of the fantasy therapy, we have sufficient evidence from psychologists to assert that positive attitudes emerge and multiply between parties who engage in exchange behavior that is mutually rewarding (Byrne and Rhamey 1965).

The above creative synthesis, in trying to grapple with pathology and disordered states, contrasts with our (American) system, in which many consult chiropractors, osteopaths, and others who are not in the standard referral system and whose healing techniques have a history of conflicting claims to legitimacy (Morley and Wallis 1978).

Festinger (1957) held that when several conflicting cognitions are held at the same time, an individual or group is motivated to abolish or weaken the dissonance. Actually, the contrary may obtain, as demonstrated by research on religious cult behavior in Melanesia (Schwartz 1962), where it was shown that dissonance (i.e., ritual observed but no promised cargo) only served to fortify an even stronger belief in the eventual arrival of the cargo. The total commitment of believers was put in doubt by failure, not the relationship between the ritual behavior and the material goods that should have appeared because of it. We can transfer this lack of falsifiability of the tenets of a belief system to the belief of the patient in the healer, regardless of results. But, in addition to such adherence to faith in all cultures, we find the resort to curative practices fluid and vacillating for an even more pragmatic reason: The parameters of assessment are many, and an outcome may or may not be related to following or not following the doctor's advice.

So, too, in this Italian community, the failure of cure did not call into question any of the components of the constantly emerging system, or the manner in which the elements were articulated. Information on health and illness in this culture is structured from metaphors in Catholicism and the language of science as it appears in newspapers, magazines, film, and theater. In this manner the nodes (a node is a nexus of information) provide centers for linkages of information systems for the new grammar to be used in the emergent discourse about health and illness. Included are the results of inductive, deductive, and analogic methods from medical science, as well as the revisionist thrust of alternative healing systems. Neologisms accrue throughout the entire network of the referral system.

The result is both agglutinative and assimilative, but the method represents a pulling away from the power holders of allopathic medicine. It is a centrifugal model and much like the model for local politics. It is good, it is thought, when no one gets the absolute majority of votes. It is good that no one school has the monopoly on restoring health to the body or the mind.

Folk practitioners aid communication between patients and modern providers of health care as the latter try to interpret the way patients report symptoms as well as responses to diagnoses and prescriptions. Folk practitioners do this through the referral system, of which they are a part, and thus lessen the burden of the health care providers. Along with the patient they explore feedback loops linking new knowledge systems to the old ones; when the new and the old are similar, this validates the entire system of the old.

Unlike health care providers in the United States, neither the healers nor the allopathic physicians have strategic resources to employ as a political pressure group, as the latter group has in the United States. Yet the health seeker and the health care provider in our Italian model are more aware than their American counterparts that medicalization implies social control and that science is a socially negotiated and politically contested enterprise. Confronted with the discourse and the knowledge structures for management of health, the folk of this area, informed by tradition and the media, continually create an event-based grammar. New information about health and illness stimulates continuous restructuring of all the information, slowly changing the discourse as grammatical elements are added, deleted, or reenvironed. As knowledge structures are dismantled, their complexity is ignored and the discourse surrounding them is mapped onto new events, as we have described for evolving therapeutic choices in diagnostics, in ethnopharmacology, in psychoanalytic therapies, and in modifications of notions of nutrition and of preventive medicine.

At any point in time the health care system for any individual or group is metastable. What remains relatively stable is the mechanism that generates change. For Ascoli Piceno and environs these generators are grounded in the religion (Catholicism), in attitudes toward authority, and in the cultural-historical substratum of ideology and values regarding health and illness. Since January 1980 all Italians have been entitled to health insurance under the provisions of the Servizio Sanitario Nazionale. The persistent distrust of government, indifference to politics, and lack of belief in the honesty and capability of bureaucrats (Banfield 1958) should interest observers as physicians, patients, and their families negotiate the new health care system.

NOTES

1. For examples of uses of herbs as medicinal plants, see mint, rosemary, sage, basil, coriander, majoram, and mallow in Table 1.1.

2. "One who knows" and shared his knowledge with me was Gaetano Mari, who in daily life is an agricultural worker for an order of *frati* (brothers) in the city. In preparing a compress for rheumatic pains he will take equal parts of corn flour, mustard seeds *(Brassica nigra L.)*, juniper *(Juniperus communis L.)*, dried figs, and the flax plant *(Linum angustifolium Huds)*, boil them in vinegar, and apply the compress. Men who are thus afflicted should also eat celery leaves; women, parsley. For eczema he will burn grapevines, boil the ashes, and apply them. As gargle for a sore throat he boils the tender needles from the tip of the pine tree. He has many other such remedies that he assured me are effective; he has "believers" in the city and the country who follow his advice, as well as the advice they receive from physicians.

3. I am grateful to Dr. Francesco Giovanozzi, psychologist and psychoanalyst in Ascoli Piceno and Pedana, for giving me access to professional reports and discussing, in a general way, the nature of his relationship with his patients.

REFERENCES

Balena, Secondo. 1979. *Ascoli nel Piceno*. Ascoli Piceno: Edizioni Turistiche, 97–100.
Banfield, Edward. 1958. *The Moral Basis of a Backward Society*. Glencoe, Ill.: Free Press.
Berselli, Aldo. 1961. "La Restaurazione e le società Segrete nelle Marche." In *L'Apporto delle Marche al Risorgimento Nazionale. Atti del Congresso della Storia*.

30 Settembre–2 Ottobre 1960. Ancona: Comitato Marchigiano per le Celebrazioni del Centenario dell Unita d'Italia, 69–91.

Byrne, D., and R. Rhamey. 1965. "Magnitude of Reinforcement as a Determinant of Attraction."*Journal of Personal and Social Psychology* 2:889–99.

Cohen, Marcine. 1983. "Medical-Social Movements in the United States (1840–1980): The Case of Osteopathy." Ph.D. dissertation, University of California, San Diego.

De Martino, Ernesto. 1961. *La Terra del Rimorso: Contributo a una Storia Religiosa del Sud*. Milan: Il Saggiatore.

Fabiani, Giuseppe. 1958. *Collana di Pubblicazioni Storiche Ascolane. Ascoli nel Quattrocento*. 2 vols. Ascoli Piceno: Societa Tipolito-grafica Editrice.

Festinger, Leon. 1957. *A Theory of Cognitive Dissonance*. Evanston, Ill.: Row, Peterson.

Foster, George M., and Barbara Gallatin Anderson. 1978. *Medical Anthropology*. New York: John Wiley and Sons.

Landy, David. 1977. *Culture, Disease and Healing*. New York: Macmillan.

Logan, Michael H., and E. E. Hunt, Jr. 1978. *Health and the Human Condition: Perspectives on Medical Anthropology*. North Scituate, Mass.: Duxbury Press.

Lott, B., and J. Lott. 1969. "Liked and Disliked Persons as Reinforcing Stimuli." *Journal of Personal and Social Research* 11:129–37.

Monografia Regionale per la Programmazione Economica Marche. 1977. Coordinated by Vincenzo de Nardo. Varese: Editrice Giuffre.

Morley, Peter, and Roy Wallis. 1978. *Culture and Curing*. London: Peter Owens.

Moss, Leonard W., and Stephen C. Cappannari. 1953. "The Black Madonna: An Example of Culture Borrowing." *Scientific Monthly* 73:319–24.

———. 1960. "Folklore and Medicine in an Italian Village." *Journal of American Folklore* 73(288):95–102.

Pelto, Pertti J., and Gretel H. Pelto. 1983. "Culture, Nutrition and Health." In *The Anthropology of Medicine: From Culture to Method*. Lola Romanucci-Ross, Daniel E. Moerman, and Laurence R. Trancredi, eds. South Hadley, Mass.: Bergin & Garvey.

Pulgram, Ernst. 1958. *The Tongues of Italy*. Cambridge, Mass.: Harvard University Press.

Reich, Wilhelm. 1969. *Character Analysis*. T. Wolfe, trans. New York: Farrar, Straus and Giroux. 1969.

Romanucci-Ross, Lola. 1982. "Medicalization and Metaphor." In *The Use and Abuse of Medicine*. Marten W. de Vries, R. L. Berg, and Mack Lipkin, Jr., eds. New York: Praeger Scientific, 171–82.

———. 1983. "Italian Ethnic Identity and Its Transformations." In *Ethnic Identity: Cultural Continuities and Change*. George de Vos and Lola Romanucci-Ross, eds. Chicago: University of Chicago Press, 198–226.

Schwartz, Lola Romanucci (aka Lola Romanucci-Ross). 1969. "The Hierarchy of Resort in Curative Practices: The Admiralty Islands, Melanesia." *Journal of Health and Social Behavior* 10:201–9.

Schwartz, Theodore. 1962. *The Paliau Movement in the Admiralty Islands: 1946–1954*. Anthropological Papers of the American Museum of Natural History 49, pt. 2. New York: The Museum.

Sebald, Hans. 1980. "Franconian Witchcraft: The Demise of a Folk Magic." *Anthropological Quarterly* 53:173–87.

2

AZTEC AND EUROPEAN MEDICINE IN THE NEW WORLD, 1521–1600

CLARA SUE KIDWELL

Spanish settlers in the New World came bringing with them their customs, their foods, and their diseases. The New World represented a strange and even exotic place. It was primarily of interest to the Spaniards because of the material wealth of gold and silver that they dug from its bowels. However, although the gold and silver of the New World mines had a tremendous impact upon the role of Spain as a world power and upon the course of European history, the most lasting contributions of the North and South America continents to the European civilizations were not the minerals that represented wealth. Instead, it was the plants, primarily in the form of foodstuffs but also in the form of herbs for medical use, that were ultimately to provide a wealth far greater than the mineral wealth of the New World continents.[1]

In return for that wealth, the Spaniards gave to the native peoples of the New World many diseases (e.g., smallpox, typhus, cholera, and measles) and a life of slavery in the mines that largely decimated the Indian populations within approximately 50 years of the conquest.[2] Although there are many problems in calculating exact numbers of native populations at the time of conquest from which to calculate a rate of decline, the fact of the population decline due to disease is readily apparent.

The Spaniards, in their turn, suffered from what is often called "Montezuma's revenge," that is, gastrointestinal distress, as well as respiratory ailments induced by the living conditions in the New World. Agustin Farfan, a Spanish physician writing in Mexico in 1579, listed the principal afflictions of the Spanish residents of the New World as "flaqueza y indigestión del estómago" (weakness and indigestion of the stomach), "tauardete" [*sic*] (typhus), "dolor de costado" (tuberculosis), and "de la colica passion y del dolor de Ijada" (appendicitis).[3] Juan de Cardenas also devoted a chapter to the subject of Spanish ills in his *Primera Parte de los Problemas y Secretos Maravillosos de la Indias*. Those ills included stomach problems, menstrual difficulties, rheumatism, liver trouble, and urinary difficulty.[4] Native populations were also subject to respiratory and gastrointestinal diseases, of course, but the Spanish seemed much more susceptible to the illnesses of the New World.[5] One disease with major social and economic importance for the Spanish was syphilis.[6] One of the important export items from New Spain to Europe was guaiacum, highly touted in Europe as a cure for syphilis.[7] The theory seemed to be that syphilis was indeed a New World disease, and thus its cure should be a New World plant.

ACCULTURATION AND MEDICAL PRACTICE

It was in the area of medical practices that early forces of cultural assimilation began to affect both cultures, European and native. The tradition of medical "simples" was well known to European settlers in the New World, and since herbal medicines formed an important part of the medical practices of the Aztecs, Incas, and other native peoples with whom the Europeans were coming into contact, it can reasonably be assumed that at least some of these herbal remedies were adopted by the Spanish colonists and thus constituted a case of reverse acculturation, the adoption of native practices by the conquering civilization.[8] But the basic premises of culture underlying the methods of treatment in the European and the Aztec societies were so different in so many respects that one would expect much less exchange of therapeutic methods outside of herbal medicines.

A body of writings by European physicians and Aztec writers (or information supplied by Aztecs) concerning materia medica in sixteenth-century New Spain shows some of the processes of acculturation that were going on in medical practice. These writings are sources of medical information that demonstrate the differing viewpoints of two cultures toward medical practices (and, as well, the viewpoint of one culture toward another). From these writings one can determine the interaction that was going on between native and European physicians, the differences and similarities of their viewpoints, and the extent to which any true influences were being exchanged in the first 80 years of contact between the cultures.

The body of writings under discussion comprises the following: from the Europeans, the *Opera Medicinalia* of Francisco Bravo (1525?–1594?), published in 1570 in Mexico;[9] the great work on New World plants compiled by Francisco Hernández (1517–1578) and published in part in 1628 under the title *Rerum Medicarum Novae Hispaniae Thesaurus . . .* ;[10] the *Tractado Breve de Anathomia y Chirugia . . .*, published in Mexico by Agustin Farfan (1531?–1604?) in 1579 (with a second edition, *Tractado Breve de Medicina*, in 1592);[11] and *Summa y Recopilacion de Chirugia . . .*, by Alonso López de Hinojosos

(1535–1597), published in Mexico in 1578 (with a second edition in 1595).[12] And from the Aztecs, *Libellus de Medicinalibus Indorum Herbis* . . . , written by Martin de la Cruz and translated from Aztec into Latin by Juan Badianus (both authors were Aztecs),[13] and the *Historia General de las Cosas de Nueva Espana*, compiled by Bernardino de Sahagun, a Franciscan priest, from Aztec informants.[14] The intricate relationship among these various works provides a fascinating insight into the differences between New World native medical practices and European concepts of medicine, and the bases upon which exchanges of information could be made. The convergences and divergences of viewpoints constitute an important chapter in the development of medicine in sixteenth-century colonial America.

COMMUNICABLE CONCEPTS IN AZTEC AND EUROPEAN MEDICINE

Aztec medicine was deeply embedded in the matrix of a culture that was highly religious in nature. Erwin Ackerknecht has commented on so-called primitive medicine that it is based essentially on supernaturalism, with some rational elements, whereas modern medicine is based essentially on rationalism in spite of its magical elements.[15] An important aspect of medical practice among the Aztecs, for instance, was the ascription of causes of disease to the wrath of various deities. Xipe Totec caused skin diseases and was appeased in a yearly ceremony in which sufferers of skin diseases walked in procession wearing the skins of sacrificial victims who had been flayed.[16] European medicine, on the other hand, was firmly rooted in the rational traditions of the Greeks, and the Galenic theory of the mechanism of the four humors and their balances in the body prevailed among European physicians. Attribution of qualities of hot and cold, wet and dry, was part of the Galenic tradition and linked European medicine with Aristotelian thought. Certainly all of the European physicians discussed here—Bravo, Farfan, López de Hinojosos, and Hernández—were firmly within the Galenic tradition of medicine. The Aztec writers, Badianus and de la Cruz, and the Aztecs upon whose information Sahagun based his work, represented a worldview based on the actions of the deities and their role in causing disease, as well as certain definite Aztec cultural values concerning fear, anxiety, and other emotional states that might be said to constitute illness.

Of the possible points of communication between the two systems of medical thought, two seem to be particularly important. The most obvious point of communication was a common belief in herbal medicines. The tradition of medical simples was well established in Europe, and the use of New World plants for therapeutic purposes would seem obvious. A second point of communication, which bears on the first, is the pragmatic nature of medical practice in the New World, where there were few physicians and where the Spaniards were confronted with new conditions relating to their health. Of the works under consideration, those of Bravo and Hernández are the most strongly based in the theoretical Galenic and Aristotelian tradition of European thought, whereas those of Farfan and López de Hinojosos, although they subscribe to Galenic doctrines, represent more the orientation of the practicing physician confronted with new situations in a land where traditional European physicians were not readily available to large parts of the colonial population. In many ways the Badianus-de la Cruz manuscript, with its almost cookbooklike approach to medical prescriptions, is closer to the Farfan and López de Hinojosos books than it is to the work by Sahagun, which sought to reflect the Aztec worldview as a whole, which devotes limited attention to specific medical practices (book 10), and which treats the role of physicians (book 10), the nature of herbal medicines (book 11), and the role of deities as causes of illness (book 1) in different parts of the final version of the work.[17]

In terms of the historical connections among all of the works under discussion, there is evidence that the writers could have been in contact with one another in various ways, either directly or indirectly. Connections among the works by Bravo, Farfan, and López de Hinojosos are established in the prefatory material of the three books. Bravo wrote endorsements for both Farfan's *Tractado Breve de Anathomia y Chirugia* and López de Hinojosos's *Summa y Recopilacion de Chirugia*.[18] His endorsements may have been sought because of his reputation, which had been established with the publication of his *Opera Medicinalia* (generally considered the first medical work published in the New World). Farfan also endorsed López de Hinojosos's work.[19] López de Hinojosos, in turn, was associated with Francisco Hernández at the Royal Hospital for Indians in Mexico, where he practiced for 14 years.[20] The connection between Hernández and Bernardino de Sahagun is very tenuous, but it appears that Hernández might have used a section of Sahagun's work in his own book (although without proper attribution).[21] Sahagun, in his turn, was for a time associated with the College of Tlalolco, where Juan Badianus and Martin de la Cruz were students. Sahagun was at the college from 1536 to 1540, and again in 1545. There is no indication that he was directly associated with de la Cruz and Badianus, whose work, the *Libellus*, was completed in 1552.[22] However, Sahagun's interest in the collection of Aztec materials may well have indicated a more general interest in writings by Aztecs at the college.

Despite the historical conjunction of these writers, there is very little evidence that transmission of knowledge from Aztec to European sources, or from European to Aztec sources, was taking place during the first century of contact. Rather, the conjunction is more evidence that differing cultural traditions were coming into contact but that, except in the area of herbal medicine, little exchange was taking place between the two cultures in medical practices.

European Physicians and Their Interpretations

Of the writers under consideration, Francisco Bravo seems most clearly the European physician. His work is divided into four major parts: a discussion of typhus (which he calls "tauardeste" [*sic*] and its treatments; a disputation in the form of a dialogue concerning the uses of venesection to treat disease; a discussion of the doctrine of critical days in the treatment of disease; and a description of sarsaparilla, with a discussion of its qualities (Bravo maintained that the plant is hot and dry, rather than being cold, as some maintained).[23] Bravo makes numerous references to Galen, and also to Arabic writers—Avicenna and Rhazes—as well as to Fracastorio and Laguna, his closer contemporaries.[24] He makes no mention of native medical practices, and the herbal remedies that he does mention (except sarsaparilla) are of European origin. For example, a remedy for plague includes "rosis, violis, hordeo, lactucis, capitiabus papaveris, soliis salicis, et cannarum et cucurbitae" mixed in water.[25]

Francisco Hernández, physician to Philip II of Spain, was sent by Philip to the New World to collect material on natural history. His work is more in the encyclopedic tradition of natural histories and herbals that were appearing in Europe during the sixteenth and seventeenth centuries. Although he used the Aztec names of plants, reflecting a classification system based on use (*quilitl* as a suffix referred to plants used as foods; *yochitl* referred to ornamental plants; *patli* referred to medicinal plants; and economic plants useful for building and material objects were referred to by several suffixes),[26] Hernández introduced his discussion with reference to the classification system of Theophrastus, who classified plants according to form: *arbor*, *herba*, *suffrutex*, and *frutex*.[27] Hernández is much more concerned with description of the form of plants, although he does include medicinal properties in some descriptions (*texaxapotla*, for example, when burned and its vapors breathed, cured sneezing and dried up phlegm in the eyes, nose, and mouth).[28] The drawings of plants in his work are much more naturalistic than those in the *Libellus* of Badianus and de la Cruz. His work is an important source of information on Aztec plants and, in some cases, their medicinal uses. However, it remained very much in the European tradition of descriptive natural history.

Farfan and López de Hinojosos both follow European traditions in their references to humors, and to Galen and Guido as authorities.[29] However, both also made reference to herbal medicines used by Aztec healers. In the 1579 edition of Farfan's work, he mentions, for instance, xoxocoyoles (for stomach disorders),[30] mechoacan (*iopmoea jalapa*, *Bryonia mechoacana*, as a purgative),[31] guayacan (*guaiacum officinale*, for "mal de Bubas"),[32] and sarsaparilla (which, in agreement with Bravo, he describes as hot, its heat moving vapors in the body).[33] In the 1592 edition of the work, which is indeed more a major expansion of the section of medical practices than simply a new edition, he includes 59 native plants as remedies.[34]

López mentions remedies newly described and discovered by experiments.[35] He mentions specifically guayacan, sarsaparilla, canafistola, and chichimecapatle as ingredients in a cure for *alferezia* (epilepsy).[36] In regard to specific medical practices, both Farfan and López mention bleeding as a curative technique, but López says that he has not seen bloodletting as a practice among the natives.[37] However, specific mention of bleeding as a practice in the cure of headaches is made in Sahagun's work.[38]

As their treatises indicate, both Farfan and López de Hinojosos are much more concerned with experience than theory. The endorsements for Farfan's book speak of his long years of experience as a physician (he evidently obtained his medical degree on 20 July 1567 from the Real y Pontificia Universidad de Mexico).[39] Farfan and López both describe their books as being intended for those who are far from cities and need to learn about remedies for illness and medical practices.[40]

In its general nature, the *Libellus de Medicinalibus* of Badianus and de la Cruz is similar to the works of Farfan and López de Hinojosos. It, too, is a description of medical practices, primarily based on herbal medicines. Its intended audience was Don Francisco de Mendoza, son of the viceroy of New Spain. The title of the book can be translated as "A Little Book of Indian Medicinal Herbs Composed by a Certain Indian, Physician of the College of Santa Cruz, Who Has No Theoretical Learning, but Is Well Taught by Experience Alone."[41] The emphasis is upon experience rather than upon theory, and the approach of the book is purely descriptive, including extensive recipes of herbal medicines. The book is organized in a straightforward head-to-foot manner, following the organization of the human body. The dedication of the work is very revealing in the attitudes of native physicians toward their Spanish overlords. Badianus and de la Cruz were, of course, educated at the College of Santa Cruz at Tlaloco, which was established by Franciscan missionaries to educate the sons of Aztec nobles. De la Cruz includes in the dedication the following statement:

Indeed I suspect that you ask so earnestly for this little book of herbs and medicaments for no other reason than to commend us Indians, even though unworthy, to His Holy Caesarian Catholic Royal Majesty. Would that we Indians could make a book worthy in the King's sight, for this is certainly most unworthy to come before the sight of such great majesty. But you will recollect that we poor unhappy Indians are inferior to all mortals, and for that reason our poverty and insignificance implanted in us by nature merit your indulgence.[42]

The *Libellus* is enlivened with colored drawings of the herbs that are described, and the work contains such typical Aztec remedies as acozoyatl for treatment of one affected by a whirlwind.[43] It is interesting to note that conditions such as "fatigue, . . . lassitude suffered by officials holding public office," "fear . . . or faintheartedness," and "mental stupor"[44] are included as conditions to be treated with herbal remedies. Although the work reflects Aztec traditions, it contains nothing of the rich religious traditions that underlay the practice of Aztec medicine. It reflects a European bias in its statements concerning the lowly status of the natives. Its concern for practical treatment rather than theory may represent a European orientation (Sahagun's book 10 follows the same head-to-foot orientation and statement of specific treatments) that ignored the religiously based aspects of Aztec medicine, but it may also reflect a kind of pragmatic orientation toward treatment of illness that is somewhat similar to the works of Farfan and López de Hinojosos.

Conflict between Rationality and Religion

If Bravo and Hernández represent the purely rational and theoretical tradition of European medicine, and Farfan and López de Hinojosos represent both the rational and pragmatic aspects, Bernardino de Sahagun represents the conflict of rational thought and religious belief, belief in both Christian and Aztec culture. The initial charge to Sahagun, given by the provincial father Francisco de Toral, was that Sahagun should write in the Nahuatl language those things that he considered useful for the maintenance of Christianity and the work and ministering of Christian doctrines.[45] Sahagun gathered information from Aztec informants and cross-checked his information with Aztecs in various parts of the country. But his original intent was to use the information to convince the Aztecs of the errors of their past ways. He thus included after his description of major deities a tract condemning the worship of those deities:

My children, perceive God's word, which is God's light. Thus will see those who live in darkness, who have lost the way; those who worship idols, who go with the sins of the devil, who is the father of lies. And thus will be known to them their gods and their lords which the word of God, which here, lying unfolded, revealeth how idolatry began. Likewise here are revealed many things concerning the error, misery, and blindness into which the worshippers of idols fell.[46]

Sahagun's work remains the standard source for descriptions of Aztec medical practices. It is interesting to note, however, that like the work by de la Cruz and Badianus, Sahagun's work was not published in his lifetime. Indeed, it was not until 1830 that even a partial edition of the work was published.[47]

Medical Knowledge from the New World

In the contacts between medical practices in the New World and the Old, the major point at which exchange of information took place was in the area

of herbal medicines. Indians were certainly treated by European practitioners in hospitals such as the Royal Hospital for Indians, where Hernández
and López de Hinojosos worked together. But in terms of the overall structure of medical practices, European physicians did not adopt any of the
religiously based ideas of the Aztecs concerning medical practices, and Aztecs did not immediately adopt any European practices that they did not
already have.

An interesting example of the transmission of knowledge from Aztec to
European sources is the plant *cacaloxochitl*, which is mentioned in Hernández's *De Rerum Medicarum*, the *Libellus*, and Sahagun's *Historia General*. The
physical description of the plant differs in the *De Rerum Medicarum* and the
Historia General. The physical description in Hernández reads as follows:

It is a tree of medium size with leaves like citrus, but much larger and with abundant
veins which run from the center vein to the edges. The fruits are one pod, very large
and red; the flowers are large, beautiful and of pleasing, pleasant scent, and are the
only part that is used; they are used to make nosegays, garlands and crowns, things
much used among the Indians and held in such esteem that they never appear before
a head person without offering beforehand some of these offerings. It makes milk.
Cooled and congealed, and applied, it is a cure for the illness of the breast which
comes from heat. Its marrow, taken in a dose in two drachms, cleanses the stomach
and the intestines.[48]

Sahagun describes the plant in the following terms:

It is a bush that they call cacaloxochitl; it has leaves that are somewhat broad, and
somewhat long, and downy. It has branches straight and spongy, and the leaves and
branches sometimes make milk, and this milk is sweet as honey. The flowers of this
tree are beautiful. They are called also cacaloxochitl. They are bronze colored, of
red, yellow and white. They have a delicate odor, and they comfort the spirit with
their odor. Through the districts of Mexico one has these flowers, but those which
come from warm lands are better; some are black. In former times these flowers were
reserved for the lords.[49]

Badianus and de la Cruz do not give a written description of the plant, but
their drawing shows a plant with red flowers and long, slender leaves. The
veins mentioned in Hernández's description do not appear in the drawing.[50]
The flowers of the plants are part of a very elaborate herbal formula entitled
"Trees and Flowers for the Fatigue of Those Administering the Government and Holding Public Office."[51] That the plant is the same in all three
sources, despite the discrepancies in written description, can be determined
primarily by the fact that all three sources mention the same use for the
plant, that is, in relation to lords or high government officials. However,
Badianus and de la Cruz mention a specific condition of those persons, fatigue related to holding high office, and the plant is thus treated as part of

a remedy that would drive weariness away and would drive out fear and fortify the heart.[52] Hernández and Sahagun do not attribute any medicinal properties to the plant in its use as an offering to high officials. They do mention other medicinal uses, however.

In the contracts between medical practices in the New World and the Old, the only major point at which exchange of information took place was in the area of herbal medicines. Those were adopted by Europeans seemingly as a matter of the practical necessities of dealing with the diseases and health conditions in the New World. Interest in Aztec culture was primarily ethnographic in nature (as in Sahagun's work), or was firmly embedded in the natural-history tradition of European academic inquiry (as in Hernández's work). The very pragmatic nature of medical practice provided the only real point of contract between two very disparate systems of medical treatment. The importation of New World plants (such as guaiacum) to the Old World, and of Old World plants to the New World, and a mutual concern with the efficacy of herbal remedies, provided the only substantial evidence of cross-cultural medical practices.

NOTES

1. See Alfred W. Crosby, Jr., *The Columbian Exchange: Biological and Cultural Consequences of 1492* (Westport, Conn.: Greenwood Press, 1972), 165–208, for a discussion of New World plants and Old World demography. See also Francisco Guerra, "Drugs from the Indies and the Political Economy of the Sixteenth Century," *Analecta medico—historica* 1 (1966):29–54.

2. William M. Denevan, ed., *The Native Population of the Americas in 1492* (Madison: University of Wisconsin Press, 1976), 7.

3. Agustin Farfan, *Tractado breve de anathomia y Chirugia, y de algunas enfermedades, que mas comunmente suelen hauer en esta nueua Espana. Compuesto por el muy reuerendo padre Fray Augustin Farfan, Doctor en medicina, y religioso de la orden de Sant Augustin. Dirigido al muy reuerendo padre maestro Fray Martin de Perea, Provincial de la dicha orden de Sant Augustin* (Mexico: Casa de Antonio Ricardo, 1579), 223–64.

4. Juan de Cardenas, *Primera parte de los problemas y secretos maravillosos de las Indias* (Mexico: Casa de Pedro Ocharte, 1591; reprinted Mexico City: Imprenta del Museo Nacional de Arqueologia, Historia y Etnologia, 1913), 185–86, 191, 193.

5. See Sherburne F. Cook, "The Incidence and Significance of Disease among the Aztecs and Related Tribes," *Hispanic American Historical Review* 26 (1946):320–35.

6. Crosby, *Columbian Exchange*, 122–64; Francisco Guerra, "The Problem of Syphilis," in Fredi Chiappelli, ed., *First Images of America* (Berkeley: University of California Press, 1976), 2:845–51.

7. Charles H. Talbot, "America and the European Drug Trade," in Chiappelli, ed., *First Images of America*, 2:834–36.

8. Juan Comas, "Influencia Indigena en la medicina hipocratica en la Neuva Espana del siglo XVI," *America Indigena* 14 (1954):329.

9. Francisco Bravo, *Opera medicinalia in quibus plurima extant scitu medico necessaria*

in 4 li. digesta, que pagina versa cotinentur, Authore Francisco Bravo Ofunesi doctore, ac Mexicano Medico (Mexico: Apud Petrum Ocharte, 1570). A facsimile reprint edition of Bravo's work, *The Opera Medicinalia* (Folkestone and London: Dawsons of Pall Mall, 1970), with an introduction by Francisco Guerra, makes the work available for scholarly study. Guerra cites the *Opera* as the earliest medical work published in the New World (see his introductory statements, p. 2).

10. Francisco Hernández, *De Rerum Medicarum Novae Hispaniae Thesaurus seu Plantarum Animalium Mineralium Mexicanorum Historia ex Francisci Hernandi Novi Orbis Medici Primarij relationibus in ipsa Mexicana Urbe conscriptis a Nardo Antonio Recchio Monte Coriunate Cath. Maiest. Medico et Neap. Regni Archiatro Generali Iussu Philippi II Hisp. Indar. Regis Collecta ac in ordinem digesta a Ioanne Terrentio Lynceo Constantiense Germ. Pho. ac Medico Notis illustrata Nunc primum in Naturaliū rerū Studiosor gratia et utilitatê studio et impensis Lynceorum. Publici iuris facta Philippo IV Magno Dicata* (Rome: Iacobi Mascardi, 1628). A new printing of the work, with a new title page, appeared in 1651. See Francisco Hernández, *Nova Plantarum, animalium et mineralium mexicanorum historia A Francisco Hernández primum compilata, dein a Nardo Antonio Reccho in volumen digesta, a Jo. Terentio, Io. Fabro, et Fabio Columna Lynceis notis, & additionibus longe doctissimis illustrata. Cui demum accessere aliquot ex principio Federici Caesi frontispiciis Theatri naturalis phytosophicae tabulae una com quamplurimus iconibus ad octigentus, quibus singula contemplanda graphica exhibentur* (Rome: V. Mascardi, 1651). The 1651 printing is much more readily available than the 1628. Hernández, during his stay in Mexico, collected 17 volumes of material, which he transmitted to Spain, where Philip II deposited them in the Escorial. A fire in the Escorial destroyed the manuscript in 1671. A version of the manuscript was derived from a copy left in the mission at Huaxtepec and was published in 1615 by Francisco Ximenez under the title *Quatro libros de la naturaleza, y virtudes de las plantas, y animales que estan recevidos en el uso de Medicina en la Neuva Espana, y la Methodo, y correccion y preparacion, que para ad mimmallas se requiree con lo que el Doctor Francisco Hernandez escrivio en lengua Latina. Muy util Paratodo Generode gente q vive en estacias y Pueblos, de no ay Medicas, ni Botica. Traduzido y aumentados muchos simples, y compuestos y muchos secretos curativos, por Father Francisco Ximenez, hijo del Conuento de S. Domingo de Mexico, natural de la Villa de Luna del Reyno de Aragon. A Nro R. P. Maestro Father Hernando Bazan, Prior Provincial de la Provincia de Sactiago de Mexico, de la Orden de los Prelicadores, y Cathedratico Iubilado de Theologia en la Universidad Real* (Mexico: Casa de la Viuda de Diego Lopez Davalos, 1615). Further published versions of Hernández's work are based primarily on the 1628 (or 1651) edition of the summary by Reccho. The two modern editions of the work are *Historia de las plantas de Nueva Espana*, 3 vols. (Mexico: Imprenta Universitaria, 1942–46); and Francisco Hernández, *Obras completas*, 5 vols. (Mexico City: Universidad Nacional de Mexico, 1960), which includes not only the Mexican work but Hernández's translation of Pliny's *Natural History*. In 1790, an edition of Hernández's work, based on the Reccho manuscript, appeared as *Opera, cum edita, tum inedita, ad autographi fidem et integritatem expressa, impensae el jussu regio* (Matriti: Ibarrae Heredum, 1970).

11. Farfan, *Tractado Breve*. The 1595 edition is *Summa y recopilación de chirugia, compuesto par mestro Alonso López de Hinofosos, con un arte para Sangrar, y examen de Barberos, va anadido en esta segunda impression el origen y nascimientes de las reumas y las enfermedades que dellas proceden, con otras cosas muy provechosas para acudir al remedio dellas, y del otras muchas enfermedades* (Mexico: Pedro Balli, 1595).

12. Alonso López de Hinojosos, *Summa y recopilacion de chirugia, con un arte para sagrar muy util y prouechosa. Compuesta por maestre alonso Lopez, natural de los Inojosos. Chirugano y enfermero del Ospital de S. Iosephus de los Indios, destra muy insigne Ciudada de Mexico. Dirigido al Lii. Y. R. S. Don P. Moya de Contreras, Arcobispe de Mexico y del cocejo de su Magest* (Mexico: Antonio Ricardo, 1578). See note 11 for 1595 edition.

13. *Libellus de medicinalibus Indorum herbis, quem quidam Indus Collegii sancte Crucis medicus compusuit, nullis rationibus edoctus, sed solis experimentis edoctus, Anno domini sexuatovis 1552.* The manuscript was discovered in the Vatican library and finally published, first as *The de la Cruz-Badiano Aztec Herbal of 1552,* trans. William Gates (Baltimore, Md.: The Maya Society, 1939), and then as *The Badianus Manuscript (Codex Barberini, Latin 241), Vatican Library, an Aztec Herbal of 1552,* introduction, translation, and annotations by Emily Walcott Emmart (Baltimore, Md.: Johns Hopkins University Press, 1940).

14. Bernardino de Sahagun, *Historia general de las cosas de nueva España,* 5 vols. (Mexico: Editorial Pedro Robredo, 1938). See also Fray Bernardino de Sahagun, *A History of Ancient Mexico (1547–1577),* trans. Fanny R. Bandelier, from the Spanish version of Carlos Maria de Bustamenta, vol. 1 (Nashville, Tenn.: Fisk University, 1932). Subsequent editions of the work include *Historia general de las cosas de nueva Espana, escrita por Fr. Bernardino de Sahagun Franciscano y fundada en la documentacion en lingua mexicana recogida por los mismos naturales. La dispuso para la prensa en esta nueva edicion, con numeracion anotaciones y apendices Angel Maria Garibay K.,* 4 vols. (Mexico: Editorial Porua, 1956); *Historia general de las cosas de nueva Espana,* 5 vols. (Mexico: Editorial Pedro Robredo, 1938); and *General History of the Things of New Spain,* trans. Charles E. Dibble and Arthur J. Q. Anderson. Monographs of the School of American Research and the Museum of New Mexico, part 13 (Santa Fe, N.M.: 1950–1965).

15. Erwin H. Ackerknecht, "Problems of Primitive Medicine," *Bulletin of the History of Medicine* 2 (1942):504.

16. Sahagun, *General History,* 2:16. See also Francisco Guerra, "Aztec Medicine," *Medical History* 10 (1966):320, for a general discussion of Aztec medical practices.

17. Sahagun, *General History,* part 11:53, 139–63; part 2:1–24.

18. Farfan, *Tractado breve* (1579), 17; and López de Hinojosos, *Summa y recopilación* (1578), 1–2.

19. López de Hinojosos, *Summa y recopilación* (1578), ibid., 3.

20. Joaquín García Icazabalceta, *Bibliografia mexicana del siglo XVI. Catalogo razonado de libros impresos en mexico de 1539 a 1600 con biografias de auteres y otras ilustraciones* (Mexico: Fondo de Cultura Economica, 1954), 235–36.

21. The connection between Hernández and Sahagun is established in Ioannis Nieremberg's *Historia naturae maxime peregrinae: Libris XVI distincta: In quibus rarissima Naturae arcana, etiam astronomica, & ignota Indarum animalia describuntur; Accedunt de miris et miraculosis naturis in Europa libri duo; item de iisdem in terra Hebraeis premissa liber unus* (Antverpiae: Ex Officina Plantiniana Balthasaris Moreti, 1635). Nieremberg attributed part of his book 2 directly to Hernández. The manuscript source from which he drew these chapters seems to be no longer extant. However, the chapters in Nieremberg's book are virtually identical to the appendix to book 2 of Sahagun's *Historia general.* The material is a listing of religious ceremonies. See Nieremberg, 142–44, and Sahagun, *General History,* 3:165–71. Leon Portilla asserts that Nieremberg took the material from Hernández without realizing that Hernández had in turn

copied it from Sahagun's manuscripts. It is surprising then that there are not more correspondences between the descriptions of plants in the Hernández and Sahagun works. See Miguel Leon-Portilla, *Ritos, sacerdotes y atavios de los dioses: Introduccion, paleografia, version & notas de Miguel Leon-Portilla* (Mexico: Universidad Nacional Autonoma de Mexico, Instituto de Historia, Seminario de Cultura Nahuatl, 1958), 21.

22. Sahagun, *History of Ancient Mexico*, 3–9.

23. Bravo, *Opera medicinalia*, 2v–3, 167v, 273–74, 295v.

24. Ibid., 4, 8, 273–74.

25. Ibid., 79.

26. De la Cruz, *The de la cruz-Badiano aztec herbal*, xvii.

27. Hernández, *De rerum medicarum*, 8–9.

28. Ibid., 29–30.

29. See, for example, Farfan, *Tractado breve* (1579), 2, 4v, 107; López de Hinojosos, *Summa y recopilación* (1578), 1, 2.

30. Farfan, *Tractado breve* (1579), 7r.

31. Ibid., 55v.

32. Ibid., 217v.

33. Ibid., 87.

34. Comas, "Influencia indigena," 345–61.

35. López de Hinojosos, *Summa y recopilacion* (1578), 16.

36. Ibid., 70.

37. Farfan, *Tractado breve* (1579), 77; López de Hinojosos, *Summa y recopilación* (1978), 34v.

38. Scarification and bleeding were known to the Aztecs. The Badianus manuscript mentions a cure for veins swelling because of bloodletting (p. 281) in the heading of chapter 10, but the text does not include a specific cure as indicated by the heading of the chapter. Sahagun, *General History*, mentions bleeding the scalp as a cure for headache (2:140).

39. Farfan, *Tractado breve* (1579), 1–2; Comas, "Influencia indigena," 344.

40. López de Hinojosos, *Summa y recopilación* (1578), 16; Farfan, *Tractado breve*, 17.

41. De la Cruz, *Libellus*, 205.

42. Ibid.

43. Ibid., 306.

44. Ibid., 207–8.

45. Sahagun, *History of Ancient Mexico*, 3–9.

46. Sahagun, *General History*, 2:34.

47. Sahagun, *History of Ancient Mexico*, 13–14.

48. Hernández, *Historia de las plantas*, 3:806.

49. Sahagun, *Historia general*, 3:276.

50. De la Cruz, *Badianus Manuscript*, 276–77.

51. Ibid.

52. Ibid.

3

PHANTOMS AND PHYSICIANS: SOCIAL CHANGE THROUGH MEDICAL PLURALISM

LIBBET CRANDON-MALAMUD

Vicente Callisaya, an elderly rural Bolivian Aymara man, was obviously sick in 1977, but everyone in town had a different opinion about what he had. He himself considered all possibilities, and finally determined he had a fatal disease that, according to local belief, affects only Indians. Another opinion was anemia that, consensus had it, cosmopolitan medicine could cure; but he rejected it. Why he made such a choice had little to do with his frame of mind, his access to medicine, or with Aymara beliefs as such. Nor was it due to race, although Doña Teresa, the self-appointed town aristocrat, held that it was. Rather, Vicente's choice was related to the use of the concept of ethnicity and race in Bolivian society and history, and to the use of medicine to create social change.

Doña Teresa's convictions about the "Indian race" are hardly peculiar. In the Bolivian popular mind, as throughout much of the Western world, ethnically defined indigenous populations are considered racially distinct.[1] On those grounds, Indian labor has been exploited since the conquest. Those segments of Bolivian society that have regarded the nation as backward have blamed the lack of national progress on the Indian—along with U.S. imperialism when the Indian vote was desirable. Although there is much to support the latter assertion, its periodic appearance contrasts with the consistency of the former explanation.[2]

This chapter is an expanded version of "Medical Dialogue and the Political Economy of Medical Pluralism: A Case from Rural Highland Bolivia." Reproduced by permission of the American Anthropological Association from *American Ethnologist* 13(3) (August 1986). It includes text from my *From the Fat of Our Souls* (Berkeley: University of California Press, 1991). Clotilde in this chapter is Doña Antonia de Villazon in *From the Fat*; Vicente Callisaya and Doña Teresa are Edegon and Doña Ana in "Medical Dialogue."

Following the concept of ethnicity as racially based, *mestizos* are thought to be of mixed Spanish and Indian ancestry. Among the Aymara and Quechua Indians and the *mestizos* of the highlands, medicine supports these racial categories when indigenous medical ideology defines certain illness as visited solely upon Indians, and when cosmopolitan medical records confirm that Indians suffer greater incidence of disease than *mestizos* or elites. When indigenous medical ideology ascribes disease suffered by Indians to *mestizo* and upper-class elements, however, medicine does just the opposite: Because it can conquer the disease, it thereby empowers resistance to oppression. Thus medicine plays a role in the formation (and reformation) of the meaning of ethnicity, and in effecting social change, particularly in an environment that is medically pluralistic and socially diverse. One way to examine how medicine can both reinforce social structure and support social change is to examine the changes in medical ideology itself. The history of the *karisiri* is a case in point.

MEDICAL IDEOLOGY AS HISTORY: THE *KARISIRI*

The *karisiri*, or *karikari*, and the illness it causes have been noted in Andean chronicles and by priests and anthropologists in the region since the colonial conquest (Oblitas Poblete 1963;[3] La Barre 1948;[4] Tschopik 1951;[5] Aguilo 1982[6]). It is the robed and bearded apparition of a Jesuit priest that, for over four hundred years, was said to inflict death upon the Aymara and Quechua by stealing the fat from their kidneys. Such fat was given to the bishop, who made holy oil from it that sanctified the non-Indian population.

During the 1960s and the Alliance for Progress years, when much of the blame for the failure of the 1952 Movimiento Nacional Revolucionario (MNR) revolution to modernize the country was placed on U.S. imperialism, some anthropologists and priests[7] reported that the *karisiri* was said to sell the oil to North Americans, who used it to generate electricity.

In the village on the Bolivian altiplano where I did my research for eighteen months between 1976 and 1978, Indians and *mestizos* alike agreed that the *karisiri* is not an apparition but, rather, a skill that any village *mestizo* can learn. Such a *mestizo* steals the fat with instruments clandestinely obtainable in pharmacies in La Paz. The fat is sold at huge profits to factories that make perfumed luxury soaps for the European and North American markets. Significantly, the affliction is no longer considered fatal.

In this explanation of illness,[8] what people say about their social world through the idiom of medicine are statements about political and economic realities and the meaning of ethnic relations; the shifts in that explanation, or medical theory, reflect changes in Bolivian society. Since the Bolivian revolution of 1952, which instituted a land reform and destroyed the hacienda system established under colonialism, landownership and increased market participation among the Aymara have resulted in decreasing rates of malnutrition and consequent reduction in mortality from infectious diseases and parasites. To be Indian is no longer to be completely at the mercy of demonic beings, the agricultural or mining elite, and the rural *mestizos* who served the interests of those elites in the countryside before 1952. Among the *mestizos*, however, the revolution and land reform took away the land and the power they had wielded over the Indians. The loss of rural power led to divisions among the *mestizos* as they suddenly found it necessary to compete against one another for the few resources that could be used for social mobility and eventual migration to the city. Within the village this once cohesive and locally powerful group is now politically and economically marginal.

Following the theoretical contributions of such authors as Emily Martin (1987), Susan Sontag (1978), and Nancy Scheper-Hughes and Margaret Lock (1987), the *karisiri* myth is another example of medicine as metaphor for social relations. The *karisiri* example, however, is more amenable to Foucault's line of reasoning (e.g., 1965, 1973) insofar as changes in its interpretation can be seen over time as concurrent with changes in the political economy, in ethnic affiliation with that economy, and in the effects of that political economy on the content of ethnic identity. The significance of the *karisiri* belief, then, is the question it raises: How medicine as metaphor changes over time, and what role it plays in interethnic relations and in the formation of social relationships.

MEDICAL PLURALISM, SOCIAL DIVERSITY, AND SOCIAL CHANGE

In an environment that is diverse in ethnicity and class, and is also medically pluralistic, people draw on multiple medical ideologies. As they do so, their medical dialogue reflects, involves, and contributes to the construction of political, economic, ideological, and social relations. Through medical dialogue, ethnic groups negotiate the meaning of ethnic identity and affiliation, and therefore of interethnic relations.[9] Consequently, medical dialogue is a medium through which we can see political and economic processes as they pertain to the nature of interethnic relations. Simultaneously it is an arena in which those interethnic relations are negotiated and played out. Hence medical ideology and dialogue are both an arena for change and a window on the politicoeconomic relationship between medicine and ethnicity (and social class).

An examination of actual use of medical ideology and medical dialogue between and among Indians and *mestizos* in a rural highland Bolivian village can move us beyond the view of medicine as metaphor to an understanding of how medicine changes in the short run, is constantly reinterpreted by different social segments as a means for the exchange of political and economic resources and as a mechanism to facilitate or impede change, particularly the reformation of social relations. How people talk about illness is a means by which the symbolic content of ethnic identity is interpreted and the nature of social relationships is defined.

This examination is dependent on a focus on dialogue about medical beliefs as symbols both within and between ethnic and class groups.[10] As such, the focus is not upon symbols that express group unity, but rather on symbols through which communication is made across ethnic and class lines and therefore permits or facilitates opposition, conflict, and change.

Field research took place in a small, biethnic rural Bolivian village on the altiplano that serves as the center of the canton of Omasullu. Here approximately a thousand Aymara and *mestizos* inhabit the *municipio* that serves some sixteen thousand Aymara in 36 surrounding *aldeas*. During my stay there, a number of people in the village became ill; each time, everyone in town knew every symptom and detail of the illness that the victim suffered and, as often as not, a number of details that he or she did not. People voiced their opinions vociferously as to what they thought a patient had, and consequently what ought to be done about it. To do so, they drew upon nosological and etiological categories that derive from Indian, folk, and cosmopolitan medical traditions, categories that carry social significance depending on the context in which they are used. Each diagnostic opinion was a statement about the sick person, the person delivering the opinion, and the relationship between the two. The social relationship being expressed was often that among the several parties discussing the illness and a person not present. Although conversations were ostensibly debates about what a patient suffered from, the fundamental issue under negotiation concerned the power to monopolize the construction of the meaning of the illness, and hence to define the relationship between the parties engaged in the dialogue. The outcome of the discussion had multiple political and economic implications in village life.

VICENTE

When Vicente became ill in 1977, he sought out several *yatiris*, Aymara shamans. They provided various diagnoses but did not make him feel any better. Vicente's son told me that Vicente had told him he had *limpu*, a fatal condition caused by witnessing an Indian stillbirth. The *limpu* is the soul of a stillborn who, having died before baptism, is prohibited from entering heaven and therefore seeks to continue its existence on earth. This soul enters the body of a witness to the birth, and since the soul survives by consuming the victim, the victim—or host—grows thinner and thinner until death occurs.

One analysis of this etiology discloses *limpu* as a statement of Indian identity that differentiates Indian oppression from non-Indian or *mestizo* domination and points to the inequality of access to resources of the two ethnic groups. *Mestizos* neither cause *limpu*—because they do not live like or are not Indians—nor get it—because they never attend Indian births. Further-more, the key element in the transmission of the disease—the absence of the baptism—is an element of Catholicism, and until the 1970s the local Catholic church was controlled by *mestizos* and elites, served their interests at the expense of those of the Aymara, and subsisted on Indian labor. More-over, Indians do grow "thinner and thinner" and die from anemia or mal-nutrition much more often than do *mestizos*.

The *mestiza* Clotilde, mother of four, wife of an itinerant schoolteacher, and landless, agreed with Vicente's son that Vicente probably had *limpu*. She allowed that her judgment rested on the fact that she herself had had experience with the illness in her family. However, she urged Vicente to see the physician just in case it was something that a physician might treat. She appeared concerned about his health and agreed that his own choice of diagnosis was reasonable. She further shared the sense of victim implied by the illness even though, as a *mestiza*, she belonged to a class of people who deny vulnerability to Indian illnesses such as *limpu*.

Over the many years they had known each other, Clotilde had frequently sympathized with Vicente when he recalled the brutality of hacienda life before 1952. The patron of the hacienda to which Vicente had been at-tached, a wealthy *mestizo* who was able to migrate to the city after the land reform, is now a professional in La Paz and calls himself white. He has spurned Clotilde's family's overtures for aid, which were first made on the basis of old *compadrazgo* (fictive kin ties).[11] His denial was based on the defense that the ties were his father's, not his, and were therefore no longer valid. Clotilde's family, reasonably well-to-do in 1952, had by the 1970s dropped into the village's lowest socioeconomic stratum. Now landless, Clo-tilde is unable to support her four children on her husband's salary, much of which goes for his own support away from home.

In 1977, Clotilde increased her contact and exchange with Vicente's fam-ily, initially on the basis of *compadrazgo* ties and later on a vague claim to kinship. However, unlike the earlier *mestizo*-Indian *compadrazgo* bond that had joined the two ethnic groups in a dependent relationship of unilateral exploitation, Clotilde and Vicente's relationship is equilateral. Clotilde's *mes-tizo* class no longer has the power to sanction labor exploitation, and Vi-cente's fellow Aymara have the freedom to bypass many local *mestizos* in order to get access to resources from the urban or national domain. Indeed, Clotilde needs Vicente and access to his agricultural produce as much as he needs her for the social ties he can gain through her. Hence, when he falls sick, Clotilde delivers an opinion and a little aid in mode that denotes the egalitarian nature of their relationship, and aligns herself with Indian eth-nicity.

The one physician in town was from La Paz and an aspirant to the urban elite serving his year of required rural duty. He examined Vicente and de-scribed his health as "perfect." Vicente was "old and anemic," he explained, and he prescribed vitamins and rest. Of significance, however, is the similarity between anemia and *limpu*; the symptoms are identical. The significant difference is that *limpu* is usually fatal, as is implied by its etiology, adding a political dimension to the illness by underlining Indian/*mestizo* inequality.

The *mestiza* Doña Teresa, keeper of the town archives, virtual head of the most prestigious *mestizo* family in town, godmother to perhaps a hundred Aymara children, and *comadre* or godmother to a number of well-placed families in La Paz, thought that both diagnoses were preposterous. She found Clotilde's medical opinions scandalous, although they confirmed what she had suspected all along: that there were Indians in Clotilde's family. That would account for Clotilde's degenerate behavior of associating beneath her class and ethnic group, disgracing the *gente decente*, as well as her lack of wealth, power, and good connections. Teresa determined to cease extending credit to Clotilde or even selling her items from Teresa's family's *tienda*.[12]

Teresa also knew better than the physician. He was, she claimed, a young fellow from the city who lacked her experience with Indians in the countryside. Her family had been godparents to Vicente's family for many generations. Yet in recent decades his family had not honored the *compadrazgo* relationship sanctioned before 1952 by providing her family with agricultural goods and services. This delinquency had produced a hardship on Teresa's household, which had lost much of its land to the reform. Teresa sees Vicente as lazy, poorly behaved, and sick because of the degeneracy of his moral constitution. Moral decrepitude leading to poor health is a folk illness derived from Euro-Christian folk tradition, and is a form of moral retribution for which there is no remedy. Consequently, Teresa had no therapeutic recommendation to offer. In her opinion, Vicente ate quite adequately. At least he had sufficient resources on his land. Her medical opinion makes it quite clear and nonnegotiable that she no longer has any obligation to Vicente.

Vicente died twenty-four hours after his visit to the physician, convinced that he had *limpu*. The cause of death was never determined in a manner that would be satisfactory to this audience, although I noted he was quite elderly and suspect he died of heart failure. As in the process of diagnosis, everyone in town held an opinion about the cause of Vicente's death. The *limpu*/anemia/moral decrepitude complex employed in this case and the particular issues involved are merely examples of a variety of options and issues employed in a given illness incident by which individuals define and display their relationships to each other. The potential of such medical dialogues for the reformation of social relations is always manifest.

UNDERSTANDING THE DIALOGUE ABOUT VICENTE

An explanation of how and why this dialogue exposes social processes requires an understanding of five dimensions of Bolivian social life that, according to popular belief, do not exist: (1) the social construction of ethnicity and race; (2) the political economy of Bolivia that facilitates or compels social mobility across ethnic boundaries; (3) the downward as well as upward social movement as a consequence of that political economy[13] (4) the confluences of culture that are shared by different ethnic groups[14] and permit that movement; and (5) the political economy of medical pluralism that facilitates that movement. The argument here is not that medicine is a metaphor for social relations embedded in a political economy, as has been argued elsewhere (e.g., Sontag 1978; Taussig 1980). Rather, medical dialogue is a means by which political and economic resources are exchanged, and is thus a mechanism that facilitates or inhibits change.

The Social Construction of Ethnicity

Contrary to Doña Teresa's convictions, racial integrity never existed in Upper Peru[15] or Bolivia. During the colonial era, many descendants of the Spanish experienced downward economic mobility and some were even designated Indians, while many Indian elites wore European dress, were educated in Europe, and married the Spanish (Abercrombie 1986; Crandon-Malamud 1991; Platt 1978a, 1978b, 1982a, 1982b; Rasnake 1988). *Mestizos* constituted that population—both Spanish and Indian—which served the interests of the elite by controlling Indian labor, particularly in the rural areas, until the MNR revolution of 1952.[16] Today they compose the middle classes—the working classes and the service sector—who are excluded from the moneyed elite. Neither Indian nor elite, they were, and remain, despised by both (Carter 1958:52).

Ethnicity is thus the product of class conflict, exploitation, and resistance, justified by concepts of race, to permit the mobilization of labor on behalf of the state or the elite. For the agriculturally based Aymara and Quechua who maintain an indigenous social organization, legal system, and economy—albeit within the national domain—the construct of ethnicity has facilitated their oppression, opposition, defiance, and survival. For Spanish *and* Indians who became *mestizos*, the myth that they were a mixed race justified their exclusion from the elite but their social class position as supervisors of Indian labor. Since both *mestizos* and Indians managed to join the ranks of the elite over the past four centuries, and many of the elite lost wealth and position and were excluded from that social class, Indians, *mestizos*, and elites all share confluences of the same culture; and a principal cultural domain they all share is medical ideology.

Thus, contrary to popular opinion, an enormous amount of shift in ethnic and class membership has taken place since the sixteenth century, and medical ideology has facilitated that social change as much as it has supported the myth of race. A brief reference to Bolivian political and economic history[17] and an analysis of interethnic relations reveals why this movement takes place. Specifically, it shows why Clotilde wants to befriend Vicente on the basis of mutual friendship and give up the privileges of her superordinate ethnic group.

Political Economy and Movement across Ethnic Boundaries

Seen as a nation of two distinct cultures—the "traditional Indian" and the "modern"—Bolivia has fallen prey to the "dual economy" dichotomy and related concepts that mask the essentiality of Indian labor, first to the colonial crown and then to the nation-state; the participation of both in the world economy (Dunkerley 1984; Wallerstein 1974; Wolf 1982); the links that articulate them; and the consequent confluences of culture that they of necessity share. The two primary related concepts are modernization and development, both of which obfuscate the confluences of culture that Indian, *mestizo*, and elite share.

"Modernization" refers to the transformation of social organization and worldview into that of an industrialized middle class (e.g., Valenzuela and Valenzuela 1978). "Development" refers to economic diversification, industrialization, and participation in a world market in a manner that is decreasingly "dependent" or "peripheral" (Muñoz 1981). The general position is that development, if it does not destroy indigenous culture, at least modernizes it in such a way that—if it is Western-oriented—the population should increasingly aspire to the principles of science and commerce, court modern medicine, and decry the "superstition of magic."[18]

However, the political economy that articulates Bolivian elites, *mestizos*, and Indians is as much a product of the detrimental effects of efforts to modernize and develop as it is of Bolivia's colonial and prerevolutionary legacy. That legacy was a political arena in which caudillismo (rule by a strongman) was the principle by which power was obtained, and *personalismo*, or privilege, that by which access to resources and power was gained. Ever since the Spanish conquest Bolivia has been a country characterized by extreme poverty of the vast majority of the population, scarcity of resources[19] caudillo rule,[20] and the exchange of goods and power through *personalismo*.

Personalismo ties are established through kinship and *compadrazgo*. They do not follow ethnic or class divisions but are specifically constructed to crosscut them, vertically linking segments of all social sectors. They thus oppose ethnic and class interests as players struggle to create and manipulate ties to gain access to limited resources and to reinforce highly centralized rule.

Contemporary Bolivia's political economy continues to be based on an increasing scarcity of resources that perpetuates those very principles. This is so in spite of many attempts to create class interests and political parties based on a more equitable distribution of wealth and the destruction of the principle of *personalismo*, particularly since 1952. In that year the MNR revolution destroyed the hacienda system, initiated an agrarian reform, armed the peasant masses, established unions (including peasant unions), and instituted universal suffrage.[21] The hacienda Indian attachment to a patron through labor obligations in exchange for rent was transformed into a landowning peasantry of campesinos that now has access to some education and some economic, even entrepreneurial, opportunity.[22] By the 1970s postrevolutionary colonization and development of the state of Santa Cruz had led to exports of gas, cotton, and sugar that appeared to be benefiting the middle and upper classes.

In spite of these great economic and social changes, a commercial class has not been able to establish itself as a dominant sector in Bolivia, and proletarianization of the peasantry on the altiplano has been slow or absent (Mendelberg 1985). Only the mining unions were able to unify a socioeconomic sector with a political platform that reflected its social interests as a class (Nash 1979). The unions accounted, however, for only 3 percent of the population and dispersed when the mines were closed in the mid-1980s.[23]

Virtually none of the development activity had a negative effect on *personalismo*, and the particular formation of the contemporary cocaine economy may well be a product of it. *Personalismo* and caudillo activity undermined the campesino unions established in the 1950s by the revolution, as campesino leaders competed for scarce resources within a divided government; these unions were dismantled before the campesinos ever perceived themselves to be in any way unified (Heath 1969b). By 1980 gas, cotton, and sugar had failed to accumulate capital. On the contrary, they escalated an already extraordinary national debt, and in the 1980s they were replaced by cocaine as Bolivia's principal export (Canelas O. and Canelas Z. 1983; Dunkerley 1984). Since the late 1970s, Argentina has virtually inhaled Bolivia's gas exports, the price of which, General Videla pointed out as he tore up his gas bill in November 1982, did not cover the interest on the loan that Bolivia received from Argentina in 1980. While the development of the lowland area has indeed diversified national production that had previously been limited to tin, the benefits have accrued solely to a particular segment of the lowland society and to the military, and have rarely, if ever, been reinvested in Bolivia. Between 1980 and 1983 national production decreased between 2 and 10 percent annually. The national debt is so great that what production there is does not begin to erase it.

In the spring of 1984, Bolivia was the first developing country to default on its loans. The government declared that it would pay nothing toward the interest until 1987; and North American banks, terrified of the precedent this would set, quietly let it pass (Gwynne 1987).[24] Although the subject of considerable debate, it appears that the cocaine economy has benefited no sector of Bolivian society except the narcotraffickers and those segments of the military that are involved with them. Most evidence reveals its social, economic, and politically destructive, if not devastating, consequences

(Aguilar personal communication; Malamud-Goti 1990). Ecologically and environmentally it has been catastrophic. Initially the major economic impact from increased coca production was inflation, calculated for 1983 at 25,000 percent.[25] During most of this time, salaries—except those of the military—were frozen.[26] Consequently, both economic and political resources are scarcer than ever for the vast majority of the Bolivian population, and *personalismo* remains the most effective, if not the only, means by which one gains access to resources.[27]

Concomitantly the democratic experiment degenerated into military rule in 1964, and although democracy appeared momentarily for elections in 1978, 1979, and 1980, the latter election resulted in the flight of the elected president and congress from military coups engineered by fortune-seeking caudillos. Although Hernán Siles Suazo, after coming in first in all those elections in the 1970s, finally took office in 1983, he held it for less than the full term and with considerable difficulty.[28]

This situation has impeded any political unification of classes, and the rigidity of ethnic boundaries remains a useful myth to explain the limited strategies available for gaining access to resources in such a system. Little remains changed or exchanged, from onions to presidents, except through *personalismo*. Among kin and *compadres*, aid, security, wealth, and privilege are exchanged for loyalty. Certainly employment in the public sector and political power are contingent on personal ties. So it is that when interim president Lydia Gueiler Tejada reprimanded her renegade nephew Luis Garcia Meza for attempting a military coup in 1979, she did not take strong legal action against him, such as imprisonment or exile. Likewise, when he successfully seized the government a year later, he liberally supplied his followers and relations with contracts in the cocaine trade and exclusive rights to diamond fields in the interior, manipulating the legislative process for his personal interests much like his caudillo predecessors.[29]

Even the Bolivian military does not compose a class or body with shared interests. Rather, it is composed of a loosely connected series of pyramidal structures, each internally organized according to the principles of *personalismo*, and each led by a general who competes with the other generals to dominate military and political activities for his own economic gain and for the benefit of his relatives and his followers, according to the ideal of the good patriarch. Such a system provides upward mobility only to the privileged—those with the right connections. For those without those connections, not only is downward mobility a necessity, but affiliation with Indian ethnicity is an advantage.

Upward and Downward Mobility

Following the myth that ethnic boundaries are rigid—a myth that is being unmasked and addressed in some contemporary anthropological literature on the area (e.g., Abercrombie 1986; Platt 1978a; Rasnake 1988)—is the further assumption, both popular and anthropological, that what social movement does occur across ethnic lines is only upward from Indian to *mestizo* to white. This assumption emerged from the belief in Western hegemony and faith in "modernization" and "development" ubiquitous among non-Indians, and is reinforced by the presence of both indigenous and national economies and modes of exchange and the nature of their articulation. To the crises of history, Bolivia has adapted by continuing to maintain the indigenous peasant economy.[30]

The peasant or *ayllu* economy of the agriculturally based Aymara and Quechua campesino is a precolonial structure: a subsistence agricultural economy that articulates multiple ecological zones through reciprocity of goods and labor. It lies primarily outside the cash economy, although it supplies much of Bolivia's domestic agricultural produce, and is locally governed or facilitated by its own elected officials (Abercrombie 1986; Buechler and Buechler 1971; Carter 1982; Rasnake 1988). It thus can provide subsistence when the national economy collapses.[31] Within and between Aymara and Quechua communities, exchange is based on egalitarian social relations and reciprocity usually defined by the *ayllu*—the extended family in which reciprocity of productive labor is obligatory.

Although *ayllu* is based on a fundamentally different mode of production relations (see Wolf 1982:23) than that of the national economy, these two economies are tightly integrated; the dominance and wealth of the non-Indian domain have been, and remain, based on the oppression and isolation of the Indians, particularly as agricultural producers. Indian participation in the cash economy as agricultural producers is limited to favor the urban sector and elites and to subsidize their modernization and development. At least through the 1970s,[32] the price of all domestic agricultural goods was fixed by the government, inhibiting the development of both the market sector of Aymara and Quechua entrepreneurs and the new campesino landowners who, long since abandoned by the government as a sector worthy of investment or support, cannot make a meaningful profit by marketing or producing agricultural goods at levels much greater than subsistence (International Work Group on Indigenous Affairs 1978; Morales 1966; Malloy 1970; Nash 1979. See also Alexander 1958; Arnaude 1957; Heath 1969a; Malloy 1971; McEwen et al. 1969; Preston 1969).

On the one hand this policy accentuates the dependency of the national economy on that of the Indian. Taken together, they constitute a single system at the political and economic peripheries of the world economic system (Dunkerley 1984; Frank 1966, 1971; Mayorga 1987; Quiroga Santa Cruz 1973; Roxborough 1979). The myth that ethnic boundaries are rigid and permit only occasional upward mobility structures economic relations and exchange between these two economic domains hierarchically along ethnic and class lines and reinforces the principle of privilege as a means of access to resources and power within the national domain.

On the other hand, this policy is facilitated by the fact that the *ayllu* economy, being independent of cash and highly adapted over thousands of years to the Andes, provides subsistence to its participants and affiliates when the national economy collapses—which it has on many occasions over the last four centuries. As the peasant economy coexists with Bolivia's non-industrialized and frequently ailing economy, the peasant economy is discerned, particularly by the poorer classes, as a flexible resource that enables one to ride out a national economic crisis. Thus in spite of continued oppression of the Indians and the use of ethnicity to justify and perpetuate it, being Indian, or being accepted by Indians, has its advantages. Downward mobility is a serious option for many poor *mestizos* like Doña Clotilde.

Crossing ethnic boundaries in Bolivia is overtly prohibited but covertly institutionalized and follows a specific set of rules. Rules for upward mobility include the change in language, dress, and comportment that Harris refers to in his seminal work on race in Latin America (1964), and the mythification of one's heritage, as Teresa's comment about Clotilde's genealogy indicates. Downward mobility requires involvement in campesino production and egalitarian social relations with campesinos. However, accessibility to it is problematic: one has to enter the peasant economy by its own social rules of egalitarianism. Movement in either direction is not achieved by the individual but negotiated within the community. One must convince the others to treat him or her accordingly. A principal way to do so is through the use of medical dialogue and the manipulation of ideologies inherent in medical pluralism. This is possible because everyone in Bolivia shares confluences of the same culture.

Confluences of Culture

As we are here conceiving of Bolivia as a single population organized into a series of interrelated hierarchical sectors corresponding to access to economic and political resources, which sectors in turn define ethnic identities between which there is bilateral movement, we are necessarily presupposing confluences of culture that are shared by all three ethnic and class groups in spite of separate ethnic, political, and social identities. This view permits one to examine how a society that perceives itself as rigidly divided ethnically has such considerable movement across ethnic boundaries, and to incorporate the data that a llama fetus and other magical items are buried under the four corners of the foundations of every modern building in downtown La Paz, including the Chase Manhattan Bank and the old Gulf Oil building,[33] that the wealthy often trust the reading of the coca leaves more than their financial advisers (Bastien 1981; Press 1969, 1971), and that *yatiris* are including intravenous solutions and antibiotics in their treatment of "magical" disorders (Bastien 1981; see also Romanucci-Ross 1986).

While in the Indian domain the earth mother Pachamama reigns supreme over a pantheon of magical and supernatural entities that control and manipulate the destinies of human lives, Indians share with the *mestizos* and elites these same symbols, using them in different ways, often to define, create, or solidify social ties that link those domains. Actual ancestry and kinship ties are less significant than recognized heritage and kinship ties; kinship ties are manipulable (Strickon and Greenfield 1972); and heritage is constructed and mythified to fit social and political needs. Ties that are recognized or acknowledged define those social relations through which power and wealth are exchanged and, hence, ethnic identity and affiliation. One way to acquire acknowledgment is through the use of medical discourse.

More significantly, the view of Bolivia as a single system permits us to examine the movement across ethnic boundaries as a negotiated process that in turn permits the consideration of how medical dialogue plays a role in these negotiations. Hence we see in the *mestiza* Teresa's dialogue that she knows very well what *limpu* is and means, and uses that knowledge to assert her social superiority over Vicente.

Clotilde's efforts to establish an egalitarian relationship with Vicente required that she both adopt some elements of Aymara identity (vulnerability to *limpu*) and be willing to sacrifice ties with and respect from some of the more prestigious *mestizos*. Her conversation with Vicente is an example of one means by which the process of crossing ethnic boundaries and establishing affiliation takes place.

The Political Economy of the Content of Ethnic Identity

The rural *mestizos* in Omasullu who were also *mestizos* in 1952 still maintain as much as possible of the pre-1952, prerevolution colonial heritage that established them as overlords of the rural Indian population. But the foundation upon which that heritage was maintained was destroyed with the land reform of 1953 and the collapse of the hacienda system. These highland rural *mestizos* try not to work the land themselves and do not participate in the new entrepreneurial activities. They survive instead as proprietors of *tiendas* that originally operated on the principle of debt peonage; the debtors were Indians with whom the *mestizo tienda* owner had *compadrazgo* ties. The *tienda* constituted the local form of patriarchal *personalismo* exchange that has broken down since 1952.

Entrepreneurial activities are now monopolized by *cholos*, nonsubsistence-based Indians, many of whom aspire to be urban *mestizos*. Today rural *mestizos* also survive on government salaries as schoolteachers and rural officials. Their main objective, and that of upwardly mobile *cholos*, is to try, through their personal contacts in the city, to establish their children there, not only because they have always emulated the urban elite but also because the contemporary rural *mestizo* has lost almost all the means by which to directly extract a subsistence from the Indian population. Consequently, unless one is willing and able to do subsistence agriculture or to engage in entrepreneurial activities, there is little for a *mestizo* to do today on the rural Bolivian altiplano. Government salaries are paltry and are dependent upon *personalismo* ties with government officials that, if not prestigious, may result in the rural employee being sent to the least desirable region of the country.

Some *mestizos* have successfully moved to the city or, like Doña Teresa, formed ties there, while others have not. Consequently, while many rural *mestizos* look to the city to establish ties with which to improve their condition, those whose strategies have been unsuccessful, like Doña Clotilde, look down, as it were, toward egalitarian relations with Indians as a means of survival in a contracting economic environment. Such a move, toward egalitarian relations with Indians in a patriarchal society, requires a renegotiation of the content of ethnic identity and affiliation.

MEDICAL DIALOGUE AND THE NEGOTIATION OF DOWNWARD MOBILITY

In the Osmasullu village where this research was carried out, a substantial number of poor *mestiza* women whose families had lost their *tiendas* and their land since 1952 were, in 1976–1978, bartering magical and medicinal items and spices in the peasant market in return for agricultural produce and eggs. The agricultural produce was their family's source of subsistence; the eggs were sold in La Paz for cash that served as their capital with which the items and spices were resupplied. Many of these women had sought Indians as godparents to their children, looking "down" rather than "up" the *compadrazgo* network, contrary to usual *mestizo* practice. By doing so, they established egalitarian rather than hierarchal relationships with Indians.

The Indian and *mestizo* modes of existence in the rural altiplano and the political significance of their hierarchal relationship, as well as the fact that that relationship is changing, not only are expressed in indigenous medical ideology to which both Indians and *mestizos* subscribe, but also are initiated through medical dialogue. The participants thereby acknowledge that they share confluences of culture as they conflate two previously distinct domains of economy and ethnic affiliation.

Between 1970 and 1977 in this village, six *mestizo* youths in their late teens and twenties suffered severe illnesses that would appear to have, in scientific terms, both nutritional and psychological complications.[34] All six came from families that had once been among the most prestigious in the area. Since the revolution they had all lost nearly everything of value they had once owned, and were now among the poorest of village *mestizo* society.

The first four of these illnesses were treated by Western medical and psychiatric therapies based on a village consensus that the youths suffered from scientifically identifiable disorders. All four died from these illnesses. In 1976 and 1977, the last two of these six ailing youths turned instead to Aymara *yatiris*, and most villagers concurred that they suffered from Indian diseases.[35]

The last two youths survived their illnesses. Both of these youths were siblings of two of the four who had died earlier of ostensibly similar but differently diagnosed illnesses. The fathers of both youths had died years earlier and the young men were supported by mothers who were landless or nearly so, and who made a living by bartering in the Indian peasant market. Both women had established relations with Indians on an egalitarian basis, even claiming kinship. One was denounced as the town "crazy lady," the other was ostracized by the better-off *mestizos*, who continued to aspire to the economic and political life of the patriarchal domain of the urban sector. While sufficient data are unavailable to establish causes of illness in each case, the decisions made about treatment, regardless of pathology, show a group of families choosing one medical tradition over another in these specific cases. The significant variable in their condition appears to be whether they had suffered rather than gained by the revolution, whether they had been unsuccessful in the non-Indian domain, whether they had inadequate personal ties and had thus been excluded from a world to which they aspired, and whether they then perceived non-Indians as oppressing them, much as the Aymara see the *mestizos* oppressing Indians.

In all cases there had been a subtle change in ethnic identification and affiliation toward "Indianness," to participation in the Indian economic exchange, and away from dependency on *personalismo* ties in the patriarchal domain of the center. Most significantly, those who take this latter course also have a self-perception of vulnerability to Indian diseases. That is, in all cases there has been a change in the content of ethnic identity. Analysis of a conversation between Doña Clotilde and several Aymara concerning a physician reveals how medical dialogue not only reflects but also implements changes in the content of ethnic identity and, as a result, incremental social change.

HOW IT WORKS: INCREMENTAL SOCIAL CHANGE THROUGH MEDICAL DIALOGUE

Like many physicians throughout the world, Dr. Tallacagua explicitly used exclusively cosmopolitan medicine to achieve upward mobility, which for him meant crossing the ethnic boundary that divides the Aymara from the Bolivian upper classes. He had been born an Aymara Indian in one of the outlying communities, then had attended a Methodist Indian school, where he won a church scholarship that put him through medical school. In

1978 he returned for two months to the village as part of his medical training. The town clinic, founded by Methodist missionaries, is jointly controlled by the local Aymara and the Bolivian Methodist Church, and is perceived as an Indian institution that receives "gringo" financial support.

Everyone in town interpreted what Dr. Tallacagua said about medicine and how he talked in the clinic—his medical dialogue—as rejection of his Aymara ethnicity, and they resented it. As they discussed this resentment, they created an alliance between themselves that led to incremental steps in the creation of social change: Tallacagua's loss of status and early departure from town, the reinforcement of Aymara control and use of indigenous medicine in the clinic.

As Clotilde saw it, the trouble with Tallacagua was that he refused to speak Aymara at the clinic except with monolingual Aymara speakers. He was brusque and uncommunicative, and intimidated Clotilde. He had reduced her salary for washing linens from one peso per item to one peso per six items. Her work at the clinic was already a social disgrace among the village *mestizos*. But, landless and *tienda*-less, Clotilde and her four children could not subsist on the remittances her husband sent home. Ashamed that he could not send her more, her husband often called her a spendthrift and threatened to leave her for another woman who would be more financially responsible. When she took him seriously, she feared he would throw her and the children out of the house to starve. Her poverty and emotional outbursts were a source of shame to the other *mestizos*, who felt she reflected badly on them, particularly by being employed as a laundress at the clinic— even though most of them are just as poor. Doña Teresa thought Clotilde behaved like an Indian. Worse, her current employer, Tallacagua, was an Indian! Clotilde frequently had "attacks" and initially turned to the clinic for tranquilizers. In 1978, however, she was afraid to request them from Dr. Tallacagua

Clotilde received more from her association with the Aymara, in or outside of the clinic, than she did from her association with *mestizos*. They had given her a job. And as she benefited more and more from the Aymara, she found herself suffering more and more from disorders that Doña Teresa insisted afflict only Indians.

The Aymara campesino Eugenio didn't like Tallacagua at all. He said Tallacagua had mistreated him and his five-year-old daughter when he brought her to the clinic with severe pains in her lower abdomen. Eugenio complained that the doctor was apparently of the opinion that everyone should learn to speak Spanish and that Tallacagua should facilitate that by being a role model. He refused to accept payment in kind. He told his patients bluntly not to come to the clinic unless they were prepared to pay for services in cash. These policies, explained Eugenio, were condescending assertions of superiority that Tallacagua wielded now that he had a medical degree and presumably consequential access to Bolivian elite society. Previous physicians had spoken a few words of Aymara, accepted payment in kind, explained diagnoses in detail, been sympathetic to the Aymara world-view, respected indigenous medicine, and permitted *yatiris* to practice in the clinic. Tallacagua, said Eugenio in more complicated terms, was trying to negotiate a new identity, and Eugenio wasn't buying.

In this case Dr. Tallacagua had diagnosed appendicitis and strongly rec-ommended immediate surgery. Eugenio insisted on postponing such a dras-tic measure until he could discuss it with the rest of the family. Tallacagua must have been anxious for the child's health and angry that his medical authority carried so little weight when the problem was so urgent. He angrily warned that the child had only hours to live, that the operation was so serious that it would cost five hundred pesos (twenty-five dollars), an enormous sum; that the child was so sick because Eugenio had waited so long to bring her in; that surgery would be risky; and that he could not even guarantee its success at that time—let alone later if the father delayed changing his mind!

To Eugenio these words further confirmed Tallacagua's exploitative in-tents. He interpreted the doctor's words as lies designed to abuse and exploit him. He argued that as an Aymara campesino he had virtually no cash. He reasoned that being an Aymara himself, Tallacagua was fully aware of that. Cash greases the *mestizo* and elite worlds Eugenio saw as oppressing his own, and now Tallacagua asked him to deliver an outrageous sum to a man who had betrayed his Aymara identity and community to join those worlds. Given the more liberal clinic policy that had obtained before Tallacagua's arrival, his demand for cash seemed unnecessary, intended to serve Tallacagua's personal interest at Eugenio's expense, consistent with *mestizo* interests pur-sued at Aymara expense. His accusation of irresponsibility and ignorance for bringing the child in at such a late state in the illness furthered Eugenio's suspicions. The timing felt quite reasonable to Eugenio, who, like everyone else in town, could not easily afford either the clinic or a *yatiri* as a first course, and waited until home remedies proved ineffective.

Eugenio interpreted Tallacagua's warning of the child's possible death as a threat. To Eugenio, Tallacagua behaved exactly like a *karisiri*. Further-more, Tallacagua had told Eugenio that the operation might not be suc-cessful, insisting that Eugenio openly acquiesce and reaffirm Dr. Tallacagua's newfound ethnic affiliation by agreeing to accept nothing in return should the treatment fail and the child die. That the words the doctor probably intended as sincere warnings were interpreted by Eugenio as threats is based upon Eugenio's definition of Tallacagua's chosen identity— the way he discussed medicine—which Tallacagua substantiated by main-taining a social distance from the Aymara, by living apart from them, and by making no compromising gestures to reform that identity.

Miraculously, the child survived. Maybe Tallacagua's diagnosis was wrong.

From another perspective Tallacagua was not the evil character the towns-people made him out to be. They had their own reason for doing so: to create an alliance against his shift in ethnic identity through medicine, which they saw as being at their expense. Admittedly the analysis that Tallacagua was abandoning his Aymara identity to become a member of the elite appears to be correct. His implication that the local folk could not or should not understand cosmopolitan medical information is the first evidence to that effect. However, an attempt to understand Tallacagua's own strategy reveals a very different picture, and exposes another role ethnicity plays in medicine and medicine plays in ethnic identity. The use of medical ideology leads to incremental social change.

Tallacagua saw himself as an ambitious Aymara with a medical degree: as forging a new frontier, and thus an anomaly in Bolivia. The only one of his kind in medical school, he finished six years in five and graduated near the top of his class, yet friends of mine attending medical school at that time assured me that Tallacagua had not done well and was a fool. No one, least of all Tallacagua, knew what to do with a professional Indian. Upward mobility, while it occurs all the time, is covert, as was the Indians' arrangement of their entry into the town's *mestizo* class at the turn of the century. Tallacagua, however, came directly from the countryside, offending everyone by breaking the rules.

As a professional in La Paz, everything that revealed the immediacy of his Aymara Indianness worked against Tallacagua. At the same time, scientific medicine was good to him, he did well in school. One of his teachers referred to him as brilliant. He felt that were he not discriminated against, he could enjoy a successful life and help lift his family out of poverty. They were expecting him to do so, and he honored his familial obligations. However, finding himself alienated from both the Aymara and the Bolivian upper classes, Tallacagua wanted to go to Brazil, where he believed his Indianness would have no negative significance and his talents would be appreciated.

In order to do so, however, he had to play by Bolivian rules. He had to show the people with power in La Paz what he thought they wanted to see before they would help him secure a job elsewhere. So he perfected his Spanish. He distanced himself socially from the Aymara, whose association he thought would jeopardize him. He changed hospital policy to approximate as much as possible the policy of the teaching hospital in La Paz, and in ways that emphasized efficiency and the importance of scientific medicine. Aymara medicine was not tolerated. Neither was payment in kind. Given that most of the drugs in the dispensary had surpassed their stipulated shelf life, cash was desperately needed. Any step toward financial self-sufficiency would reduce dependency on "gringo charity" and make the hospital stronger. Tallacagua felt he was contributing to the modernization of the clinic. He also hoped to capitalize on those efforts. An article appeared in the La Paz newspaper referring to his work at "Tallacagua's clinic." That reference offended many in town, and after two months Tallacagua left, much to the relief of all parties, particularly himself.

In stark contrast with Dr. Tallacagua, Felipe Apaza, a proud Aymara and head nurse at the clinic, employed the ethnic dimension of medicine to his social and financial benefit by taking advantage of medical pluralism. Trained at the clinic by Methodist missionaries, he came to town from one of the surrounding communities. He maintained great respect for Aymara medicine, although he was less skilled at it than in referring patients to *yatiris*. Medicine provided him with multiple incomes at the clinic because he was administrator, nurse, radiologist, and laboratory technician. He also picked up extra cash by running a private practice out of his home for people who didn't wish to go to the clinic, either because he could treat some cases less expensively or because, unlike Tallacagua, he drew on Aymara medical ideology and incorporated indigenous medical resources into his cosmopolitan medical skills. During his long and successful career he had covertly become the primary authority at the hospital, although he carefully allowed the doctors who came and went to take credit for decisions that he himself supervised. Through the deft use of both medical traditions, he cultivated himself as cultural ambassador but definitively Aymara. As such he gained enormous stature throughout Omasullu and not a little wealth.

Everyone in town, Aymara and *mestizos* alike, looked up to Felipe. In the 1970s he was voted president of the local PTA.[36] He also was the only person in town to actively pursue the negotiation of a settlement between ethnic and religious groups, and the development of a single united community. When Father Christian called a meeting to castigate his Catholic flock for not attending church, not fulfilling their obligations to the church, and letting the building fall into disrepair, it was the Methodist Aymara Felipe who was the first to donate money to repair the padre's roof. He insisted the church repair was a community issue, not a Catholic one, and in so doing he renegotiated *mestizo*-Aymara relations so that both had equal civic responsibility—at least for a while. Facilitating that community unity was Felipe's staunch defense and use of Aymara medical beliefs. The Aymara said proudly, "Felipe Apaza is the hospital administrator." As such he wielded a lot of power in town. He is very proud of the Aymara medical tradition and wants someday to write a book on it. "Perhaps you can help me write them down," he said to me once, "I want to preserve them before they disappear." Because Felipe's strategies at the clinic were successful and Dr. Tallacagua's were not, he does not have to worry about the disappearance of Aymara medicine.

THE MORE PRACTICAL ARGUMENT

The relationship between ethnic identity and medical traditions is more than ideological. The diagnosis of an Indian illness, which today is more or less a diagnosis that involves some component of what cosmopolitan prac-

titioners might decry as "magic," has a number of implications that are related to the political economy of the *mestizo* and Indian modes of existence.

Belief in the magical component involves accepting that one shares a vulnerability with Indians and an acceptance of a sanction which ensures—that
the appropriate therapy *will* be followed. Indian illnesses are usually caused
by one of a pantheon of phantasms and spirits who are hungry, and will be
pacified only with a meal. Refusal to feed them results not only in death of
the victim but also in further inflictions on the victim's relatives. An unfed
demonic being is a public menace. Consequently, when the doctor diagnoses
anemia and insists the patient eat meat daily, the desperately poor *mestizo*
or Indian patient places his concern for personal well-being far behind the
welfare of his family and, like Vicente, does not eat the meat. Protein-rich
foods, mostly guinea pigs, eggs, chicken, and pork, are usually the only
source of cash, and there are numerous expenses that have greater priority
to the poor of the Bolivian altiplano than the vague symptoms of a chronic
illness. But when the *yatiri* says the patient is a victim of a hungry spirit
that demands to be fed, and that the patient must make a *mesa*[37] and sacrifice
pigs, guinea pigs, chickens, and eggs every Tuesday and Thursday for six
Tuesdays and Thursdays, the patient and his extended family sacrifice pigs,
guinea pigs, chickens, and eggs every Tuesday and Thursday for six Tuesdays and Thursdays. This explains in part why the doctor's diagnosis of
anemia held so little weight for Vicente.

Sacrifices are made along with a vast number of herbal treatments that
are quite likely effective because they derive from the Callaguaya medical
tradition (Bastien 1987; Oblitas Poblete 1963). The sacrificed animals are
expensive; the herbs come from all over Bolivia and are Indian property.
Treatment, then, often requires both wealth and the mobilization of social
relationships with Indians who have access to herbs. For the wealthy in La
Paz, this presents little problem; for the rural *mestizos* who are poor, despised
by elites and Indians alike, such resources may be hard to find. Isolated from
both groups in the postrevolutionary era, *mestizos* who are unable to join the
urban elite find some rewards in discarding their superordinate status and
allying themselves with the Aymara. For Felipe Apaza it is good business.
Though paradoxical from the perspectives of both modernization theory and
cosmopolitan medical wisdom, one consequence of this downward mobility
may be improved health care.

WHAT IT ALL MEANS

The focus of this study has been the anthropology of medical ideology
and medical dialogue in a medically plural environment: how such social
change takes place through medicine and how social analyses of medicine
and medical dialogues can contribute to the study of social change. This
analysis generates a reexamination of the popular dichotomy in medical an-

thropology between traditional and modern medical systems and the relatively new notion of medical pluralism.

The dichotomy between traditional and modern medical systems still obtains in the anthropological literature in spite of its inaccuracies (cosmopolitan medicine has a tradition; the *yatiri's* medicine is modern) and misleading connotation (not all traditional systems are alike). It implies that the two are discrete and that the latter will eradicate the former over time (Foster and Anderson 1978). This study is one of many that have demonstrated the fallacy of that assumption. The concept of medical pluralism (e.g., Leslie 1979; Elling 1980) refers instead to an environment in which there is more than one medical tradition. This conceptual change has permitted a shift toward examination of several coexisting medical traditions and how they interact. Nevertheless, within this concept the focus remains on medical traditions as bounded systems rather than as social institutions (Paul Unschuld is a noted exception—e.g., 1975, 1985). The major questions in this area today include the following: What is of medical or therapeutic value, and hence what is retainable of traditional systems according to cosmopolitan standards? How can medical systems that are of nationalistic or symbolic value be upgraded to meet Western standards through education, licensing, and incorporation into the Western medical model? How can such systems coexist and interact with cosmopolitan medicine?

While these are essential questions, they cannot adequately explain the persistence of medical traditions, their significance, the ways in which they change, and their relations to other dimensions of social change. An understanding of the political economy of medical traditions in a pluralistic environment, however, reveals something about the composition and dynamics of social change within that environment, and hence the nonmedical significance of medical traditions. Because of the politicoeconomic nature of the Bolivian indigenous medical tradition and the cosmopolitan medical tradition as it exists in Bolivia, the deployment of those medical traditions, the use of medical ideology, and medical dialogue—how people talk about who has what disease or illness and what should be done about it—all constitute a social idiom through which Bolivians negotiate the content of ethnic identity, and thereby facilitate or impede movement of economic and political resources across ethnic boundaries.

An analysis of the political economy of Bolivia at large, of the relations between *mestizos* and Indians within that context, of the contemporary directions that social change has been taking in Bolivia, and of the way that affects community life, clarifies the parameters of the negotiation of identity that takes place through the idiom of medicine. If we look at the confluences of culture in Bolivia, we see a population that encompasses several economic and ethnic domains, but also shares the same symbolic system, in such a way that symbols can be manipulated and negotiated. The use of ideologies that pertain to medical pluralism then becomes both a reflection of social

processes taking place as well as a means by which they do so. And medicine
is also a necessary idiom with which to negotiate identity, because the political economies of the various medical traditions involve the same social
relations that define a person's identity and social and economic standing on
the altiplano of Bolivia.

NOTES

1. Marvin Harris's seminal treatment of race in Latin America (1964) argues that
the concept there differs fundamentally from that in the United States. In Latin
America race is culturally based, defined by language, dress, and comportment, not
by phenotypic or genetic characteristics, as it is in the United States. All evidence I
encountered leads to the somewhat different interpretation that, while ethically
speaking, Harris is right, discourse engages the concept of genetics. In this article I
contend that there is no "racial integrity" whatsoever in Bolivia, that race is a mask
for social class, but that the genetic or racial argument inherent within the concept
of ethnicity is ubiquitously evident, particularly in medical ideology.

2. The most comprehensive histories of twentieth-century Bolivia are Dunkerley
1984; Klein 1969; and Kelley and Klein 1981. All three cover the rise of American
imperialism as an issue in the MNR revolution of 1952 and its aftermath for very
concrete reasons, including the manipulation of the world tin market by the United
States to the detriment of Bolivia just after the nationalization of the Bolivian tin
mines in 1953. They argue as well, however, that blaming U.S. imperialism for Bolivia's poverty was effectively employed to deflect attention from the demands of
the Indians and from the resistance of the revolutionary government to meeting
them.

3. Oblitas Poblete 1963, 112: the *khariciri* takes the image of a priest, steals fat
from the navel, and sells it to indigenous medicine men *(callaguayas)*, who can cure
or ensorcell with it.

4. La Barre 1948, 167: the *q'ariq'ari* is "an evil spirit incarnated in a body, with
a penchant for cutting open the neck of a person and stealing his soul, after which
that person sickens and dies." Another version, he says, is that it is "frequent in
August . . . steals the heart and puts sand in its place."

5. Tschopik 1951, 204: the *karikari* "are spirits of deceased Catholic priests . . .
[who] take away all of a man's fat and make soap out of it. They look like Franciscan
Fathers."

6. Aguilo 1982, 122: the "Karisiri" is a white man, a priest or engineer who at
night steals blood or fat, for holy oil and for curing.

7. Personal communication with anthropologists and priests in Peru and Bolivia.
Bastien came across the *kharisiri* among the Kallawaya (1987:71) but limits his discussion to how the fat is believed to be extracted.

8. Here and throughout most of the chapter, the dialogue presented constitutes
statements made by individuals, rather than linguistic interchanges between two or
more people. That is, the data presented here are statements rather than discussions.
However, the fact that these statements are "consumed" or accepted by the parties
to whom they are directed implies the nature of the response to the statements
presented here and of the discussions that ensued. On that basis I use the term

"dialogue." I thank Alexander Alland, Jr., for bringing the possible ambiguity of my usage to my attention.

9. The same argument can be made for class. While the focus of this article is ethnicity, its premise is that ethnicity in Bolivia is in fact a mask for social class.

10. I am arguing here that ethnicity is a mask for social class. However, not all social classes are distinguished by ethnicity. Ethnicity permits both oppression and resistance. Thus, while one often constitutes the other, the two terms are not synonymous.

11. The significance of fictive kin or *compadrazgo* ties in Bolivia and throughout most of Latin America is its subscription to patronage and clientage; godparents serve as patrons to the parents of godchildren *(compadres)*, who in turn—in Bolivia—provide the godparents with agricultural resources and services. This obligation was often inherited over several generations (see Strickon and Greenfield 1972).

12. A *tienda* is a small store that sells the same items that all other *tiendas* sell: canned goods, noodles, sugar and other staples, alcohol, beer, and magical items for curing. Running a *tienda* is a *mestizo* occupation and, until recently, one of a very few ways of generating some cash. Since all the *tiendas* sell the same items, customers are won through *compadrazgo* ties and goodwill, not through competitive marketing.

13. Some people might find my description of shifts between Indian, *mestizo*, and elite as upward and downward mobility offensive. Economically and politically, however, the use of these terms is accurate.

14. Since the argument here is that ethnicity is a mask for social class, what pertains to ethnicity, such as social movement and use of medical ideology and dialogue, also pertains to social class.

15. Until independence from Spain, what is now Bolivia was referred to as Upper Peru.

16. The revolution of 1952, engineered by the Movimiento Nacional Revolucionario (MNR) under the leadership of Victor Paz Estensorro and Hernán Siles Suazo, brought an end to the hacienda system instituted under colonialism, nationalized the mines that supported the state, and transformed the rural countryside. It was unable, however, to modernize Bolivia as it intended.

17. The intent of this chapter is not to do an analysis of Bolivia's political economy or to review the outcome of the 1952 revolution, except insofar as some analysis and review will clarify the context of medical dialogue. Hence this analysis and review are considerably simplified to suit the purposes of the chapter. Those interested in such an analysis are referred to Kelley and Klein 1981.

18. This is, naturally, the basis of all efforts in applied medical anthropology. For a splendid example of effective work, see World Health Organization 1975, concerning the Carroll Behrhorst program in Chimaltenango, Guatemala, and publications of the National Council for International Health. The Andean Rural Health Care Program in Bolivia is introducing revolutionary changes in the delivery of health care to the rural sector.

19. Though Bolivia is rich in natural, particularly mineral, resources, these have always been expensive to tap.

20. Caudillos were strongmen who cultivated and developed power domains based on personal favors and loyalty and who fought one another to expand their spheres of influence. This decentralized and competitive political structure was originally encouraged by the Spanish crown as a means of maintaining royal control over an

independent-minded population far from home. Upon independence, the competitive caudillo structure merely fitted itself to the new parameters of independence. Between 1825 and 1984, Bolivia experienced over 260 successful coups d'état. Many of the early presidents who seized office looked on Bolivia as their personal property (Carter 1971:39); Garcia Meza's behavior from 1980 to 1982 strongly suggests that he felt the same way.

21. Many of these gains, particularly universal suffrage, have had very little exercise since 1952.

22. One response to this change was the development of peasant entrepreneurs and middlemen *(cholos)*, who dominate the internal market for small goods and agricultural produce and transportation.

23. The most recent and valiant attempt to organize a political platform and pursue economic goals for political (in this case national) rather than personal ends was President Hernán Siles Suazo's presidency. Prevented from carrying out needed reforms in a divided nation under severe strain, he resigned halfway through his presidency. The Reagan administration's grinding pressure on Siles to take action against the drug trade came at a time when the state's economic resources were thoroughly depleted and social needs were at an all-time high. Further, Siles had just been kidnapped by the special drug forces—the Leopardos—that the Reagan administration, through the Drug Enforcement Agency, had organized. Indeed, the history of that administration gives solid credence to the argument that much of Bolivia's inability to modernize is related to U.S. policies.

24. This policy was reversed under Paz Estensorro, elected president in 1985, who immediately approached the International Monetary Fund to resume negotiations.

25. The dollar, worth 20 pesos bolivianos in 1979 after nearly a decade of stability, and 25 pesos bolivianos from 1979 to 1982, was being bought officially for 1,500,000 in September 1985. Whether inflation was due to the booming cocaine economy or to other factors is the subject of great debate.

26. President Siles, upon taking office in 1983, reduced government salaries; when President Victor Paz Estenssoro assumed office, he froze all wages until 1986.

27. The United States and the world economy played major roles in Bolivia's economic crisis during the 1980s. The return to democracy in 1983 also occurred under extraordinary circumstances.

28. Referring to Bolivia's history before 1952, Carter wrote that "for many decades it was a notable event for a Bolivian president to finish his term of office alive" (1971:39). Possibly the one achievement of the replacement of caudillo rule by military dictatorship is the contemporary fate of deposed presidents: exile instead of execution. However, Siles Suazo's successor, Paz Estenssoro, elected in 1985, was successfully succeeded in 1989 by Jaime Paz Zamora.

29. Historian Herbert Klein situates the end of caudillismo in Bolivia in the last century with the rise of republicanism. I do not dispute him in any way by pointing out that contemporary politics maintains many of the characteristics of its heritage. Klein has agreed to let me get away with this interpretation.

30. There is yet another mode pertaining to the *cholo* population that has developed since 1952. Likewise, yet another mode has recently developed in the Santa Cruz and Chapare areas that pertains to the cocaine economy. Neither is relevant to the case discussed here.

31. These two economies, the national or cash economy and the *ayllu*, do, of

course, articulate in multiple arenas. During the colonial era they were specifically articulated to serve the interests of capital accumulation and labor (Ainger 1990).

32. They may still be; I have not investigated this issue since 1978, at the conclusion of the research discussed in this chapter. Shifts in the 1980s in many Latin American economies toward unfettered free market principles have led to the elimination of such controls. Peru is a case in point (Ainger 1990).

33. Personal communication with numbers of members of the commercial and elite classes in La Paz.

34. I have written on this series of cases elsewhere: see Crandon 1983; Crandon-Malamud 1991: chs. 9–11.

35. One of these cases is the focus of Crandon 1983; two more, of Crandon 1986. All are examined in Crandon-Malamud 1991.

36. The local PTA is called the Padres de Familia.

37. A *mesa* is the prepared offering to the designated spirit and is composed of a variety of items carefully arranged on a cloth or table.

REFERENCES

Abercrombie, Thomas, 1986. "The Politics of Sacrifice: An Aymara Cosmology in Action." Ph.D. dissertation, University of Chicago.

Aguilar, Anibal. 1990. Personal communication.

Aguilo, Federico. 1982. *Enfermedad y Salud*. Sucre, Bolivia: Los Talleres Graficos Qori Llama.

Ainger, Hilary. 1990. "Agrarian Structure and Local Experience: Continuity and Change in Peru's Southern Sierra 1560–1982." Ph.D. dissertation, Teacher's College, Columbia University.

Alexander, Robert J. 1958. *The Bolivian National Revolution*. New Brunswick, N.J.: Rutgers University Press.

Arnaude, Charles. 1957. *The Emergence of the Republic of Bolivia*. Gainesville: University of Florida Press.

Bastien, Joseph. 1981. "Evaluation of Herbal Curing among the Callawaya Indians." Paper presented at the 41st meeting of the Society for Applied Anthropology, Edinburgh.

———. 1987. *Healers of the Andes: Kallawaya Herbalists and Their Medicinal Plants*. Salt Lake City: University of Utah Press.

Buechler, Hans, and Judith-Maria Buechler. 1971. *The Bolivian Aymara*. New York: Holt, Rinehart and Winston.

Canelas Orellana, Amado, and Juan Carlos Canelas Zannier. 1983. *Bolivia: Coca Cocaina*. La Paz: Los Amigos del Libro.

Carter, William. 1958. "Kachitu: Change and conflict in a Bolivian Town." Master's Thesis, Columbia University.

———. 1971. *Bolivia: A Profile*. New York: Praeger

———. 1982. *Irpa Chico: Individuo y Communidad en la Cultura Aymara*. La Paz, Bolivia: Libreria Editorial "Juventud."

Crandon, Libbet. 1983. "Between Shamans, Doctors and Demons: Illness, Curing and Cultural Identity midst Culture Change." In *Third World Medicine and Social Change*. John Morgan, ed. Lanham, Md.: University Press of America, 69–84.

———. 1986. "The Political Economy of Medical Dialogue in Rural Highland Bolivia." *American Ethnologist* 13(3):463–76

———. 1989. "Changing Times and Changing Symptoms: The Effects of Modernization on Mestizo Medicine in Rural Bolivia." *Medical Anthropology* 10(4):255–64.

Crandon-Malamud, Libbet. 1991. *From the Fat of Our Souls: Social Change, Political Process, and Medical Pluralism in Bolivia.* Berkeley: University of California Press.

Dunkerley, James. 1984. *Rebellion in the Veins: Political Struggle in Bolivia 1952–1982.* London: Verso Press.

Elling, Ray, ed. 1980. "Medical Sociology: Traditional and Modern Medical Systems." Special Edition of *Social Science and Medicine* 15A(2).

Foster, George, and Barbara Anderson. 1978. *Medical Anthropology.* New York: Wiley.

Foucault, Michel. 1965. *Madness and Civilization: A History of Insanity in the Age of Reason.* Translated by Richard Howard. New York: Random House.

———. 1973. *The Birth of the Clinic: An Archaeology of Medical Perception.* Trans. A. M. Sheridan Smith. New York: Vintage.

Frank, Andre Gunder. 1966. "The Development of Underdevelopment." *Monthly Review* 18:17–31.

———. 1971. *Capitalism and Underdevelopment in Latin America.* New York: Monthly Review Press.

Gwynne, S. C. 1987. *Selling Money.* New York: Viking Penguin.

Harris, Marvin. 1964. *Patterns of Race in the Americas.* New York: Walker.

Heath, Dwight. 1969a. *Land Reform and the Social Revolution in Bolivia.* New York: Praeger.

———. 1969b. "Bolivia: Peasant Syndicates among the Aymara of the Yungas: A View from the Grass Roots." In *Latin American Peasant Movements.* H. Landsberger, ed. Ithaca, N.Y.: Cornell University Press, 170–209.

International Work Group on Indigenous Affairs. 1978. *The Indian Liberation and Social Rights Movement in Kollasuyu (Bolivia).* Copenhagen: IWGIA.

Kelley, Jonathan, and Herbert Klein. 1981. *Revolution and the Rebirth of Inequality.* Berkeley: University of California Press.

Klein, Herbert. 1969. *Parties and Political Change in Bolivia 1880–1952.* New York: Cambridge University Press.

La Barre, Weston. 1948. "The Aymara Indians of the Lake Titicaca Plateau, Bolivia." *American Anthropologist* 50(1, Pt. 2).

Leslie, Charles, ed. 1979. "Medical Anthropology: Medical Pluralism." Special Edition of *Social Science and Medicine* 14B(4).

Lomnitz, Larissa. 1977. *Networks and Marginality.* New York: Academic Press.

McEwen, William, et al. 1969. *Changing Rural Bolivia.* New York: Research Institute for the Study of Man.

Malamud-Goti, Jaime. 1990. "Politics, Cops, Soldiers and Drugs in Bolivia." Department of Anthropology, Columbia University. Unpublished manuscript.

Malloy, James M. 1970. *Bolivia: The Uncompleted Revolution.* Pittsburgh, Penn.: University of Pittsburgh Press.

———. 1971. *MNR: A Study of a National Popular Movement in Latin America.* Council on International Studies. Buffalo: State University of New York.

Martin, Emily. 1987. *The Woman in the Body: A Cultural Analysis of Reproduction*. Boston: Beacon Press.

Mayorga, Rene A. 1987. *Democracia a la Deriva: Dilemas de la Participación y Concertación Social en Bolivia*. La Paz: CERES.

Mendelberg, Uri. 1985. "The Impact of the Bolivian Agrarian Reform on Class Formation." *Latin American Perspectives* 46(12):45–58.

Morales, Ramiro Condarco. 1966. *Zarete el "Temible" Willka, Historia de la Rebelion Indigena de 1899*. La Paz: Talleres Graficos Bolivianos.

Muñoz, Geraldo. 1981. *From Dependency to Development*. Boulder, Colo.: Westview Press.

Murra, John. 1975. "El Control Vertical de un Maximo de Pisos Ecologicos en la Economia de las Sociedades Andinas." In *Formaciones Economicas y Politicas del Mundo Andino*. Lima: Instituto de Estudios Peruanos, 59–116.

Nash, June. 1979. *We Eat the Mines and the Mines Eat Us*. New York: Columbia University Press.

Oblitas Poblete, Enrique. 1963. *Cultura Callaguaya*. La Paz: Talleres Graficos Bolivianos.

Platt, Tristan. 1978a. "Symetries en miroir. Le concept de yanantin chez les Macha de Bolivie." *Annales, E.S.C.* (Paris) 33(5–6):1081–1107.

———. 1978b. "Acerca del sistema tributario pre-toledano en el Alto Peru." *Avances* (La Paz) no. 1:33–46.

———. 1982a. *Estado Boliviano y Ayllu Andino: Tierra y Tributo en el Norte de Potosí*, Historia Andina 9. Lima: Instituto de Estudios Peruanos.

———. 1982b. "The Role of the Andean Ayllu in the Reproduction of the Petty Commodity Regime in Northern Potosí (Bolivia)." In *Ecology and Exchange in the Andes*. David Lehmann, ed. Cambridge: Cambridge University Press, 27–69.

Press, Irwin. 1969. "Urban Illness: Physicians, curers and Dual Use in Bogota." *Journal of Health and Social Behavior* 10(3):209–18.

———. 1971. "The Urban Curandero." *American Anthropologist* 73:741–56.

Preston, David. 1969. "The Revolutionary Landscape of Highland Bolivia." *The Geographic Journal* 135:1–16.

Quiroga Santa Cruz, Marcelo. 1973. *El Saqueo de Bolivia*. La Paz: Ediciones Puerta del Sol.

Rasnake, Roger. 1988. *Domination and Cultural Resistance: Authority and Power Among an Andean People*. Durham, N.C.: Duke University Press.

Romanucci-Ross, Lola. 1986. "Creativity in Illness: Methodological Linkages to the Logic and Language of Science in Folk Pursuit of Health in Central Italy." *Social Science and Medicine* 23(1):1–7.

Roxborough, Ian. 1979. *Theories of Underdevelopment*. Atlantic Highlands. N.J.: Humanities Press.

Scheper-Hughes, Nancy, and Margaret Lock. 1987. "The Mindful Body: A Prolegomenon to Future Work in Medical Anthropology." *Medical Anthropology Quarterly* 1(1):6–41.

Sontag, Susan. 1978. *Illness as Metaphor*. New York: Farrar, Straus and Giroux.

Stein, Stanley J., and Barbara H. Stein. 1970. *The Colonial Heritage of Latin America*. New York: Oxford University Press.

Strickon, Arnold, and Sidney Greenfield, eds. 1972. *Structure and Process in Latin*

America: Patronage, Clientage and Power Systems. Albuquerque: University of New Mexico Press.

Taussig, Michael. 1980. *The Devil and Commodity Fetishism.* Chapel Hill: University of North Carolina Press.

Tschopik, Harry, Jr. 1951. *The Aymara of Chucuito, Peru.* Anthropological Papers of the American Museum of Natural History. New York: The Museum.

Unschuld, Paul. 1975. "Medico-cultural Conflicts in Asian Settings: An Explanatory Theory." *Social Science and Medicine* 9:303–12.

———. 1985. *Medicine in China: A History of Ideas.* Berkeley: University of California Press.

Valenzuela, J. Samuel, and Arturo Valenzuela. 1978. "Modernization and Dependency: Alternative Perspectives in the Study of Latin American Underdevelopment." *Comparative Politics* 10(4):535–57.

Vincent, Joan. 1974. "The Structure of Ethnicity." *Human Organization* 33(4):375–79.

Wallerstein, Immanuel. 1974. *The Modern World-System: Capitalist Agriculture and the Origins of the European World Economy in the Sixteenth Century.* New York: Academic Press.

Wolf, Eric. 1982. *Europe and a People Without History.* Berkeley: University of California Press.

World Health Organization. 1975. *Health by the People.* Geneva: WHO.

PART II

EMPIRICAL ANALYSES OF NON-WESTERN MEDICAL PRACTICES AND MEDICAL ECOLOGY

Non-Western folk or tribal medical systems use a broad range of botanical and other elements in the treatment of the sick. That these herbal systems may reside within complex and medically significant ideologies in no way mitigates the fact that the herbs themselves are significant as medicines.

Humans have been experimenting with medicinal plants for a long time. Indeed, although one cannot be certain that they were used medicinally then, the fact that most of the pollens found by Solecki with the middle Paleolithic burial of Shanidar IV were from plants still in use medicinally by the local Iraqi population suggests that they were so used. One of the plants identified was *Ephedra*, source of ephedrine, a substance widely used in modern medicine as an antihistamine. Several of the other plants also have substantial demonstrable active principles (Solecki 1975).

That cases like these are not simple luck, that people carefully select medicinal plants and do not merely choose them at random, has been demonstrated twice, by independent researchers, in analyses of different continents. But, Hu, and Kong (1980), analyzing the use of 4,941 species of Chinese medicinal plants, and Moerman in Chapter 4, analyzing the use of 2,143 species of North American medicinal plants by Native Americans, have both concluded (by somewhat different techniques) that medicinal plants used are nonrandom selections of plants available. In addition, Moerman has shown that the plants selected tend to come from groups that produce biologically active substances to protect themselves against competition from other plants or from browsing by insects or vertebrates. At another analytical level, Michael Heinrich worked closely with Mixe healers in southern Mexico to determine how they selected plants for their medicinal value. His account tells us of their intimate knowledge of the natural world and how they exploit this knowledge to cure. Even so, the Mixe sense the limits of such a phytotherapeutic approach; any illness that causes chronic pain and is debilitating calls for supernatural intervention.

Bogin, in his comprehensive review of the evolution of human nutrition, demonstrates clearly that human health is a consequence of culture. He also demonstrates the much less obvious notion that changes in the human diet since the end of the Upper Paleolithic, and especially since the development of agriculture and the consequent reduction in both the variety and the quality of foodstuffs, have led to a general decline in the state of human health. Similarly, Van Blerkom shows how the great preponderance of infectious diseases were transferred from animals, primarily domesticated animals. This argument follows from a comparison of the extraordinarily different disease histories of Europeans and Asians, on the one hand, and Native Americans, on the other; the latter suffered very few infectious diseases because they had no domesticated animals of significance.

In a closer analysis of one West African society, Etkin and Ross argue that diet is tied not only to the maintenance of health but also to the amelioration of disease, as they argue that a number of elements in the Hausa diet can actually affect the course of malaria. The difference between "drugs" and "food" is ultimately one of concept, not of content. The empirical aspect of non-Western curing and healing, as we here exemplify, may have something to teach us.

REFERENCES

But, P. P., S. Y. Hu, and Y. C. Kong. 1980. "Vascular Plants Used in Chinese Medicine." *Fitoterapia* 51:245–64.

Moerman, D. 1979. "Symbols and Selectivity: A Statistical Analysis of Native American Medical Ethnobotany." *Journal of Ethnopharmacology* 1:111–19.

Solecki, R. 1975. "Shanidar IV, a Neanderthal Flower Burial in Northern Iraq." *Science* 190:880–81.

4

POISONED APPLES AND HONEYSUCKLES: THE MEDICINAL PLANTS OF NATIVE AMERICA

DANIEL E. MOERMAN

Some time ago, I reported a statistical analysis of the medicinal uses of plants by Native Americans (Moerman 1979). This chapter updates that analysis on a much larger sample, using data very nearly comprising a census of the medicinal plants of North America. In 1979 it seemed reasonable to focus on the issue of "efficacy," to attempt to demonstrate that Native American botanical medicine was not "only placebo medicine," that it was not simply a sort of random activity. While this is still a useful exercise, the field of ethnobotany and the world around it has changed enough in a decade that other emphases now seem more interesting. The primary question addressed here is, given the mass of available data, what sorts of plants were Native Americans most or least likely to select for use as medicines, and what can we learn from this about the human process of making choices—how did people learn which plants to use?

THE DATA BASE

My earlier analysis was based on a sample of 4,869 uses of 1,288 species of plants. That database is referred to as American Medical Ethnobotany (AME) (see Moerman 1977). Since then a much larger database referred to as Medicinal Plants of Native America (MPNA) has been constructed (Moerman 1986); the complete data set includes 17,634 uses of 2,397 taxa. The present report is based on an analysis of 15,843 uses of 2,143 species, for which complete taxonomic and botanical data are available (See Table 4.1).[1] As in the earlier paper, botanical information is derived from the provisional checklist of species from the Flora North America (FNA) (Shetler and Skog 1978).

Table 4.1
Comparison of the Data Bases

	American Medical Ethnobotany	Medicinal Plants of Native America	MPNA AME
Items	4,869	15,843	3.25
Cultures	48	123	2.56
Species	1,288	2,143	1.66
Genera	531	735	1.38
Families	118	141	1.19

MPNA includes all the data in AME (all checked against the original sources and corrected accordingly). It is worth noting that tripling the number of items in the database increased the number of species by only 66 percent and the number of genera by only 38 percent. This can be taken as evidence of the notion that MPNA is less a sample than a census of the medicinal plant species of the continent. Substantially increasing the number of items would be unlikely to markedly increase the number of medicinal taxa.

This chapter displays a technique of regression residual analysis for selecting portions of the data for further examination. A particular benefit of this method is that it allows us a means of observing not only the plants that are used frequently, but also the ones used infrequently or not at all, hence permitting a kind of controlled comparison.

ANALYSIS

The data were subjected to regression and residual analysis; the results are shown in Tables 4.2 and 4.3. The number of species per family used medicinally (MPNASPE) is regressed on the total number of species in each family according to FNA (FNASPE).

There are three primary elements in a regression analysis, these are the intercept or constant (a), the coefficient (b), and the correlation coefficient (r). The analysis generates a linear equation of the form

$y = a + bx$

which allows us to predict the value of y given the value of x. In the current case, the regression equation is:

$MPNASPE = 1.21 + .111 \times (FNASPE)$
with $r = .876$.

To predict the number of species used medicinally from a given family, multiply the number available by .111 and add 1.21. The analysis indicates

Table 4.2
Subsequent Regressions of Number of Species in MPNA on Number of
Species in FNA

Case	N	r	Coeff	Const	S.E.	Min	Max	Residuals	
								Skewness	Kurtosis
1	232	0.87	0.11	1.21	13.20	-129	95	-2.43	52.10
2	226	0.89	1.12	0.96	5.40	-15	25.3	1.81	7.39
3	209	0.91	0.12	0.67	2.80	-8.2	11.2	0.93	2.62

that this is a "good" regression because the correlation is high. This means
that the number of species in a family used medicinally is well predicted
by the number of species in that family. This could be taken as evidence
that the selection of medicinal plants was more or less random, that is, it
was not very selective at all.

However, an analysis of the residuals shows that selection was *not* random.
In a regression analysis, the residual is defined as the actual value of the
dependent variable minus the predicted value of the variable. Consider a
case: the very large Asteraceae (sunflower) family has 2,231 species in North
America according to FNA. Multiplying the number of species by .111 and
adding 1.21 we get 250 as the predicted number of species used medicinally;
MPNA indicates however that 345 species were used medicinally. The residual then is

$$\text{actual} - \text{predicted} = 345 - 250 = 95$$

Ninety-five more species were used medicinally than the regression predicted.

Another measure of a "good" regression is one where these residuals are
all small; a standard measure of this is, essentially, the standard deviation of
the residuals, called here the "standard error of the regression." In addition,
to be confident of the predictive value of a regression, the collection of
residuals should be distributed "normally" about the mean. Two measures
of normality are "skewness" and "kurtosis." Skewness measures whether
values are distributed equally about the mean, while kurtosis, roughly speaking, measures the shape of the distribution. Kurtosis of 0 represents a normal
distribution; positive values indicate sharply peaked distributions while negative values indicate flat distributions. These values are shown in the first
row of Table 4.2; they indicate some skewness and a high value for kurtosis,
indicating a peaked distribution. These cases with particularly large residuals
(positive or negative) indicate plant families that are selected for medicinal
usage far more or less often than is ordinarily the case. The great value of
residual analysis is that we can easily identify these important "outliers."

Table 4.3
Families by Residual from Regression Analysis

Case	Family	FNA		MPNA		MPNA Species	
		GEN	SPE	GEN	SPE	Predicted	Residual
High Use Families							
1	Asteraceae	296	2231	99	345	250	95.1
	Rosaceae	53	577	28	115	66	49.4
	Lamiaceae	56	320	30	64	37	27.1
2	Ranunculaceae	24	294	17	60	34	26.0
	Pinaceae	7	71	6	35	9	25.8
	Caprifoliaceae	7	77	7	35	10	25.2
	Salicaceae	2	131	2	40	16	24.1
	Liliaceae	59	393	27	67	45	21.9
	Apiaceae	79	319	30	58	37	21.2
	Corylaceae	5	33	5	21	5	16.1
	Saxifragaceae	34	260	17	46	30	15.8
	Ericaceae	30	180	16	36	21	14.7
	Solanaceae	23	129	6	28	16	12.4
3	Cupressaceae	5	27	5	15	4	10.7
	Fagaceae	5	140	4	26	17	9.1
	Cornaceae	1	17	1	12	3	8.8
	Polypodiaceae	44	215	17	33	25	7.8
	Pyrolaceae	12	27	5	12	4	7.7
	Berberidaceae	7	29	6	12	4	7.5
	Aceraceae	1	15	1	10	3	7.1
	Polygonaceae	20	413	5	54	47	6.7
Low Use Families							
1	Poaceae	206	1477	24	37	166	-128.8
	Cyperaceae	27	718	5	22	81	-59.2

Table 4.3 (Continued)

2	Fabaceae	118	1225	39	108	138	-29.7
	Caryophyllaceae	36	287	7	22	33	-11.2
3	Juncaceae	2	123	2	4	15	-10.9
	Agavaceae	9	86	0	0	11	-10.8
	Boraginaceae	33	304	12	25	35	-10.1
	Hydrophyllaceae	16	183	5	12	22	-9.6
	Scrophulariaceae	66	632	17	63	72	-8.6
	Acanthaceae	19	65	0	0	8	-8.4
	Euphorbiaceae	33	264	10	23	31	-7.6
	Cactaceae	22	180	6	14	21	-7.2

Note that the predictive value of regression is not of great interest here. We have little need to predict how many taxa from some family will be used medicinally, because we already know that; the data are very nearly a census of the situation, and prediction is not really necessary. The analysis of residuals, however, gives us an elegant way to identify families that are particularly interesting in one way or another.

Given this, a simple iterative process was used to identify and subdivide the "most used" and the "least used" families. Families with residuals more than (less than) twice the value of the standard error were eliminated from the sample, and the regression was repeated. This was done three times, yielding four regression equations on successively smaller samples (shown in Table 4.2), and three sets each of low-use and high-use families (shown in Table 4.3).

DISCUSSION

The 23 "high-use" families in Table 4.3 compose 37 percent of the species in FNA but 55 percent of the species used medicinally by Native Americans. The 13 "low-use" families likewise compose 37 percent of the species in FNA but only 18 percent of species in MPNA. What differences exist between the high-use and low-use families? This is not the place to consider all 36 of these families in detail, but some observations bear notice.

The Edible Grasses

The Poaceae, the grass family, stands apart from the rest as being by far the least used medicinally. This is a very large and complex family; in North

America, it has some 206 genera and 1,477 species, nearly 10 percent of the species of the continent. Only 24 of the genera and 37 of the species are used medicinally (in 107 ways). A number of these uses are quite distinctive. The Blackfeet, Cheyenne, Dakota, Omaha, Pawnee, Ponca, and Winnebago all use *Hierochloe odorata*, sweet grass, as an incense to purify, beautify, or otherwise enhance a variety of healing and other activities. The Thompson Indians of British Columbia used an infusion or decoction of the plant as a pleasant wash for the body or hair. Other grass species are used similarly, thus while these plants take their part in medicine, the grasses are rarely used as internal medicines. Simultaneously, we note that the grass family is the source of the vast majority of human food—wheat, corn (maize), oats, rye, and barley are only a few of the many seed grains that feed most people barley and their domesticated animals.

One may now raise the more general question, Why do plants produce medicines? What is it that leads poppies to produce chemicals that mimic the biological activity of the vertebrate endorphins? Generally, why do plants produce substances that have biological activity? In detail this is a very difficult question to answer, although in broad strokes it seems apparent that most such substances are designed to minimize browsing or to enhance pollination or seed dispersal. Speaking ecologically, these botanical activities can be seen as similar to a K-strategy of investment where animals devote energy to enhancing the survival of individual offspring (MacArthur and Wilson 1976); most botanical medicines are toxic and are only of value in moderation. The grasses, it seems, do not produce a significant number of these chemicals and are, therefore, not useful sources of medicines—the reaction of many grasses to being browsed (or mowed) is to grow back. One might note that the grasses seem to adopt an r-strategy rather in the manner of oysters, producing a great many seeds and investing little in them. Alternately, some species of this great family have made themselves so non-toxic and nutritious that a curious vertebrate species has for the last 8,000 years made it its business to tend these grasses until they have become the dominant plant species over vast regions of the temperate zones.

Given that the grass family is such a large one, it is not surprising to find exceptions to the general principle, as in the case of several species of the genus *Andropogon*, bluestem, which are used internally by the Chippewa, Omaha, Comanche, Houma, Catawba and others, formulated as analgesics, diuretics, stimulants and the like. At least one species of this genus *(A. nardus)* produces the fragrant oil citronella, which is to some degree toxic or noxious to insects (Claus, Tyler, and Brady 1970:179). Related species may produce similar substances.

Poison Apples

What is hinted at by the Poaceae is much clearer elsewhere—the Rosaceae demonstrates this same point in a very intriguing way. This family, which includes apples *(Pyrus)*, pears, peaches, cherries, and almonds (all-*Prunus*), seems to combine both of these strategies, creating what we can refer to as the "poisoned apple syndrome." Many members of the rose family produce nutritious and attractive fruits, as do the grasses; they produce quite toxic substances as well, which occur in the leaves, bark, and pits of many species. Amygdalin is one of a number of cyanogenetic glucosides produced by various species of Rosaceae that can give rise to cyanide poisoning. Usually this is only moderate, with distress, but occasionally more serious poisoning gives rise to loss of consciousness and serious respiratory trouble. Apnoeia and fatal collapse are exceptional but have occurred (Bodin and Cheinisse 1970:162).

People have died eating apple pits; poisoned apple is redundant. In this manner, these plants can attract various browsers to them to aid in dispersion of the seeds while simultaneously protecting the seeds from being destroyed. At the same time, in moderation, people have made medicinal use of these chemicals, as this is one of the primary sources of plant medicines. Appearing second in Table 4.3, 20 percent of the species of Rosaceae are used medicinally by Native Americans (in 1,038 ways in MPNA), notably for treatment of gastrointestinal, gynecological, and otorhinological problems of many sorts.

The Honeysuckle Family

Useful as such an approach is, no ethnobotanist is going to be surprised to see Asteraceae, Rosaceae, and Lamiaceae (mints) on a list of medicinal plants. More valuable is the presence of less obviously useful taxa, like the Caprifoliaceae (the honeysuckle family). All 7 genera in this family were used medicinally by Native Americans, as were 35 of its 77 species, in nearly 450 ways (see Table 4.4). Looking at the table it is apparent that elder *(Sambucus)* is the most heavily utilized of the seven genera. Were it not quite as apparent, one could use the same sort of regression/residual analysis as earlier. In this case, regressing the number of USES on the number of species used medicinally (MPSPE) gives

$$USES = 6.5 + 11.5 \times MPSPE,$$
$$r = .79$$

The predicted number of uses for elder by that equation is 98.5; the actual value is much greater:

$$residual = 170 - 98.5 = 71.5.$$

Table 4.4
Characteristics of Genera in Caprifoliaceae

Genus	FNA species	MPNA species	Uses	
Diervilla	2	1	18	Bush honeysuckle
Linnaea	1	1	8	Twinflower
Lonicera	29	8	77	Honeysuckle
Sambucus	14	8	170	Elder
Symphoricarpos	10	7	70	Snowberry
Triosteum	2	1	26	Feverwort
Viburnum	19	9	79	Viburnum

Elder is an interesting genus. Like members of the Rosaceae, this genus provides edible berries. The earliest recipe I am aware of using elder is from Apicius's cookbook, written during the reign of Tiberius in the first century. He recommended a sort of omelet of eggs, elderberries, and liquamen (a sauce made of fish and salt, on the order of Worcestershire), with pepper and wine (Flower and Rosenbaum 1958). Yum. Most elderberries must be cooked, dried, or fermented before they are eaten to ameliorate the effects of several emetic alkaloids that they contain, probably acting for the plant to inhibit excessive browsing by birds. These substances and others are responsible for the preponderant usage of the genus as an emetic, cathartic, and laxative (making up 40 of the 170 uses in MPNA). The next major grouping of uses is in various preparations for external applications to sprains, bruises, or swellings (by the Cherokee, Delaware, Houma, Iroquois, and Paiute), on cuts, wounds, boils, or sores (by the Iroquois, Rappahannock, Makah, and Pomo), and to the head for headaches (by the Chickasaw and Iroquois). While the basis for this sort of action is not as clear as the plant's emetic qualities (it probably produces tannin), many other peoples around the world have discovered these properties as well, whatever their origin. Hartwell (1982:105–6) lists two pages of similar topical usage of *Sambucus* from sources ranging from Chile to Belgium, and from Dioscorides to Lord Bacon, while Duke and Ayensu (1985:236) note the use of the genus in China for, among other things, "injuries, skin diseases, swellings . . . sprains . . . and traumatic injuries" in addition to its use as an emetic and diuretic.

Moreover, these two major categories of use (laxative/emetic and discutient) are the same as the recommended uses in the U.S. Pharmacopoeia, in which elder was listed one way or another from 1820 until 1905, and in the National Formulary from 1916 until 1947. For instance, the first revision of the USP said of *Sambucus canadensis*: "The flowers, are diaphoretic and discutient; the fruit, laxative, and sudorific." (USP 1830:55).

CONCLUSION

There is no single explanation for how Native Americans or others learned the medicinal values of plants. But at least one category of biologically active plants comprises those that have produced substances to protect themselves from browsing. Clearly the effectiveness of such protections would be enhanced if the plants could somehow signal, and browsers could somehow detect, their presence—perhaps through a distinctive odor or taste—before too much was eaten.

It seems likely that people have used these same signals as evidence of potentially valuable medicines and, over millenia, human knowledge of the subject accumulated. "Knowledge" is a complex phenomenon with both historical and cultural dimensions: "In their practical projects and social arrangements, informed by the received meanings of persons and things, people submit . . . cultural categories to empirical risks" (Sahlins 1985:ix). In the process, the explanations for things may change; but a kernel of truth, a sort of natural object (e.g., *Sambucus* heals sores) may remain, even though it may be accounted for in a multitude of ways. The initial experiments by which this natural object became "known" need not have been repeated many times; things only have to be learned once. The same may be true for *Pyrus* and *Prunus* and perhaps even for sweet grass.

ACKNOWLEDGMENTS

The database MPNA was produced with the support of the National Endowment for the Humanities, grant number RT-20408–04. The current paper was written with support from the National Science Foundation, grant number BNS-8704103. Stanwyn Shelter of the Smithsonian Institution Museum of Natural History provided the computer tape with the indispensable Flora North America data. Special thanks to Barry Bogin, Katie Anderson-Levitt, Charlotte Gyllenhaal, and Sally Horvath for providing extremely helpful criticisms of earlier drafts of this chapter. The University of Michigan-Dearborn has supported me in uncounted ways for over a decade.

NOTE

1. Several hundred items in MPNA, identified only to the genus, are excluded here as are a small number of domesticated species with anomalous distributions, like chamomile, mustard, cabbage and cotton.

REFERENCES

Bodin, F., and C. F. Cheinisse. 1970. *Poisons*. Trans. H. Oldroyd. New York: McGraw-Hill.

Claus, Edward P., Varro E. Tyler, and Lynn R. Brady. 1970. *Pharmacognosy*. Philadelphia: Lea and Febiger.

Duke, James, and Edward Ayensu. 1985. *Medicinal Plants of China*. 2 vols. Algonac, Mich.: Reference Publications.

Flower, Barbara, and Elisabeth Rosenbaum. 1958. *The Roman Cookery Book*. London: Harrap.

Goodman, Louis S., and Alfred Gilman. 1970. *The Pharmacological Basis of Therapeutics*. 4th ed. New York: Macmillan.

Hartwell, Jonathan L. 1982. *Plants Used Against Cancer*. Lawrence, Mass.: Quarterman Publications.

MacArthur, Robert H., and Edward O. Wilson. 1976. *The Theory of Island Biogeography*. Princeton, N.J.: Princeton University Press.

Moerman, Daniel. 1977. *American Medical Ethnobotany: A Reference Dictionary*. New York: Garland Publishing.

———. 1979. "Symbols and Selectivity: A Statistical Analysis of Native American Medical Ethnobotany." *Journal of Ethnopharmacology* 1:111–19.

———. 1986. *Medicinal Plants of Native America*. 2 vols. Technical Reports, Number 19. Research Reports in Ethnobotany, Contribution 2. Ann Arbor: University of Michigan Museum of Anthropology.

Sahlins, Marshall. 1985. *Islands of History*. Chicago: University of Chicago Press.

Shelter, Stanwyn G., and L. E. Skog, eds. 1978. *A Provisional Checklist of Species for Flora North America*. Monographs in Systematic Botany, Vol. 1. St. Louis: Missouri Botanical Garden.

Solecki, Ralph. 1975. "Shanidar IV, a Neanderthal Flower Burial in Northern Iraq." *Science* 190:880–81.

United States Pharmacopoeia. 1830. *The Pharmacopoeia of the United States of America*, 2nd ed. New York: S. Converse.

5

HERBAL AND SYMBOLIC FORMS OF TREATMENT IN THE MEDICINE OF THE LOWLAND MIXE (OAXACA, MEXICO)

MICHAEL HEINRICH

One of the central aspects of any culture is its medical system. In non-Western cultures, "indigenous," "traditional," or "non-western" forms of treatment are still of enormous importance. There are estimates that "perhaps 80% of the . . . inhabitants of the world rely on traditional medicines for their primary health care, and it can safely be presumed that a major part of traditional therapy involves the use of plant extracts or their active principles" (Farnsworth et al. 1985).

Although there are numerous studies that document Mexican medicinal plants from a botanical point of view (e.g., Amo 1979; INI 1994) and studies that describe and analyze the Mexican indigenous medical systems (e.g., Rubel 1960; Young 1981; for two examples of specific aspects of medical systems in Mexico, Aguirre Beltran 1986; Foster 1976; Greifeld 1982; Logan 1977), the integration of these two approaches is still scarce (Ramirez 1978). But, an integrated study ought to be a principal focus of anthropologically oriented ethnopharmacological research (cf. Etkin 1988, 1993). Thus, the goal should be twofold: to comprehend the sociocultural basis for indigenous therapies and to evaluate these therapies for their medical and pharmaceutical potentials and risks. The approach to the latter goal will then be interdisciplinary in itself, requiring collaboration between pharmaceutical biologists, pharmacologists, botanists, phytochemists and anthropologists.

In our research, we attempt to achieve this by combining methods of anthropological and botanical fieldwork with a subsequent phytochemical and pharmacological-microbiological evaluation of the plants most commonly used (Heinrich et al. 1992a, 1992b, 1992c; Hoer et al. 1995; Kuhnt et al.

An earlier form of this chapter was published in *Anthropos* 89 (1994):73–83. Permission to include that material here granted by *Anthropos Redaktion*, Sankt Augustin, Germany.

1995). Plants and their medical uses are documented during field studies of 14–16 months. We try to understand the concepts that form the basis of these uses. We then evaluate a selection of important plants using several pharmacological and (micro-)biological methods in order to obtain information on the potential effects of these plants with respect to the uses as reported by the healers. The most active plants are subsequently studied phytochemically in order to isolate the bioactive compounds.

In this chapter I analyze the sociocultural basis of the indigenous plant use as part of the medical system of the Lowland Mixe of Oaxaca (Mexico), especially as it relates to the roles of the healers. The discussion is subdivided into five sections: (1) the role of the healers within the community and their forms of treatment; (2) the concept of diseases prevalent (see also appendix and Heinrich 1985, 1989); (3) treatment strategies; (4) the importance of plants within the medical system; and (5) the availability of plants as a medical resource in the ecological zones around the Mixe house as they are described locally. The interplay of herbal and symbolic forms of healing is discussed using two examples: the treatment of snake bites and the use of preventive ritual medicine for newborns.

ETHNOGRAPHIC BACKGROUND AND METHODS

Ethnographic Background

The land of the Mixe extends mostly through the cool and humid mountains of the Sierra de Juarez in the Mexican state of Oaxaca; San Juan Guichicovi is the only Mixe-speaking community belonging to the subtropical Istmo de Tehuantepec. San Juan is the principal community *(cabecera)* of a subdistrict *(municipio)* of the same name. In 1980, 20,000 people lived in the *municipio*, approximately 5,500 to 6,500 of them in the *cabecera* (Censo General 1980:145–46; and unpublished data). Seventy-five percent of the population in the *cabecera* is bilingual. A minute fraction of the population speaks only Spanish. The economy is based on subsistence agriculture (mostly maize) and on the production of coffee and citrus fruit.

No detailed monograph on the Lowland Mixe is available. Brief accounts are given by Foster (1969) and Nahmad (1965). The only cultural aspects that have been dealt with in detail are the ritual calendar, which is still in use in some parts of the *municipio* (Carrasco et al. 1961; Lipp 1991; Weitlaner and Weitlaner 1963), and the relationship of religious ritual and medical concepts (Lipp 1991).

The language belongs to the macro-Mayan stock. Mixe vowels are generally pronounced as in Spanish. Additionally, *ë* is used, pronounced as a nasalized Spanish *o*. The consonants are pronounced as in Spanish. A glottal stop(') and palatalized consonants and vowels are frequently written as *ay*, *ky, my,* and so forth. In this article, the Mixe words are transcribed as used by the bilingual teachers in the community.

Methods

The data presented here were collected during four stays in the community totaling a period of 19 months (November 1992, December 1989–January 1990, November-December 1988, November 1985–December 1986). We interviewed a total of 15 specialists in medicinal plants and/or healing, who accompanied us on excursions to the surrounding countryside to collect plants, identified by them as medicinal. For each plant, detailed information on its uses, preparation, and application were solicited. We observed the healers during their healing sessions and asked them in open interviews to describe various illnesses and their treatments.

We conducted structured interviews with a total of 185 inhabitants of the community on the treatment strategies known to cure eight culturally salient illnesses and on the plants most frequently used as medicinals. The illnesses were chosen to represent both illnesses (or syndromes) also recognized in Western medicine (*të'ënëë*—diarrhea, *kopt ba'am*—headache, *jo'ot ba'am*—stomach pain) and so-called culture-bound syndromes (*tsëkë'ë*—sudden fright, *tsubox wiintoy*—illness caused by the bad winds of the night, *wiintoy*—evil eye). One ambivalent category (*joxk ba'am*—pain of the whole body) was also included for comparison with *tsubox wiintoy*, which is said to be associated with pain all over the body. The treatment forms and modes of application (e.g., tea, rectal application, limpias, religious acts) had first been elicited in open interviews. In addition, we conducted unstructured interviews and open discussion on medicinal plants or treatment methods with a very large proportion of the population.

We collected voucher specimens of the plants indicated as medicinals and identified them by comparison with authenticated specimens at the National Herbarium of Mexico (MEXU). Some difficult species were identified by specialists for the respective taxa. A complete set of the specimens is available at MEXU and at the Institut für Pharmazeutische Biologie (FB) in Freiburg, Germany.

RESULTS

The Healers and Their Specializations

There are at least 15 different healers known in the community. Healers are generally referred to as *pa'am iixyp'*. The literal translation of this phrase is "the one who sucks out an illness." Fairly large differences exist between the various groups of healers in the community. The largest groups are "specialists in home remedies." Other important groups are midwives (*ma uunk wixyp'* or *parteras*), *chupadores* (*pota'ak ixyp'* or *ma'ixyp'*-those who suck), prayer makers (*rezadores*), Spiritists (*espiritistas*) and Spiritualists (*espiritualistas*).[1]

The "specialists in home remedies" are a group of practitioners who do not consider themselves healers, but who "only give some plants or a *limpia* (ritual cleansing)" if a person is ill. These persons are generally knowledgeable with respect to plants that can be used in the treatment of common, minor illnesses and ailments. Any person who has a "cooling hand" (*këtoxk*) is capable of performing a *limpia*. If an illness is severe or difficult to treat, the patient may be referred to other healers, especially those who are ritual specialists.

Midwives assist pregnant women, women in labor, and mothers with children during the first few weeks of the life of the newborn. During pregnancy, the midwife sees the pregnant woman at least two or three times, more frequently if there are problems with the pregnancy. The midwife palpates the belly and checks the position of the child. If necessary, the patient is asked to use special teas or is given massages. There are several midwives in the community who claim to be able to change the position of the child in the womb if this is necessary. During labor, the midwife oversees the birth, frequently together with female relatives of the woman in labor. The birth usually takes place in the home of the parturient. The newborn is bathed and rapidly given back to the mother. After a few days or weeks, the midwife returns to the home of the mother and the rite, *jekëëny tsiiny*, is performed (see under "Special Preventive Ritual Medicine," below). Midwives frequently give other forms of health advice or treatment. They are generally knowledgeable about medicinal plants and sometimes advise young mothers on how to treat their children. Many of the specialty areas discussed in the following paragraphs are held by women who also work as midwives. Many midwives have had intensive contact with doctors, nurses, and midwives of the Mexican national health service and now have some basic training in gynecology and pediatrics.

The *iixy poxujp* (persons who blow away an illness) also cleanse a person with *limpias* and perform rituals. The name refers to the blowing of alcohol (*aguardiente*) on the patient during the healing ceremony.

Chupadores specialize in "sucking out" an illness. If there is pain at a certain part of the body, they suck at these regions. The cause of the pain is usually a part of a bone, a little pebble, or a potsherd. This fragment is spit out and declared the causal agent of the illness. With additional massages and recommendations for herbal preparations, the treatment is terminated. Each treatment may be repeated if necessary. This form of treatment is used especially when supernatural causes are suspected.

The *amamabie* know how to perform the oracle using maize kernels. Its use is restricted to situations in which an illness is considered very heavy and/or painful, or when evil spirits or witchcraft are suspected. Using this rite, the healer predicts the future of the patient and indicates whether a treatment is going to be successful. The healers in the community who know these rites are usually midwives, but occasionally they may be some other type of healer.

Prayer makers (*rezadores*) ask forgiveness, or *nu'ux tak*. According to local perception, this rite (called *koxtenabie*) is (or, for more and more people, was) an essential part of many interactions between humans and nature. Cleaning a forest, sowing seeds, and building a house, as well as asking for health, are examples of situations in which this rite is considered necessary.

If an illness is considered to be very severe, a prayer maker is asked to perform the healing ceremony. Following his advice, the rite may be performed in front of the house altar, in front of the altar of the local patron saint (San Juan Bautista) or one of the minor saints (San Juan Degollado, Santa Cruz) of the main church, or in front of the altar of San Martin Caballero, which has its own chapel. Frequently, if such a rite is performed, two or more saints may be addressed one after the other.

An example of such a prayer (used in a healing ceremony) is given in the following:

yaaxy wiin nëwa'ats	save and heal
miixy yaaxy oy'it	we ask so that you will be well
ya nëwa'ats	so that you will be well
ya kuwa'ats	unbottle it[2]
yaaxy oy'it	so that you will be all right
yaaxy wiinit	so that you will be well

Spiritists and spiritualists are a fairly recent phenomena in the region. Spiritualists are members of a Mexican religious movement that started at the end of the last century and that now has temples in many areas of rural and urban Mexico. There are several studies of this religious movement from other areas of Mexico, most of which focus on its medical aspects (Finkler 1985). This cult is distinct from Roman Catholicism. Each temple is structured hierarchically with a head, a guardian, several pillars, and other religious functionaries. According to spiritualist beliefs, the founder of the movement was the son of an Otomi Indian mother from Hidalogo and a *mestizo* father of Spanish and Jewish descent. He proclaimed himself the incarnate of the Holy Ghost, and is generally referred to as "Father Elias." He is frequently regarded as being identical with the Holy Spirit (at least by the spiritualists from San Juan) and thus one of the three principal figures in the spiritualist pantheon (together with God Father and God Son).

Locally, the movement was started in 1962 when a person, who had been ill for several years, visited a spiritualist temple in the *mestizo*/Zapotec city of Tehuantepec. He had very severe convulsions, frequently became unconscious, and was aggressive. The treatment lasted for several months and one essential part of the curing process was the requirement by the spiritual leader of the Tehuantepec temple to start "la obra" in Guichicovi, too. Therefore, he began to build a temple and to cure.

On rare occasion, healing ceremonies are conducted by a medium who is possessed by a spirit. In earlier years one or two persons from the temple in San Juan were mediums themselves. Nowadays such healers come once or twice a year from Tehuantepec. This is different than in other areas of Mexico, where the spiritualistic leader of a temple and the healer usually work as a medium.

Today, there are several temples of this medico-religious group in San Juan. The original founder in the community treats a large variety of illnesses and uses symbolic as well as phytotherapeutic and physiotherapeutic forms of treatment. Most of the more recently founded temples use largely symbolic forms of treatment (e.g., prayers, spiritual cleansing ceremonies), and have in recent years been influenced by Mexican government organizations, who try to promote "indigenous" forms of treatment (see below).

Spiritists are a possession cult, which is still strongly associated with the Catholic Church. According to spiritist belief, the healer is only a medium for a spirit; the spirit is the actual "spiritistic healer." Usually it was a more or less well-known clergyman, medical doctor, or indigenous healer, who during his lifetime performed miraculous healings or lived a particularly "holy life."

In previous decades, several other groups of specialists practiced in the community, for example bone setters and *culebreros* (healers of snake bites). However, none of them was still working at the time of the study. Recently, traveling salespeople (most of whom speak Mixe), people with some minimal experience in Western medicine, helpers of the local Roman Catholic priest and of various Protestant groups, and some trained nurses are offering their help to heal the ill. The differences between these groups and also between the various individuals are enormous. Some (especially among the traveling salespeople and the people with some minimal experience in Western medicine) are charlatans, but others have a sound background in basic medical therapies.

The last group that should be briefly mentioned is university-trained medical doctors. The first ones were working in San Juan in the early 1960s, but no permanent clinic was opened until the late 1970s. At this time, two government institutions—the Instituto Nacional Indigenista (INI) and the Instituto Mexicano del Seguro Social (IMSS)—opened one clinic each, staffed with a medical doctor who usually is available from Monday to Friday. Two trained nurses work in the IMSS. The INI additionally provides dental care. A private medical doctor started working in San Juan in the mid-1980s. A detailed discussion of these groups would be beyond the scope of this paper (see also under "Recent Changes").

Disease Concepts

To the Mixe, minor ailments of relatively short duration are of little concern. Such illnesses include superficial cuts, bruises, and other minor dermatological conditions, and coughs and other respiratory illnesses (see appendix). They are generally treated with medicinal plants. These diseases are thought to be caused by natural forces. Cuts, bruises, and burns need no further explanations, since the physical impact on the person is obvious. In the case of colds, the coldness of the season (e.g., December) and the lack of proper clothing or "una infección" (an infection, a Spanish loan word in Mixe) are blamed.

There are three important reasons for an illness to be considered more severe: if it is seen as debilitating, dangerous or even life-threatening to the patient, if it is associated with severe pain, or if it is long lasting (chronic).

These illnesses require an explanation as to their cause. Such explanations frequently refer to supernatural powers that transmit an illness onto a patient who has been careless and did not pay attention to the proper forms of protection. Several Mixe illnesses are widespread in Latin America. One example is the exposure to the evil winds of the night (*tsubox wiintoy*). The night wind carries with it a large number of evil forces, especially spirits, that may steal a soul or cause other malevolent results. Another explanatory model is *tsëkë'ë* (susto, or sudden fright). A sudden fright causes a loss of the soul and thus leads to illness (Rubel 1964, 1988; Rubel et al. 1984; Klein 1978).

Wiintoy (evil eye) is another illness that is known in a large number of Mesoamerican cultures. This is an illness that especially afflicts persons who are not very resistant to illness. It is caused by adults—frequently by those with a "strong eye." By being too kind and friendly to a child who is not a relative, "heat" is "injected" into the child. Occasionally, a weakened adult may also be the victim. In a few cases *wiintoy* may lead to death.

Treatment of these conditions requires an approach based on more than simply the utilization of medicinal plants. Depending on the "patient," one of the above-mentioned sorts of healers will be consulted; if the first treatment is not successful, a new medical choice is often made (Young 1981). The explanations for such illnesses frequently refer to supernatural phenomena (see translations in the Appendix).

Treatment Strategies

Obviously the strategy a person chooses for the treatment of his or her illness or that of a relative depends on personal experiences and preferences. Table 5.1 summarizes the data from interviews conducted with 182 inhabitants of the community. Each informant was asked to list the form or forms of treatment that he or she found most appropriate to cure each of eight

Table 5.1
The Preferred Forms of Treatment of Eight Popularly Recognized Illnesses Elicited in
Interviews with 182 Inhabitants of San Juan Guichicovi

Illness category / Mode of application	tsĕkĕ'ĕ (susto)	wintoy (evil)	tsubox wiintoy (malaria)	tooy (fever)	tĕ'ĕnĕš (diarrhea)	joxk pa'am (body pain)	kopt pa'am (head ache)	joot pa'am (stomach pain)
1. External								
limpias	36.8% (85)	82.7% (158)	48.5% (80)	13.4% (36)	0.9% (2)	1.4% (3)	3.5% (7)	0.0% (0)
massages	35.9% (83)	11.5% (22)	15.1% (25)	39.0% (105)	1.9% (4)	57.6% (122)	51.0% (101)	7.5% (17)
sucking	3.0% (7)	1.0% (2)	3.6% (6)	0.7% (2)	0.9% (2)	1.4% (3)	0.0% (0)	2.2% (5)
2. Oral Applications								
tea	3.5% (8)	0.0% (0)	2.4% (4)	3.3% (9)	64.3% (137)	2.4% (5)	0.5% (1)	49.1% (112)
drops	0.0% (0)	0.0% (0)	0.0% (0)	0.0% (0)	6.1% (13)	0.0% (0)	0.0% (0)	2.6% (6)
purging	4.3% (10)	0.0% (0)	0.6% (1)	0.7% (2)	3.3% (7)	1.4% (3)	0.5% (1)	20.2% (46)

tablets	0.4%	0.0%	0.0%	10.4%	18.3%	30.2%	42.9%	9.6%
	(1)	(0)	(0)	(28)	(39)	(64)	(85)	(22)
3. Rectal Applications								
'lavados'	7.4%	1.0%	0.6%	32.0%	4.2%	2.8%	1.5%	8.8%
	(17)	(2)	(1)	(86)	(9)	(6)	(3)	(20)
4. Injections								
injections	0.4%	0.0%	0.0%	0.0%	0.0%	2.4%	0.0%	0.0%
	(1)	(0)	(0)	(0)	(0)	(5)	(0)	(0)
5. Religious Acts								
corn oracle	7.4%	1.0%	17.6%	0.0%	0.0%	0.0%	0.0%	0.0%
	(17)	(2)	(29)	(0)	(0)	(0)	(0)	(0)
rites in the church	0.4%	1.0%	4.2%	0.0%	0.0%	0.0%	0.0%	0.0%
	(1)	(2)	(7)	(0)	(0)	(0)	(0)	(0)
other rites*	0.4%	1.6%	7.2%	0.4%	0.0%	0.5%	0.0%	0.0%
	(1)	(3)	(12)	(1)	(0)	(1)	(0)	(0)

Table 5.1 (Continued)

Total number of positive responses**							
99.9%	99.8%	99.8%	99.9%	99.9%	100.1%	99.9%	100.0%
(231)	(191)	(165)	(269)	(213)	(212)	(198)	(228)
Number of "know" responses							
90.7%	92.3%	74.7%	95.1%	95.6%	97.3%	95.6%	94.0%
(165)	(168)	(136)	(173)	(174)	(177)	(174)	(171)
Number of "don't know" responses							
9.3%	7.7%	25.3%	4.9%	4.4%	2.7%	4.4%	6.0%
(17)	(14)	(46)	(9)	(8)	(5)	(8)	(11)

*These are mostly rites involving the burning of incense, chile, and so on in front of the house altar or ritually "fumigating" the house.

**The number of responses is higher than the number of interviewees, since each informant was asked to list all forms of treatment which he/she finds appropriate.

common illnesses. Afterward, these answers were divided into five groups, based on the mode of application used (four groups) or whether ritual forms of curing were used (one group). The four modes of application are external, oral, rectal, and injection (mostly intramuscular). This Western form of therapy is only rarely regarded as useful. The category "religious acts" includes the corn oracle rites in the church (*koxtenabie*) and rites in front of the house altar and elsewhere. Additionally, Table 5.1 lists the number and percentage of the 182 informants who knew none, one or more forms of treatment.

For each of the eight illnesses, a culturally preferred form of treatment is known by the Sanjuaneros. *Tsë'ënëë* (diarrhea), is generally treated with herbal teas. These are largely based on plants with astringent properties (Heinrich et al., 1992c). *Jo'ot ba'am* (stomach pain) usually is also treated using teas. The qualities of the plants are usually bitter, aromatic, or bitter-aromatic. In this case, two additional forms of application, rectal application (*lavados*) and the use of purgatives (*pixk*), are important. The latter two forms of treatment are important because they are said to "cleanse the body internally."

With illnesses associated with pain (*joxk ba'am*, pain of the whole body; *kopt ba'am*, headache), the use of tablets is increasingly important. This is especially the case with headache, where 43 percent of all respondents indicate tablets as an appropriate form of treatment. The tablets are usually a commercial preparation of acetylsalicylic acid (ASA/aspirin). It is not surprising that a high percentage of the respondents find external rubbing and massage to be the appropriate form of treatment for *joxk ba'am* (pain of the body). Especially the affected parts of the body are massaged (e.g., the leg).

If none of the culture-bound syndromes is suspected, oral forms of treatment (including, nowadays, tablets) are usually regarded as appropriate. The culture-bound syndromes (*tsëk'ëë*—sudden fright, *tsubox wiintoy*—illness caused by the bad winds of the night, *wiintoy*—evil eye) are generally treated using *limpias* (ritual cleansing ceremonies with aromatic herbs and eggs) or by rubbing or massaging the body. Of particular interest is *tsubox wiintoy*. This is the illness for which the lowest number of informants knew a treatment (75% compared to more than 90% for the other seven illnesses.) Since we did not ask for treatments the informant had received (or given), the answer refers to the knowledge that a person has about a specific treatment. This knowledge may be based on observation, personal experience as a patient, or by having heard about it. *Tsubox wiintoy* is clearly something for which one must consult a specialist. At the same time, this illness (together with *tsëk'ëë*) is frequently seen as requiring religious acts in front of the house altar (*namabie*), in the church (*koxtenabie*), or the maize oracle (*contar maize*).

This ritual was observed with a female healer who was approximately 70 years old. She had been ill with headaches for some time and used the oracle to find out whether she would get well again or die. The corn oracle is a rite in which a corn cob with 12 rows of kernels is selected; 102 kernels are removed from the lower half of the cob. The kernels are blessed, passed over incense, and put on a chair. A handful of the kernels is taken into one hand and the rest put aside. The kernels are then grouped into heaps of five. These heaps are arranged in a circle. If less then 10 kernels remain, they are partitioned in two equal portions and put into the center of the heap. The kernels have to be in pairs, otherwise the process has to be repeated. If there are two heaps of four kernels each, the patient will get well. If there are two groups of three kernels the patient will die. In the case of the above-mentioned healer, she determined that the illness would disappear soon.

Today, the rite *pa'am exkopy* is used only by a few persons in the community. Old clothes, candles and some mescal are deposited in a hidden spot, usually a place that is not frequented by people. It is usually performed in case of *tsubox wiintoy* (malaire). The goal is to leave an illness far away from the home.

Plant Use

The species used have been described in detail elsewhere (Heinrich 1989; Heinrich et al. 1992b, 1992c). Plants are generally used in the treatment of minor illnesses such as cuts and skin infections. The medicinal plants that are regarded as potentially helpful are sought as soon as the person notices an infection or a cut. No healers or ritual specialists are consulted in these cases.

There are a large number of illnesses where oral (or less frequently rectal) applications of herbal preparations are a frequent part of the treatment (stomach pain, diarrhea, see Table 5.1; dysentery, intestinal parasites, various liver disorders). Consequently, plants used for these illnesses are ideal candidates for a pharmaceutico-botanical evaluation.

In order to understand the criteria that are used to characterize and select a medicinal plant, the informants were asked *why* a specific plant is considered to be medicinal. The Mixe distinguish a large number of properties of smell and taste of medicinal plants (Table 5.2). Odor and taste of a plant or its parts are the most important criteria for deciding which illnesses a plant may cure. To treat infections of the skin, plants with any of the qualities summarized in Table 5.2 are used. The only exception is *pa'ak*. Aromatic (cooling) plants are considered very useful in treating illnesses that are associated with fever (Heinrich 1988) and are mostly applied externally (shower baths, rubbing, and massages using alcoholic preparations of the plants). Astringent drugs (especially the bark of various trees) are valued to treat diarrhea and dysentery. Additionally, bitter plants are employed as a supplemental therapy for these indications. Bitter, aromatic, and aromatic-bitter plants are valued in the treatment of gastrointestinal cramps and pain. Cough and other respiratory system complaints are treated mostly with sweet

Table 5.2
Important Qualities of Medicinal Plants According to Mixe Indian Criteria

Mixe	English
jajp	hot (like onions)
jamuup	hot (like chile)
pa'ak	sweet
ta'am	bitter
ti'ity	astringent
tsu'tsp	burning
u'ty	gelatinous (also called tëmnë)
xajts oo'ts	foaming ('forms foam when rubbed')
xun	sour
xuup	aromatic (cooling)

(and sometimes sour) drugs. A special category is *xajts oo'ts* ("makes foam"). The foam that forms when one rubs the plant is seen as a hint of its medicinal properties. These qualities also guide the search for new medicinal plants. Systems of plant classification based on taste and smell are also reported from other regions of Oaxaca. Ortiz de Montellano and Browner (1985) describe the significance of astringent plants in the popular medicine and botany of a Chinantec-speaking community. The importance of taste and odor is also stressed by Messer (1991) using a Zapotec community as an example.

A plant may also have other qualities that prevent its usage or make it dangerous to touch. The most important ones are *ke'ep* (burning), *no'op* (burning-itching), *taamts* (salty), *xi'ip* (hot-itching), and *u'xp* (itching).

The hot/cold dichotomy, widespread in Latin America (Foster and Anderson 1976; Logan 1973b), is of little importance in San Juan Guichicovi. In fact, asking whether a plant ought to be considered as hot or cold does not make sense to many informants. The terms collected in interviews (see Table 5.3) suggest a different understanding of the thermal character of plants.

Plants, then, are a very important resource in treating minor illnesses and ailments. Healing in these situations signifies the use of medicinal plants. The picture changes somewhat if one looks at severe illnesses. While ritual is considered central to *healing* severe illnesses, plants are salient in the process of *treatment*. Ritual and empiric forms of curing are integrated. After a cleansing ceremony, a tea or another form of phytotherapeutic treatment is frequently recommended, especially in the case of more common infectious illnesses. Consulting the corn oracle or another diagnostic means may also result in the recommendation to the patient of a certain plant.

Table 5.3
Thermal Qualities of Medicinal Plants

Mixe	English (*Spanish*)
aan	hot (*caliente*)
jokx	lukewarm (*tibio*)
nik	fresh (*fresco*) or humid
tëtxk	cold (*frio*) as weather, or an object
tsuxt	cold, or green, if it refers to an animal that recently died

Generally, these herbal remedies are not prepared by the healer; instead, the patient is asked to look for the appropriate plants and is instructed how to prepare and use them. Commercial plants may be purchased in the nearby city of Matías Romero (Heinrich et al. 1992b), or are stored by the healer and sold in the required amount. A few shops in the community also sell two or three of the most important commercial medicinal plants (*Matricaria chamomilla, Eucalyptus spp., Cinnamomum ceylanicum*). In some cases a healer may put together the appropriate remedy, and especially prepared ointments are given away by a few healers. Usually these are alcohol extracts of one or more (up to approximately five) medicinal plants.

Medicinal Plants Available in the Ecological Zones of the Mixe

The Mixe divide their environment into areas depending on the type of management these zones receive and on the distance from the house. These "ecological zones" do not necessarily correspond to a scientific ecological perspective.

The closest and most important area where plants grow is the house yard (*tsëwa'ant* Spanish: *solar*). Another nearby area where plants grow is the area in the village, especially along roadsides (*mëj tu'u*). A third area where plants grow is along the paths that lead out of the village, for example the paths to the wells (*në na tu'uj*) or to neighboring communities. The fourth area are the fields already cleared (*yuik*), burned (*të'x mo'ok*), sown (*kam*), or once again abandoned (*pë'ëts kekooyk*). Fifth, some plants grow in meadows (*por-treros* or *corales*). These are larger plots maintained for keeping and breeding cattle and donkey at some distance from the village (the two Spanish terms are also used in Mixe to refer to these zones). The last area from which plants are obtained is the "wilderness" or *monte* (Mixe: *yuk*). This is largely secondary vegetation found in areas that have no use except the occasional collection of fire wood. (Commercially available plants, which are largely bought in the nearby city of Matías Romero, are also of importance, but

Table 5.4
Medicinal Plants in the Ecological Zones of the Mixe

	Number	Percent
Grown in the "house yard," (Spanish: *solar)*	67	31.5%
Weed in the village	28	13.1%
At the outskirts of the village	56	26.3%
In the milpa, pasture land, or old fields	18	8.5%
(Sp: *terreno trabajado)*		
In the mountains	33	15.5%
Commercial plants (plants available to the	9	4.2%
community in nearby city or community		
markets)		
Total	213	

Source: based on data in Heinrich (1989).

obviously these are not part of the ecological zones in a strict sense of the word.)

The center of the Mixe habitat is the house and its yard (Table 5.4). This is at the same time the source of many items that are required daily. Corn is stored in the house or in an adjoining hut. Also, much *quehaceres del hogar* (daily housework) is performed there. Coffee is dried in the sun or on top of flat-roofed houses. In the yard, a few trees (usually no more than three to five) are planted, which give shade and are at some time of the year the source of fresh food; among them, *Annona spp.*, *Citrus spp.*, *Parmentiera aculeata* (Kunth) L. O. Williams, *Terminalia catappa* L., and others. Many of these are also used medicinally.

The largest number of medicinal plants (67, or 31.5%) are grown in the *solares* (see Table 5.4). These are mostly herbs and shrubs. Individual households may have an astounding variety of plants. The most frequent ones are *Pluchea symphytifolia* (Mill.) Gilis, *Pedilanthus tithymaloides* (L.) Poit., *Jatropha curcas* L., *Aloe barbadensis* L., *Ocimum basilicum* L. (basil), and *Piper* spp. (species of pepper). Many of these plants will not be found outside the yard, but some trees may be grown in the *corales* and *portreros*, too. Also, a few plants that are from the region but are difficult to obtain because of their distant habitat may be grown by individual healers, for example, *Ipomea alba* L., *Sinningia incarnata* (Aubl.) D. Denh. Other plants have been introduced from other regions of Mexico, including *Porophyllum ruderale* ssp. *macrophyllum* (DC) R. R. John, and *Tagetes filifolia* Lagasca. Many of the plants central to today's healing practice are grown in the *solares*. But the Mixe also conserve plants that were used in earlier times and are now becoming obsolete. An interesting example is *Pedilanthus tithymaloides*, a drug formerly used frequently for purging. The plant is (rightfully) considered to be very toxic. Today, magnesium hydroxide [Mg(OH)$_2$] is often used in place of this plant. A similar use is reported for *Hura polyandra* Baillon, a tree (also with a toxic sap) introduced around the turn of the century and now similarly being replaced by magnesium hydroxide. The hard fruits are still used occasionally as wheels of little carts made by boys. Only one tree of this species grows in the community. In earlier years it was part of the garden of a family who brought the plant at the end of the last century from a Zapotec community approximately 100 km South of San Juan. Due to the subsequent construction of a road, it is now growing at a street side.

A number of herbs are plentiful along the streets and ways in the community (ruderal plants) and are esteemed for their medicinal purposes. Twenty eight (13.1%) medicinal plants grow in these open spaces, for example, *Capraria biflora* L., *Chaptalia nutans* (L.) Pollack, *Helio-tropium indicum* L., *Hyptis verticillata* (Jacq.) Roem & Schlecht., *Sida* spp. The area along the roads and ways are cleaned once or twice a year (usually during the dry season). Little attention is paid to these plants, but they are a handy resource if suddenly needed. A few people prefer to have these plants right at hand in their yards. Such plants are considered "cleaner" because no pigs or other domestic animals eat or urinate/defecate on them.

The next group comprises 56 plants (26.3%), which are numerous in the immediate surroundings of the community outside the inhabited area. Most are found along the little ways that lead to the wells, the fields, or to neighboring communities, and at the wells themselves. Many of these plants are trees and shrubs: *Guazuma ulmifolia* Lam., *Tithonia diversifolia* (Hemsl.) Gray, *Miconia albicans* (Sw.) Triana, *Eugenia acapulcensis* Steud, *Thevetia ahouai* (L.) A.DC., and *Malvaviscus arboreus* Cav. This area also conserves plants that were brought into the community in earlier decades and which escaped cultivation: *Boussingaultia leptostachys* Mog., introduced around 1900, was used to treat broken bones, but is no longer used. These plants grow on ground which is common property and therefore everyone is free to use them. They receive little or no attention, but some species are frequently spared from being cut down completely.

Only 18 plants (8.5%) are usually encountered in the fields, *acahuales*, *corales*, and/or *portreros*. In the *milpas*, one finds, for example, *Poiretia punctata* (Willd.) Dev. and *Cecropia obtusifolia* Bert, in the pastures (*corrales* and *portreros*) *Quercus* spp. and *Smilax lanceolata* L. Only those who have the right to utilize these grounds (*ejidatarios*) can get these plants. Some trees, which mainly grow in the village, may be grown there too. Examples are *Citrus* spp. and *Annona* spp. For medical purposes, one usually takes some leaves, fruits, or bark from plants that grow closer to the house.

Only 33 (15.5%) medicinal plants grow in the "mountains" (*monte*) outside the directly managed area (Table 5.4). Among these are several species (*Croton repens* Schldl., *Scleria nutans* Kunth, *Psidium guineense* Sw.) that are considered particularly effective in the treatment of a certain illness or are sought in severe cases. Other species of this zone are *Pinus oocarpa* Schiede and *Critonia quadrangularis* (A. M. Decandolle) R. M. King and H. Robinson (syn: *Eupatorium quadrangulare* DC).

Only two plants with medicinal uses are sold in the little shops of the community: *Matricaria recutita* L. and *Cinnamomum ceylanicum* Sw. Further plants are sold in the neighboring city of Matías Romero, approximately 33 km from San Juan (Heinrich et al. 1992b). Several of these are frequently used in the community (Heinrich 1989).

SPECIAL CASE I: THE TREATMENT OF SNAKE BITES

Snake bites are a particularly life-threatening and disturbing illness. Today, treatment by medical doctors is generally preferred. Therefore the treatment of this illness using indigenous forms of therapy is now no longer used.

It was not just the bite itself and the poisonous effects that had to be treated, but also the person as a whole who had suffered a susto (Rubel 1964; Viesca Treviño and Ruge S. 1985) by being bitten suddenly. Therefore the treatment of snake bites required special rituals and the use of some plants (Heinrich 1989) that were applied locally (*Nicotiana tabacum* L., Solanaceae, *Citrus limon* (L.) Burm., Rutaceae) and orally (*Diphysa carthagenesis* DC., Fabaceae s.str. and *Abelmoschus moschatus* Med, Malvaceae).

The rite, called *amatokëpi'*, was carried out by a specialist, the *culebrero*. First, the healer sucked at the bite, then he enlarged the wound with a knife and continued to suck. Afterward the wound was cleaned with salt and lemon water (*Citrus limon*). To cure the very heavy itching experienced by the patient, the healer repeated this treatment daily. Also, *Nicotiana tabacum* was used as a poultice to prevent the wound from becoming infected. For the ritual that followed this treatment, the healer had to choose a "good day" for curing as indicated by the "keeper of the days," or *kuxë* (Carrasco et al. 1961; Weitlaner and Weitlaner 1963). The healer made a snake using corn flour dough. Then he went to the place where his patient was bitten by the snake, left the snake, and prayed. The healer sacrificed a chicken (*amadukëpie*) and left several candles (usually nine). The blood of the chicken was sprinkled on a spot near the candles. The chicken was left for some time at the "mouth" of the cornmeal snake. Later, tamales were made and eaten by the patient and his family. Afterward, the healer went three times to pray in front of the altar of the patron saint, San Juan Bautista. Also, the patient and his family had to have a special meal together. It was essential that *all* food, which was prepared especially for this meal, had to be eaten.

Compared to other areas where *culebreros* are known, the importance of phytotherapeutic treatments of snake bites was rather low in San Juan Guichicovi (Heinrich et al. 1990).

SPECIAL CASE II: PREVENTIVE RITUAL MEDICINE

A few weeks after the birth of a child, the *jekëëny tsiiny* is performed. It is called jekëëny tsiiny ("pine [needles] for the guardian spirit") because in former times the house was adorned with bundles of pine needles and branches for the ritual. This rite ensures that the child will be strong and grow well. The *jekëëny* of the child has to leave the body and is directed out of the community. The rite must be performed on a good day, determined by the ritual calendar (Carrasco et al. 1961; Weitlaner and Weitlaner 1963). There are several known variations of the rite, and today few people use the "complete" form. Praying, the burning of candles at home and in front of the main altar, and the offering of aguardiente to *naax wiin* (the eye of the earth) are the essential parts today. Earlier, the leaves of *Pinus oocarpa* Schiede (Pinaceae, Mixe: *tsiiny*) were also offered, and the midwife had to carry some of the ritual paraphernalia to a place outside of the village.

RECENT CHANGES

The medical system is continuously changing. In recent years these changes have increased dramatically. Several state and non-government organizations have started projects on the use of medicinal plants. None of these projects looks at indigenous medicine as a whole, even though the term "traditional medicine" ("medicina tradicional") is part of the title of many of them. Usually these programs attempt to document the most important of the medicinal plants and to help in the preparation of "improved" remedies. Therefore, the healers and other interested persons in the community are shown how to prepare ointments, syrups, medicinal soaps, and even capsules (filled with dried and pulverized plant material).

DISCUSSION

This article describes the Mixe Indian medicinal system, focusing on phytotherapeutic aspects of plant use. The data presented here demonstrate the enormous importance of medicinal plants in treating a large variety of illnesses. But, the data also shows at what point the Mixe see the limits of such phytotherapeutic forms of treatment. Any illness that is associated with heavy pain, which is debilitating or long lasting, requires contact to and help by the supernatural. This is also necessary for any human activity that alters the relationship of humans to the environment such as the building of a new house, the cleaning of a future milpa, or the building of a well.

The traditional system used two cultural key expressions to integrate the various aspects of village life: the ritual calendar, and the rite of *koxtenabie*. The ritual calendar gives clear indications when certain rituals had to be performed and thus structured the time. The rite of *koxtenabie* enables the villagers to relate their ritual needs to supernatural powers and to ask for help and forgiveness. Today, in communities like the one described, there is an increasing interest in phytotherapeutic forms of curing. Many of the state programs are very well intended but lack anthropological consultation. As a consequence, one aspect of the medical system, the ritual form of curing, is slowly becoming less and less important.

While this is a special example, there are some general conclusions that can be drawn from these data. Plants are an important medical resource. They are used *as* medicine, and, as Farnsworth et al. (1985) has pointed out, a great number of people rely on medicinal plants. The importance of these plants is also demonstrated by the fact that these plants are generally either found in the immediate surroundings of the community or are grown in the *solares* (house gardens).

Medicinal plants have frequently been documented (e.g., Alcorn 1984; Amo 1979; Heinrich 1989, 1992) and put into ecological (Alcorn 1984) or cognitive perspective (cf. Berlin 1992). Other researchers are especially interested in the role of phytotherapeutic forms of treatment in primary health care (Bannermann et al. 1983; Heinrich 1992; Heinrich et al. 1992c). Some scholars have also discussed the relevance of phytotherapeutic forms of treatment and of plants in medical systems or in the treatment of specific disorders (Smet 1985; Logan 1973a). Also, there are numerous descriptions and analyses of medical systems, but these generally *do not consider medicinal plants in ethnographic detail.*

It ought to be of special interest to anthropologists and ethnologists to describe and analyze the cultural importance and role of medicinal plants in a given society in greater detail and to study the sociocultural basis of such uses. Such studies would be truly ethnobotanical in their organization and would be a much better basis for pharmacological and phytochemical research on such plants (Heinrich et al. 1992c). They should include the relative importance of the various taxa in the indigenous medical system, the concepts of plants and their properties as they relate to healing (Messer 1991), their symbolic values, their procurement from the environment, and changes in their use.

APPENDIX: MIXE TERMS FOR DISORDERED STATES

A) Skin Infection and Injuries:	
aat	affliction with lice
apu'utsp	infection of the mouth
max apu'utsp	infections of the mouth and the throat, that produce a whitening of the affected parts (algodoncillo)
axuky	heavy skin infections
cancer	long-lasting, very heavy skin infections
com	pus, abscess
jot	injury
ka'atx	bruise, produced by a stone
Ki'ix	itching, localized skin infections
kox	bruise, produced by a fist or by a blunt object
Kumy	injury produced by stabbing
max taiky	severe, not easily localized infection or inflammation of the skin
nëteto	measles
nëxiba	generalized itching over the whole skin
pi'int	infection with *Trepanoma caratum* (pinta)
ji'iny pi'int	black pinta
pux	black pinta (infective organism uncertain)
pu'uts	localized skin infections (grano)
ji'iny pu'uts	localized skin infection that produces a blackening of the affected region
pu'ts max	localized, very heavy infection of the skin
tsaj në tooy	small-pox (literally: watery fever of the heaven, referring to its introduction together with the Spanish missionaries)
tsi'ik	localized, heavily itching skin infections
tsi'naky	infections of the skin which are very dispersed and which lead to a blackening of the affected regions

APPENDIX (continued)

tsuky	cut, produced by a knife
tuk xu'um	infected insect or scorpion bites (?)
xikt	scabies
B) Other Illnesses:	
aanik xui	insolation
ajuk pu'uts	leishmaniosis (infection with *Leishmania brasiliensis*, that produces lesions
diabetis	long-lasting, consumptive, feverish illness or sometimes clinically diagnosed Diabetes mellitus
gripa	cold
joxk pa'am	pain of the muscles, e.g., caused by dengue
jo'ot pa'am	pain and cramps of the stomach
jo'ot ma'ats	"annoyance" (the belly is getting freckled, this is caused by being annoyed)
jo'ot may	depression ("the sad stomach")
jo'ot xëhë	malnutrition (literally: spastic movements of the belly, cough, key sign is the more noticeable pulsation of the artery) (Bauchschlagader)
jokëëny ixy mi'ët	illness of the stomach, caused by annoying the guardian spirit (nagual)
kopk pa'am	headache
metsk kuaay	malnutrition (literally: second skin; principal sign are hairs (="a second skin") in the region of the neck)
në'ty xye'exp	vaginal hemorrhage
ojy	cough
ni'ixy ojy	whooping-cough
ёёt	vomiting
pata'ayky	bewitchment
pa'am	pain, illness (general term)
poh	wind, that produces illness
poj	uncontrollable cramps, e.g., epilepsia

APPENDIX (continued)

Pu'uts pa'am	various illnesses of the liver (hepatitis, liver-cirrhosis)
taj tecty ba'am	madness, that leads to violent acts by the afflicted and that is caused by ingesting the hallucinogenic plant Datura stramonium L., Solanaceae, literally father-mother illness
tëënk	intestinal parasites
tooy	fever
tsubox wiin tooy	possession by spirits (malaire, ataques), caused by spirits of the night, it leads to pain in various parts of the body
wiin toy	evil eye
tëxkpa këtotsoj	muscular cramps
të'ënëë	diarrhea
në't të'ënëë	disenteria
tsa'anty tsya'tsë	snakebites
tsi'itsk ki'ix	pain of the breast (women)
tso'oy	"empacho," gastrointestinal obstruction
tsëkë'ë	"susto" (illness caused by a sudden fright)
tu'unk	intestinal parasites
wi'in pa'am	pain and illnesses of the eye
woots	malnutrition (see also metsk kuay and jo'ot xëhë)
xaam pok	parotitis (e.g., mumps)
xiim	malaria
xëhë	cough associated with cramps (Krampfhusten)

ACKNOWLEDGMENTS

This research would not have been possible without the collaboration of the numerous healers and other inhabitants of San Juan Guichicovi, who are the traditional keepers of this knowledge. I am particularly grateful to Don Abelardo Ascona and Doña Glafida Figeroa, their family and to Maestro Erasto Gonzalez. I would like to thank H. Rimpler, R. Hertel, and U. Köhler (all of Freiburg) for their continuous interest and help. The botanical identification at MEXU was performed in collaboration with the numerous specialists of this institution. I would like to thank particularly D. Lorence (now Hawaii), T. Ramamoorthy, R. Torres, and Fr. Ramos.

Financial support by the "Deutsche Akademische Austauschdienst" (Bonn, F.R.G.), the "Secretaría de Relaciones Exteriores" (México D.F.), the Freiburger Wissenschaftliche Gesellschaft (F.R.G.) and the "Deutsche Forschungsgemeinschaft" (Bonn, F.R.G.; through a grant for phytochemical research on Mexican Indian medicinal plants) is gratefully acknowledged. An earlier version of this chapter is Heinrich (1994). Permission to reproduce large parts of this publication was granted by the publisher.

NOTES

1. Note that the Mixe use Spanish loan words for these two recent types of healers.

2. The sense of the metaphor is to open, uncork, the bottle/body so the illness will leave.

REFERENCES

Aguirre Beltran, Gonzalo. 1986. *Antropologia Medica*. Mexico D.F.: Ediciones de la Casa Chata 13.

Alcorn, Janis B. 1984. *Huastec Mayan Ethnobotany*. Austin: University of Texas Press.

Amo R., Silvia del. 1979. *Plantas Medicinales del estado de Veracruz*. Xalapa (Veracruz): Institutode Investigaciones sobre Recursos Bioticos.

Bannermann, Robert, J. Burton, and Ch'en Wen-Chieh. 1983. *Traditional Medicine and Health Care Coverage*. Geneva: World Health Organization.

Berlin, Brent. 1992. *Ethnobiological Classification*. Princeton, N.J.: Princeton University Press.

Carrasco, Pedro, Walter Miller, and Roberto J. Weitlaner. 1961. "El Calendario Mixe." *El México Antiguo* 9:153–72.

Censo General. 1980a. *X Censo General de Población y Vivencia, 1980, Estado de Oaxaca*. Vol. 1 (1–3), Vol. 2 (1). México, D.F.: Instituto de Estadistica, Geografía, e Información.

———. 1980b. *Mexico, Direccion General de Estadistica, Censo General de la Republica Mexicana*. México, D.F.: Oficina Tip. de la Secretaria de Fomento.

Etkin, Nina. 1988. "Ethnopharmacology: Biobehavioral Approaches in the Anthropological Study of Indigenous Medicines." *Annual Review of Anthropology* 17: 23–42.

———. 1993. "Anthropological Methods in Ethnopharmacology." *Journal of Ethnopharmacology* 38:93–104.

Farnsworth, Norman R., Olayiwola Akerele, Audrey S. Bingel, Djaja D. Soejarto, and Zhengang Guo. 1985. "Medicinal Plants in Therapeutics." *World Health Organization Bulletin* 63(6):965–81.

Finkler, Kaja. 1985. *Spiritualist Healers in Mexico*. South Hadley, Mass.: Bergin & Garvey.

Foster, George M. 1969. "The Mixe, Zoque and Populuca." In *Handbook of Middle American Indians*. Evon Z. Vogt, ed. Vol. 7 (Ethnology Pt. 2). Austin: University of Texas Press, 448–77.

———. 1976. "Disease Etiologies in Non-Western Medical Systems." *American Anthropologist* 78:773–82.

Foster, George M. and Barbara G. Anderson. 1976. *Medical Anthropology*. New York: Wiley.

Greifeld, Katrin. 1982. "Zur Situation der traditionellen Medizin in Mexiko." *Curare* 5:163–66.

———. 1985. "The Anthropology of Malaria Control." *Central Issues in Anthropology* 6(1):27–40.

Heinrich, Michael. 1988. "Enfermedades infecciosas y conceptos populares de problemas de salud en las tierras bajas de la communidad Mixe, Oaxaca, Mexico." In *Conceptos y Tratamientos Populares de algunas enfermedades en Latinoamerica*. A Kroeger and W. Ruiz Caro, eds. Cusco, D.F.: Centro de Medicina Andina, 159–65.

———. 1989. "Ethnobotanik der Tieflandmixe (Oaxaca, Mexico) und phyto chemische Untersuchung von Capraria biflora L. (Scrophulariaceae)." *Dissertationes Botanicae* no. 144. Berlin und Stuttgart: J. Cramer in Gebr. Borntraeger Verlagsbuchhdlg.

———. 1992. "Economic Botany of American Labiatae." In *Advances in Labiatae Science*. R. M. Harley and T. Reynolds, eds. Richmond, Va.: Kew Botanical Gardens, 475–88.

———. 1994. "Herbal and Symbolic Medicines of the Lowland Mixe (Oaxaca, Mexico): Disease Concepts, Healer's Roles, and Plant Use." *Anthropos* 89:73–83.

Heinrich, Michael, Michaela Kuhnt, Colin W. Wright, Horst Rimpler, David P. Phillipson, Alfred Schandelmaier, and David C. Warhurst. 1992a. "Parasitological and Microbiological Evaluation of Mixe Indian Medicinal Plants (Mexico)." *Journal of Ethnopharmacology* 36:81–85.

Heinrich, Michael, Antonio B. Nereyda, and Michaela Kuhnt. 1992b. "Arzneipflanzen in Mexiko: Der Markt von Matias Romero (Oaxaca)." *Deutsche Apothekerzeitung* 132:351–58.

Heinrich, Michael, Horst Rimpler, and Antonio B. Nereyda. 1992c. "Indigenous Phytotherapy of Gastrointestinal Disorders in a Mixe Lowland Community." *Journal of Ethnopharmacology* 36:63–80.

Heinrich, Michael, O. Velazco, and Fr. Ramos. 1990. "Ethnobotanical Report on the Treatment of Snake-bites in Oaxaca, Mexico." *Curare* 13(1):11–16.

Hoer, M., Horst Rimpler, and Michael Heinrich. 1995. "Inhibition of Intestinal Chloride Secretion by Proanthocyanidins from *Guazuma ulmifolia*." *Planta medica* 61(3):208–12.

Instituto Nacional Indigenista. 1994. *Atlas de las plantas de la medicina tradicional Mexicana*. 3 vols. Coordinador: Argueta Villamar, Arturo México D.F.: INI.

Klein, J. 1978. "Susto: The Anthropological Study of Diseases of Adaptation." *Social Science and Medicine* 12:23–28.

Kuhnt M., Horst Rimpler, and Michael Heinrich. 1995. "Biological and Pharmacological Activities of the Mixe Indian Medicinal Plant *Hyptis verticillata*." *Planta Medica* 61(3):227–32.

Lipp, Frank. 1991. "The Mixe of Oaxaca, Religion, Ritual and Healing." Austin: University of Texas Press.

Logan, Michael H. 1973a. "Humoral Medicine in Guatemala and Peasant Acceptance of Modern Medicine." *Human Organization* 32:385–95.

———. 1973b. "Digestive Disorders and Plant Medicinals in Highland Guatemala." *Anthropos* 68:537–47.

———. 1977. "Anthropological Considerations on the Hot-Cold Theory of Disease: Some Methodological Suggestions." *Medical Anthropology* 1:89–112.

Messer, E. 1991. "Systematic and Medicinal Reasoning in Mitla Folk Botany." *Journal of Ethnopharmacology* 33:107–28.

Nahmad, S. 1965. *Los Mixes.* México D.F.: Instituto Nacional Indigenista.

Ortiz de Montellano, B., and C. Browner. 1985. "Chemical Bases for Medicinal Plant Use in Oaxaca, Mexico." *Journal of Ethnopharmacology* 13:57–88.

Ramirez, Axel. 1978. *Bibliografía Comentada de la Medicina Tradicional Mexicana (1900–1978).* Monografias cientificas 3. Mexico D.F.: IMEPLAN.

Rubel, Arthur J. 1960. "Concepts of Disease in Mexican-American Culture." *American Anthropologist* 62:795–814.

———. 1964. "The Epidemiology of a Folk Illness: Susto in Hispanic America." *Ethnology* 3:268–84.

———. 1988. "Lessons for Biomedicine from Folk Medicine." In *Rituales y Fiestas de las Americas (45° Congreso Internacional de Americanistas).* Bogota, Columbia: Ediciones Uniandes, 342–47.

Rubel, Arthur J., C. W. O'Neill, and R. Collado-Ardon. 1984. *Susto, a Folk Illness.* Berkeley: University of California Press, NA 85/611.

Smet, P. A. G. M. de. 1985. "Ritual Enemas and Snuffs in the Americas." *Latin America Studies* 33, Dordrecht Foris.

Viesca Treviño, C., and T. Ruge S. 1985. "Aspectos Psiquiatricos y Psiquologicos del Susto." *Anales de Antropologia* (Mexico D.F.) 22:475–90.

Weitlaner, J., and Roberto J. Weitlaner. 1963. "Nuevas versiones sobre calendarias Mijes." *Revista Mexicana de Estudios Antropologicos* 19:41–62.

Young, James Clay. 1981. *Medical Choice in a Mexican Village.* New Brunswick, N.J.: Rutgers University Press.

6

THE EVOLUTION OF HUMAN NUTRITION

BARRY BOGIN

During a lifetime, a human being will eat thousands of pounds of food. The body will use this food to grow, to repair damaged tissue, and to maintain organs such as the brain and heart. Some of these foods will be enjoyable to eat because they are perceived to look appetizing and taste delicious. Other foods may not be enjoyable to eat, but will be consumed anyway because they are "good for the body or the spirit." Biochemically, the body does not distinguish between foods that are liked or disliked, for the human body does not use food, rather the body requires the biological nutrients contained in food. Biology, however, is not the entire story of human nutrition. Cultural variables, such as the type of food eaten, its manner of preparation, and the social context in which it is consumed, often determine the efficacy of that food in meeting human needs for health and well-being. It is the purpose of the chapter to explore the evolution of some of the biological and cultural requirements of human nutrition. Although at times the biology and culture of nutrition will be treated separately, the major theme of this chapter is to view human nutrition holistically as a biocultural phenomenon.

The biocultural nature of people and food is shown by the following Maya story of creation.

The Conception of the People of Corn

It was night, and the gods sat thinking in the darkness. Among them were the Bearer, Begetter, the Makers, Modelers named Tepeu Gucumatz, the Sovereign Plumed Serpent. Twice before they had tried to create a human being to be servant to the gods. One time the humans were made of clay and the other time of wood; but on both occasions the creatures so formed were stupid, without any intellect and without spirit. So, they were destroyed. As the dawn approached the gods thought, "Morning has come for humankind, for the people of the face of the earth." Their great wisdom was revealed in the clear light; they discovered what was needed for human flesh— white corn and yellow corn. Four animals brought the food: fox, coyote, parrot, and crow. The animals showed the way to the citadel named Broken Place, Bitter Water Place. Here was a paradise filled with white and yellow corn and all the varieties of fruits and vegetables, including *pataxte* and *cacao*. The white and yellow corn were given to Xmucane, the divine Grandmother of the gods, and she ground the corn nine times. She washed the ground corn from her hands with water and this mixture made grease. The corn was used to make human flesh, the water made human blood, and the grease made human fat. From these staple foods were born the strength and vigor of the new beings. (From the *Popol Vuh*, the Maya book of the dawn of life and the glories of gods and kings [compiled from the translations of Tedlock 1985 and Figueroa, 1986].)

The domestication of maize, or corn, and other plants occurred in Mesoamerica about 7000 B.P. By 3000 B.P. maize-based agricultural societies were established and these developed into the state-level, hierarchical societies of the Olmec and, eventually, the Maya. The central place of maize as the staple food in Maya society is emphasized in the creation story. People are corn, in both the literary and literal sense. Today, the living Maya people of Guatemala depend on maize for 80 percent of their energy intake. It is likely that the ancient Maya also consumed a large portion of their calories from maize, or more correctly from maize-based foods. Very little maize is eaten in Guatemala today. Instead people eat *tortillas, tamalitos, tamales, tacos, enchiladas, atoles* (a beverage), and many other foods and drinks made from *masa harina*. *Masa harina* is a flour made from maize that has been dried, ground, and processed by boiling in lime water (Figure 6.1). Some of the "tortilla chips" sold in American supermarkets may be made from a flour like *masa harina*, but most brands are made from corn meal, which is ground maize without any processing. The difference is vitally important in terms of nutrition and health, for without the processing, a maize-based diet leads to death from pellagra. Later in this chapter the biochemical and nutritional properties of *masa harina* and the cause of pellagra are explained in greater detail.

The Maya, ancient and modern, do not live by *tortillas* alone. At Broken Place, Bitter Water Place (a supernatural site located inside a mountain), all varieties of fruits and vegetables were found and given to people. A visit to any Maya marketplace today in Guatemala or southern Mexico shows that dozens of species of fruits, vegetables, and dried mushrooms are sold, along with fresh and dried fish and meat. Archaeological and ethnographic fieldwork substantiates the diversity of foods in the Maya diet over the past 1,000 years or more (Saenz de Tejada 1988). Even *pataxte* and *cacao* were given to people by the gods (Figure 6.2). These are fruits from which cocoa and

Figure 6.1
Xmucane Grinding Yellow and White Corn to Make People

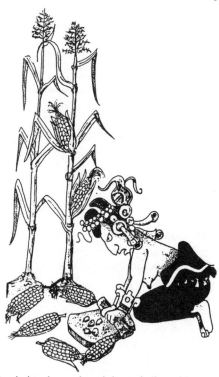

The corn is processed by drying the seeds and then grinding with a *mano* (grinder) on a *matate* (grinding stone). Xmucane's behavior is a metaphor for the Maya people's dependence on agriculture and the technology required to process corn into nutritious foods.

chocolate are made (chocoholics might recite an extra prayer of thanks to Sovereign Plumed Serpent before retiring tonight). A chocolate and hot pepper beverage was a drink used in Maya religious ritual, and was usually reserved for the royal family or other people of high status. Thus, food is used not only to sustain the body, but also to demarcate social position and as part of religious behavior.

NUTRIENTS VERSUS FOOD

Nutritional biochemists have determined that there are 50 essential nutrients required for growth, maintenance, and the repair of the body. Essential nutrients are those substances that the body needs but cannot manufacture. These substances are divided into six classes: protein, carbohydrate, fat, vitamins, minerals, and water. Table 6.1 lists the essential nutrients in these categories. One way that nutrients are shown to be essential is via experiments with non-human animals. A young rat, pig, or monkey is

Figure 6.2
Maya Priest Surrounded by Cocoa Pods

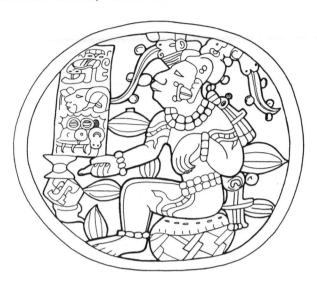

Cocoa was a sacred food, reserved for high status Maya and for religious ritual (after Caraway
    1981).

fed a diet that includes all of the known nutrients except the one being
tested. If the animal gets sick, stops growing, loses weight, or dies it usually
means that the missing nutrient is essential for that animal. Such experiments do not prove that the same nutrient is needed for people. Some
controlled experiments were done in the twentieth century with people,
such as prisoners and residents of villages in underdeveloped nations. Since
about 1980 these experiments have been considered unethical. Certain medical conditions deprive people of nutrients, and social, economic, and political conditions of life also deprive people of food and nutrients. By using
these "experiments of nature," along with past research, it is possible to
prove the necessity of the essential nutrients.

   People do not usually intake essential nutrients directly as pure chemicals,
rather we eat food. This was certainly true for all of our animal ancestors
throughout evolutionary history. Human foods come from five of the six
Kingdoms of living organisms: plants, animals, fungi (e.g., mushrooms), pro-
tists (e.g., species of algae referred to as "seaweed"), and eubacteria (e.g.,
bacteria used in fermented foods). These organisms present us with a daz-
zling array of colors, flavors, odors, textures, shapes, and sizes. The sixth
Kingdom, archaebacteria, are not eaten directly, but are essential in the diet
of other species that people do eat. Herbivores, for example, have archaebacteria in their guts to digest the plant cellulose.

Table 6.1
Essential Nutrients of the Human Diet

Carboyhdrate
Glucose

Fat or Lipid
Linoleic acid
Linolenic acid

Protein
Amino acids
  Leucine
  Isoleucine
  Lysine
  Methionine
  Phenylalanine
  Threonine
  Tryptophan
  Valine
  Histidine
Nonessential amino nitrogen

Minerals
Macronutrient elements
  Calcium
  Phosphorus
  Sodium
  Potassium
  Sulfur
  Chlorine
  Magnesium
Micronutrient elements
  Iron
  Selenium
  Zinc

Micronutrient elements *(continued)*
  Manganese
  Copper
  Cobalt
  Molybdenum
  Iodine
  Chromium
  Vanadium
  Tin
  Nickel
  Silicon
  Boron
  Arsenic
  Fluorine

Vitamins
Fat-soluble
  A (retinol)
  B (cholecalciferol)
  E (tocopherol)
  K
Water-soluble
  Thiamin
  Riboflavin
  Niacin
  Biotin
  Folic acid
  Vitamin B_6 (pyridoxine)
  Vitamin B_{12} (cobalamin)
  Pantothenic acid
  Vitamin C (ascorbic acid)

Water

Source: Guthrie and Picciano 1995.

EATING A BALANCED DIET

How does a person know which foods to eat so that all of the essential nutrients are consumed in required amounts? Children learn what to eat because they are dependent on their parents, or other older individuals, to prepare their food. By tasting these foods, and watching older people prepare them, children acquire patterns of food preferences, including what should not be eaten, under what social conditions a food should be eaten, and the ways to prepare foods. Thus people learn what they like, for not all people eat all the same foods. For instance, some people in the United States eat chocolate covered ants, but most Americans do not think of insects as food.

In parts of Africa and South America, however, insects such as ants, termites, and beetle larva are food, in fact they are considered delicacies. Yanomamo Indians of southern Venezuela cultivate certain plants in which they know beetles will lay their eggs. The Yanomamo harvest the beetle larvae and eat them raw or roasted (Chagnon 1983). From a nutritional point of view insects are excellent sources of protein, fats, and some minerals. In fact, pound for pound, grasshoppers have more protein than cattle or hogs, yet this fact is unlikely to encourage the sale of "grasshopper nuggets" at fast-food outlets in the United States.

Every group of people has developed a cuisine; that is, an assortment of foods and a style of cooking that is unique to that culture. Some examples are Italian cooking, Chinese cooking, and Mexican cooking. Even Americans have a cuisine, including foods such as corn-on-the-cob and hamburgers. Despite the differences in specific foods, the cuisine of each human culture provides all of the essential nutrients. No one knows how cuisines developed to meet human biochemical requirements. Experiments with non-human animals and with people indicate that diets, or cuisines, are developed by learning to avoid foods that produce illness or feelings of malaise and seeking foods that promote feelings of well-being (Franken 1988:107).

One fascinating aspect of food preferences in different cultures is the way two or more foods are combined and eaten together to help assure nutritional adequacy. One example is complimentary protein consumption. Table 6.1 shows that there are nine amino acids (the building blocks of proteins) that are essential nutrients. There are 11 additional amino acids in nature that are needed for life but are not essential nutrients. Not all foods contain all nine essential amino acids, so we must eat several foods to get them all—the amino acids in some foods complementing those lacking in others. Cereal grains, such as wheat and rice, lack some of the amino acids that are found in beans, peas, milk, and cheeses. Conversely, beans, peas, milk, and cheeses lack the amino acids found in cereal grains. In the Middle East, many people eat wheat and cheese in the same dish. In Mexico, beans, tortillas, and rice are popular, while on the island of Jamaica peas and rice is the national favorite. In the United States, cereal (grains) and milk are complementary protein sources popular at the breakfast meal. The biochemistry of complementary protein foods has been discovered only recently, yet the cultural history of this food practice is ancient.

Each culture developed its own cuisine for many reasons. Not all foods grow in all countries, for instance maize originally comes from Central America and rice originally comes from Asia. But most food preferences cannot be so easily explained. The isolation of many human cultures, exploration and contact between cultures, ethnic identity, and social, economic, political, and religious status are some further explanations. Hindu culture, for example, specifies different cuisines for people of different castes. According to Burghardt's (1990) analysis of Hindu dietary recommendation, not all castes can tolerate all foods. The intolerance is due to harmful reactions between the qualities of the food (such as animal meat) and the nature of the bodies of different caste members. Thus Hindu epistemology does not identify the universal set of essential nutrients recognized by Western biomedical research. Many other unknown factors occurring throughout thousands of years of human history are also responsible for the development of culture-specific cuisines.

From the foregoing, two universal observations about human nutrition can be made: (1) All people have the same basic biological requirements for nutrients; and (2) Each culture has a unique cuisine that has the potential to satisfy these nutrient requirements.

In addition some universal features of human food systems have been complied by Pelto and Pelto (1983):

1. People are extremely omnivorous, eating hundreds of different species of plants, animals, fungi, bacteria, and even algae.
2. People depend on systems of food transport from the place where foods are found or acquired to their place of consumption.
3. People make use of systems for food storage that protect the nutritional quality of foods from the time of their acquisition until the time of their consumption. That time period may last for months, even in premodern societies.
4. People expend great effort on food preparation, such as cooking, mixing, flavoring, and detoxifying natural ingredients, and depend on technology to do this preparation (e.g., the hand-axes and fire used by *Homo erectus* or the food processors and microwave ovens of *Homo sapiens*).
5. People share and exchange food regularly and have cultural rules that order such sharing and exchanges.
6. People have food taboos; that is, social proscriptions against the consumption of certain foods based on age, sex, state of health, religious beliefs, and other culturally defined reasons.

One final item must be included in this list of human food behavior.

7. People use foods for non-nutritional purposes, such as for medicine to cure or cause disease and as offerings in ritual or religious behavior (see the chapter by Etkin and Ross in this volume). In these contexts food may have some physiologic function (plants do contain active pharmaceutical compounds), but the foods also have symbolic meaning for the people using them.

Evidence from fossil and archaeological remains of human ancestors indicates that these universal features of human nutrition and food have been in existence for at least 35,000 years, and possibly more than 100,000 years. Yet, until this century, most foods were acquired locally. The most parsimonious way to account for these biological and cultural universals relating to food is to hypothesize that a common evolutionary history for all people shaped human nutritional requirements, food acquisition and processing systems, and food behavior. This is a hypothesis that can be verified or rejected by research.

SOURCES OF KNOWLEDGE

There are several kinds of data that may be considered in the study of the evolution of human nutrition. Archaeological and paleontological evidence provide the only direct data on what our ancestors ate and what effect diet may have had on our physical and behavioral evolution. However, studies of living primates and other mammals, living hunter/gatherer societies, and crosscultural comparisons of cuisines provide indirect evidence that is useful in reconstructing human nutritional history.

PRIMATE STUDIES

The living primates include prosimians, New World monkeys, Old World monkeys, Asian and African apes, and people. Fossil evidence indicates that all primates evolved from insectivorelike mammals that lived some 75 million years ago. The geological context of these fossils indicates that the general habitat was tropical forest. Primate ancestors may have been those insectivores that moved into the flowering trees of these tropical forests to exploit insects, and then the flowers, fruits, gums, and nectars of those trees (Cartmill 1974; Conroy 1990). The flowering plants and trees, called angiosperms, appear in the fossil record about 100 million years ago, and their appearance opened up new habitats and ecological niches that promoted the coevolution of other species, including the primates. The earliest primates of the Paleocence period (65–55 million years ago) exploited an insect-eating niche. Most species had jaws that moved in a scissorlike motion and teeth with pointed cusps, both features well suited for catching insects, by rapid mouth "snapping" and piercing their exoskeletons (the "crunchy" covering of the body) to extract internal tissues and fluids. By the late Paleocence many species show some dental traits indicating a mixed diet of insects, fruits, leaves, seeds, or gums. By about 55 million years ago primate fossils show changes in jaws and teeth toward those of living forms, with jaws adapted for greater power in biting and chewing. It seems that by that time most primates were eating fruits, leaves, and seeds as well as insects.

Thus, the general primate dietary pattern is ancient. That pattern is based on the ability to eat a wide variety of foods in order to meet nutritional requirements. Primate nutritional requirements are highly varied; the higher primates, including people, may be the animals with the longest list of essential nutrients. The reason for this may be our tropical origins. Today, tropical forests are characterized by having a high diversity of species, but a low density of any given species. There are thousands of species of tropical trees and at any one site there may be between 50 to 100 different species per hectare (Oates 1987), but only a few trees of the same species may be growing on that hectare. In contrast, temperate and high-altitude forests are often characterized by a few tree species, such as pine-oak forests, but large numbers of trees of those species. The diversity and density of animal species in tropical forests follows the pattern for plant life. There is no reason to expect that ancient tropical forests were different than modern tropical forests in terms of species diversity. Ancestral primates capable of eating a wide variety of foods would have had a veritable smorgasbord of choices, and judging by their descendants, the living primates, many food types were consumed.

The large number of essential nutrients required in the human diet, then, is likely a consequence of the tropical primate diet. With a wide variety of food resources, especially fruit, foliage, and insects, ancestral primates were able to obtain many vitamins, minerals, protein, carbohydrates, and fats from their diet. It is metabolically expensive, in terms of energy consumption, for an organism to manufacture its own nutrients (a process called autotrophism). Thus, through mutation and selection, those early primates that reduced autotrophism and shifted to a dependency on dietary intake to meet nutrient needs would have gained an energetic advantage, one that could be put to use, for instance, toward increasing reproduction. All mammals, for example, require vitamin C for maintenance and repair of body tissue, but only in some mammals, including all members of the primate order, is vitamin C (ascorbic acid) an essential nutrient. About 25 million years ago a mutation occurred in the metabolic pathway that produces vitamin C in primates ancestral to living monkeys, apes, and people. The glucose (carbohydrate energy) needed to convert biochemical precursors to ascorbic acid was released for use by other body systems (Scrimshaw and Young 1976). The wide distribution of vitamin C sources in tropical environments and the ability of primates to utilize these sources assured that this nutrient could be supplied by the diet alone.

Using published data, Harding (1981) divided naturally occurring tropical forest foods into eight categories and calculated the dietary frequency of each category for 131 species of primates from all families, excluding people (Table 6.2). The dietary frequency is defined as the percentage of those species surveyed "for which a given food category was listed in the diet" (p. 206). The data show that variety is the rule, and most species included seven of the eight food categories in their diets ("grasses and roots" was the category most often missing). The chimpanzee, our closest living primate relative, eats foods from all eight categories. It is worth noting at this point, that on a worldwide basis, living people eat more grasses, such as wheat and maize, and roots, such as potatoes and manioc, than any other foods listed in Table 6.2.

Table 6.2
Dietary Frequency and Major Diet Components of 131 Primate Species

Food category	Dietary frequency	Major component[1]
Fruit	90	45
Soft plant foods	79	9
Mature leaves	69	15
Invertebrates	65	23
Seeds	41	2
Hunted and scavenged vertebrates	37	0
Tree parts	34	0
Grasses and roots	13	5

[1]Percentage of species for which this category was identified as the major food.
Source: Harding 1981.

Some selectivity in diet is seen in its major components, with fruits, invertebrates, and mature leaves being the most common items. Meat from vertebrates, either hunted or scavenged, and tree parts (e.g., bark, cambium) are not reported as major components for any non-human primate species. Thus it might be best to characterize primates not as omnivores, but as selective omnivores. There are several reasons for this selectivity. First, primates are, with few exceptions, diurnal and highly active. Second, primates have brains that are about four times larger, relative to body size, than the brains of other mammals. Third, primates have relatively long gestations prior to birth and are nursed on demand for a relatively long period after birth. Each of these traits places a high metabolic demand on an animal to maintain activity, to supply the brain with energy and oxygen (the human brain uses 20% of the body's energy and oxygen), and to meet the nutritional needs of a mother primate and her fetus or infant.

Accordingly, primates must select foods that are dense in essential nutrients. Fruits and invertebrates are such foods; fruits are dense in carbohydrates, minerals and vitamins, and invertebrates are rich in fats and proteins (remember those grasshoppers!). Soft plant foods are mostly water and tree parts are mostly cellulose or lignin, all of which are low in nutrients. Grasses and roots are good foods for those species that live in savanna-woodland habitats where grasses are abundant (e.g., baboons), however most primates live in the tropical forests. Vertebrate meat and seeds are also nutrient dense, but require hunting skills or specialized mastication or behavior to make use of them. Of the 131 species surveyed, only some baboons and chimpanzees regularly hunt mammalian prey (Strum 1981; Teleki 1981), and only two monkey species, *Cercopithecus neglectus* and *Colobus satanas*, include seeds as major foods. Chimpanzees, bonobos, and baboons have been seen to use rocks to break open seeds to eat the contents, but this requires much effort and time, which takes away from feeding on more easily acquired foods.

The human primate, not included in Harding's survey, is unusual in that seeds, grasses, roots, and vertebrate meat are major components of both modern and ancient diets. Seeds, grasses, and roots have their nutrients protected by cellulose membranes that must be mechanically broken. This can be done either by mastication or by using technology. People, and our hominid ancestors dating back to *Australopithecus*, possess the anatomy (e.g., small canines, flattened molars, and enlarged pterygoid muscles—the muscles that move the lower jaw from side to side) that allows for a type of chewing called rotary grinding, which can break cellulose. People, and our ancestors of the genus *Homo*, are also dependent on technology (e.g., tools, fire) for food processing (Figure 6.1). Technology is also required for hunting at a level that makes vertebrate meat a regular part of the diet.

A second reason for selectivity is the coevolution of primates and their foods. Coevolution refers to the interactions of different species of living organisms that exist in the same community, which result in genetic change in those organisms over time. Predator-prey relationships are a common example of coevolution. Animals can move, and animal prey may run, jump, or fly away to evade capture. Over time, there will be selection for predators that are better suited to capture their prey and selection for prey that are better able to avoid capture. In contrast, plants are stationary but not defenseless. Plants produce a host of noxious or toxic substances (called secondary compounds), such as tannins and alkaloids, to discourage their predators. Plants may also evolve edible parts with low nutritional content (Hladik 1981) or seeds and fruits with coverings too hard to pierce (Kinzey and Norconk 1990), thus making those parts less attractive as food items to primates. In a review of the literature on secondary compounds, Glander (1982) found that the rich appearance of the tropical forest may be deceptive, for many primate species avoid a large percentage of potential plant foods. Glander concludes that the selectivity of primates for plant species and parts of plants must be viewed as a strategy balancing "the nutrient and secondary compound content variation in these foods" (p. 1.).

A third reason for selectivity is that primates have a worldwide distribution as an order, but are localized as genera into dozens of populations restricted to species-specific habitats. Thus it is not surprising that many primates, despite their evolutionary heritage of an eclectic food base, have, in practice, species-specific diets. The tammarins and marmosets of South America, for example, eat insects, fruits, and foliage, which are food items common to most primate diets, but also require tree sap for survival. The tree sap is the major source of calcium in their diet (Sussman and Kinzey 1984). These primates have clawlike nails used to cling to tree trunks and procumbent lower incisors used to gouge bark and release sap. No other group of primates has this set of anatomical specializations for tree sap consumption.

HUMAN DIET EVOLUTION

People also have unique requirements and specializations related to nutrition and diet. All primates require a relatively high-quality diet, but people require a higher quality diet than any other species. Leonard and Robertson (1994) compared the diet of 5 human foraging societies (!Kung, Ache, Hiwi, Inuit, and Pygmies) to 72 nonhuman primate species and found that diet quality of the human groups was almost twice that of other primates of the same body size. The human ability to include seeds, roots, and meat in the diet increases quality, as these are nutrient-dense foods. Building on the research of Martin (1983), Leonard and Robertson show that the need for high diet quality is a consequence of the human brain being several times larger than expected for a primate their size. Using estimates of brain and body size for extinct hominids, Leonard and Robertson estimate that humanlike dietary requirements evolved with the appearance of the genus *Homo*. But the only way to find out what our ancestors actually ate is to look at the evidence, which comes from the study of remains of hominids and their activities.

ARCHAEOLOGY AND FOSSIL STUDIES

Archaeological methods "include the identification of edible materials, functional analyses of artifacts employed in food preparation, coprolite [fossil feces] analysis, information on paleohabitat, and analyses of [hominid] skeletal material" (Sillen and Kavanagh 1982). Paleontological data are derived from the kinds and percentages of fossil remains found at a site. Each type of evidence contributes some knowledge, but each has serious limitations. The association of hominid fossil remains with the skeletal remains of other fossil vertebrates may result from geologic forces, such as rivers carrying dead carcasses to a central location or a volcanic eruption burying simultaneously a community of animals, rather than hominid food-gathering behavior. Early speculation by Dart (1957) that the bone accumulations at the South African cave sites of *Australopithecus* represented hominid hunting activity are now considered incorrect. Rather, Brain (1981) argues that the fossil remains, including the hominids, represent the activity of nonhominid carnivores, especially leopards, and geological forces. Dr. Brian aptly names his book on this subject *The Hunters or the Hunted*, and his conclusion is that the early hominids were the prey of the leopards.

Research conducted during the 1980s produced a 180-degree shift in the fossil evidence for the evolution of human hunting. In *The Descent of Man*, Charles Darwin (1871) proposed that hunting large game provided much of the selection pressure for human evolution. That view persisted through the 1960s, and the book *Man the Hunter* (Lee and DeVore 1968) represented majority opinion that uniquely human characteristics, such as bipedalism, large brains, division of labor, sharing, and intense parental investment in offspring, were the consequence of hunting and carnivory (see especially the chapter by Washburn and Lancaster in that volume). Implicit in this argument is the notion that the type of diet consumed by human ancestors played a significant role in the evolution of human biology and behavior. This notion is reasonable, but the explicit assumption of carnivory and hunting became less acceptable as existing evidence was reevaluated and new evidence discovered. The existing data, based on fossil and archaeological remains and the study of living hunting and gathering people such as the !Kung and Australian Aborigines, showed that gathering and processing plant foods was the main activity of tropical foragers. Moreover, women in living foraging societies provided most of the calories consumed by these people. These observations turned "man the hunter" into "woman the gatherer," and the hunting hypothesis was attacked for both lack of data and its male-biased implications (Zihlman 1981).

The new evidence is based on analyses of bone and stone tool material associated with early hominids. Potts and Shipman (1981) used scanning electron microscope images of mammalian long bones dating to 1.7 million years ago to show that cut marks produced by stone tools were incised above those made by carnivore teeth and the teeth of known scavengers, such as porcupines. Assuming that the order of markings reflects the order of use by hunters and scavengers, the hominids were the last to have at the bones—even after porcupines. Subsequent analysis shows that hominids may have been collecting bones for their marrow and brain tissue rather than for any meat still remaining on the surface of the bone (Binford 1987). Marrow and brain are high in fat and protein, but few carnivores have the morphology necessary to break open large long bones. Hyenas have the ability to exploit marrow and are formidable predators and scavengers but are most active at night (Schaller and Lowther 1969). Hominids are most active during the day and thus could scavenge for carcasses with less threat from hyenas. The invention of stone tools, first manufactured by hominids about 2.2 million years ago, may have been a dietary adaptation for extracting marrow. At Olduvai Gorge there are sites where the bones of large game animals (from gazelles to elephants) are found together with stone tools. The tools are called scrapers and choppers. Blumenschine and Cavallo (1992) report that the bones are mostly from limbs and skulls and that these are precisely the animal parts that only hyenas and tool-wielding hominids can crack open. Further, they report that one-half hour's work with a chopper can yield enough calories from the marrow and brain of a carcass the size of a wildebeest to meet an adult's daily energy requirements.

Hominids may also have scavenged for larger pieces of meat. Cavallo (1990) studied the ecology and behavior of leopards in Tanzania. Most carnivores, such as lions and hyenas, leave their prey on the ground and consume most of the internal organs and limb meat within a few hours after the kill. Leopards, in contrast, carry their kill into trees and consume their prey over several days. The kill may even be left unattended for up to ten hours, for other terrestrial carnivores ignore carcasses hanging in trees. Cavallo believes that human ancestors may have scavenged these arboreal caches of meat. This speculation is supported by the South African cave evidence of Brain (1981), which shows that australopithecines and leopards lived together and that the hominids were often the prey of the carnivores. Cavallo argues that by the time of the appearance of *Homo*, some hominids may have reversed the predator-prey relationship. There are modern-day reports of groups of baboons killing leopards as well as confirmed observations of chimpanzees scavenging tree-cached leopard kills and taking and eating leopard cubs (Cavallo 1990), stone tool–wielding hominids may have done the same on occasion.

Perhaps it was the occasional (or regular?) consumption of leopard that caused the hypervitaminosis A of the *H. erectus* individual from the Koobi Fora formation, located on the eastern shore of Lake Turkana, Kenya. The skeleton is dated to 1.6 million years B.P. (Walker et al. 1982), and analysis indicates that it was female and has "striking pathology" in the long bones of the limbs. These bones have a deposit of abnormal coarse-woven bone, up to 7 mm thick in places, above the normal skeletal tissue on the outer surface of the bone. Walker and his colleagues consider many possible causes for this pathological bone growth and conclude that an overconsumption of vitamin A (hypervitaminosis A) is the most likely cause. Similar cases of hypervitaminosis A have occurred in arctic explorers who consumed the livers of polar bear and seal. The liver stores vitamin A, and the liver of carnivores, who are at the top of the food chain, usually contain the greatest amounts of this vitamin. Walker et al. suggest that the cause of the bone pathology in this specimen of *H. erectus* was due to eating the liver of carnivorous animals.

Despite the evidence for scavenging animal carcasses and, perhaps, preying on leopards, the bulk of the hominid diet has almost always been from plants. The stone tools of the early hominids may also have been used to process plant foods that were difficult to chew, such as seeds. Walker (1981) and Kay (1985) studied the finer details of early hominid dental structure and tooth wear using the scanning electron microscope and tooth wear experiments. These researchers propose that the diet of the early hominids, including *Australopithecus* and *H. habilis*, was largely herbivorous, including softer plant foods (leaves, fruits) as well as the tougher seeds and tubers. Given all of the evidence now available, perhaps it is safest to say that the gathering of plants, insects, birds' eggs, and other relatively immobile foods along with the scavenging of marrow from carnivore kills typified early hominid food behavior.

The early hominid dietary pattern continues through *H. erectus* times. Binford (1987) reanalyzed fossil material from Torralba, a *H. erectus* site in Spain, and Zhoukoudian, a cave site near Bejing, China, spanning the period from *H. erectus* to *H. sapiens*. During the *H. erectus* period of occupation (250,000 to 450,000 years B.P.), both sites show evidence of the gathering of plant foods and scavenging, rather than hunting. The animal bones at these sites appear to have been processed and consumed on the spot, rather then carried to any sort of "base camp." If this is so, then past theories about the evolution of human biology and behavior—including bipedalism, large brains, division of labor, sharing, and intense parental investment in offspring—that depended on hunting and "family style dining" at home bases have to be rejected. Binford (1984) states that convincing evidence for the regular hunting of big game does not appear in the fossil record until 90,000 years B.P. at the earliest.

H. erectus added fire to its repertoire of technology. Fire, which may have been used as early as 1.4 million years ago and was certainly controlled by 750,000 years B.P., provided warmth, light, protection, and a new way to process foods. Where and how cooking was invented is a matter for speculation. Cooking, by roasting or boiling, increases the nutritional benefit of many vegetable foods by helping to break down the cellulose in those foods, which is undigestible to people. Fire may be used to open large seeds that resist even stone tools. Cooking, especially drying or smoking, helps to preserve foods for storage. Fire may also be used to obtain foods, especially when used to drive game toward a convenient killing site. All of these uses of fire did not appear simultaneously, and many appear to be the invention of *H. sapiens* rather than *H. erectus*. What is certain is that the controlled use of fire was a significant addition to hominid technology with profound consequences for nutritional status.

FOSSILIZED FECES

Coprolite analysis might seem to provide unequivocal evidence of dietary habits, but it too is subject to misinterpretation. First, the coprolite must be identified as unambiguously being from a hominid. Second, coprolites can only verify that a particular substance was eaten. That substance may or may not have been a food item itself, it may have been ingested coincidentally along with a food, such as a seed or insect clinging to an animal or plant. Third, only undigestible substances will be found in feces and those substances must be suitable candidates for fossilization to be preserved in a coprolite. Thus, coprolite analysis may provide a very biased picture of the true dietary intake. Even so, considerable information has been obtained about the diet of prehistoric humans, and limited information about the diet of hominid species ancestral to modern people, using coprolite analysis. The animal affinity of desiccated coprolites can be determined by placing the specimen in a trisodium phosphate solution for 72 hours. Human coprolites turn the solution an opaque dark brown or black color, no other species produces this effect (Bryant and Williams-Dean 1975). Other characteristics of human feces are inclusions of charcoal and the presence of undigested animal parts from a wide variety of species. Charcoal comes from cooking food over a wood fire. Since people cook their food and other animals do not, the presence of charcoal in feces is indirect evidence of a unique human behavior. People also have an eclectic diet compared to most other mammals, so undigested parts from a wide variety of species is another indicator of the human affinities of a coprolite. More than 1,000 paleoindian coprolites from the American southwest have been identified and analyzed. One group of specimens was collected from Texas sites that date from 800 B.C. to 500 A.D., representing the temporary camps of hunting and gathering peoples (Bryant 1974). By comparing the pollen content of the coprolites with that of the adjacent soils, it was determined that the people had consumed high quantities of flowers. Because the physical characteristics of flower pollens are unique to each species, it was possible to determine that flowers of agave, sotol, yucca, prickly pear cactus, gilia, and leadtree were popular foods. Also found were remains of wild onion bulbs, bark, grasshoppers, fish, small reptiles, and snails. Although not the current cuisine of Texas, this diet is typically human in its diversity of species. The flower pollen even provides a time frame for the occupation of the sites of spring and early summer.

Coprolites from paleoindian sites in New Mexico, Arizona, and Texas contain pollen from plants of known pharmacological value, suggesting that people have a long history of consuming plants as medicines as well as foods (Reinhard 1989). Willow, an analgesic with essentially the same active ingredient as in aspirin, *Ephedra*, an antihistamine, and creosote, an antidiarrheal, are the most concentrated pollens in the samples. Ethnographic evidence shows that these three species were, and are still, widely used as medicines by Native Americans (Moerman, 1986, 1989). Willow tea is used for the treatment of many aches and pains, *Ephedra* tea is prescribed for the stuffy noses of the common cold, and creosote is indicated for any type of loose bowls. Reinhard (1989) states that the analysis of these coprolites "demonstrates the antiquity of folk remedies and provides circumstantial evidence of certain disorders suffered by prehistoric peoples" (p. 2).

The oldest verified coprolites of a hominid species are from the *H. erectus* site of Terra Amata located on the French Mediterranean. These coprolites may be as old as 300,000 B.P., and they are heavily mineralized. They have only a slight reaction to trisodium phosphate rehydration (Bryant and Williams-Dean 1975). The specimens contain sand grains, charcoal, and mollusk shell fragments. The sand and shell are expected, since Terra Amata is a beachfront site, and the charcoal helps establish that foods were cooked before consumption (maybe evidence for a prehistoric clam bake!).

TRACE ELEMENT AND STABLE ISOTOPE
ANALYSIS

A more general picture of the relative amounts of plant and animal food in the diet may be available from chemical analyses of trace elements and stable isotopes in skeletal remains. The ratio of strontium and/or barium to calcium (Sr/Ca, Br/Ca) in animal bone is the most widely used form of trace element analysis at present. Sillen and Kavanagh (1982) and Ezzo et al. (1995) review the use of Sr/Ca, Br/Ca analysis in paleodiet research. The following is a brief summary of these reviews. Strontium, barium, and calcium resemble each other chemically, and if any or all are present in the soil, plants will assimilate and utilize them. Animals eating these plants can digest and absorb all three elements, up to 80 percent of ingested calcium, but less than 10 percent of ingested strontium or barium. Calcium is an essential nutrient for mammals, but strontium and barium are not essential. Once digested and absorbed, mammals eliminate strontium and barium from the blood circulation in two ways: excretion from the kidney and sequestration in bone where they are stored and they become inactive metabolically. Given this, the Sr/Ca or Ba/Ca ratio in organisms should decrease from plants (no discrimination against Sr or Ba), to herbivore mammals (initial discrimination against Sr and Ba), to carnivore mammals (secondary discrimination against Sr and Ba). Thus, the Sr/Ca or Ba/Ca ratio in bone from living or extinct mammals, including hominids, could serve as an indicator of the relative amounts of plant food versus meat in the diet.

The Sr/Ca and Ba/Ca method shows some promise for paleodiet research, but unfortunately there are a number of factors that can influence Sr/Ca ratios in bone that are not due to diet. The amount of calcium, barium, and strontium in groundwater affects uptake by plants and herbivores. The age of a mammal influences the absorption of these elements. Young animals, growing bone tissue rapidly, absorb more strontium and barium than older animals. Deficiencies of other nutrients, such as vitamin D, may impair digestion and absorption of all three elements. Pregnancy and lactation also are factors. Laboratory animal research and human clinical studies show that pregnant and lactating females store more strontium in bone than males or postreproductive females (Blakely 1989). Finally, the geological context of preservation and fossilization of bone may enhance or deplete the Sr/Ca and Br/Ca ratios.

Although caution must be exercised in the interpretation of Sr/Ca and Br/Ca ratios in living or fossil bone, the technique has proven useful in some cases. In archaeological samples of human skeletons from Mexico, Schoeninger (1979) found a strong negative correlation between indicators of social status and strontium in bone. Burials with greater amounts of high-status grave goods had lower Sr/Ca ratios than burial with fewer or no high-status grave goods. This suggests strongly that high-status individuals consumed more meat and lower status individuals consumed more plant foods in their diet.

Using stable isotopes preserved in human bone, a team of archaeologists and biological anthropologists found that high social status does not always lead to more meat in the diet. In highland Ecuador, in a suburb of the present capital of Quito, there is an archeological site called La Florida. The site dates from 100 to 450 A.D. and includes well-preserved burials of 9 high-status individuals of the ruling elite and 23 low-status individuals buried along with the elites. Some of the low-status people were buried alive, and historical sources indicate they were members of a hereditary servant class, essentially slaves, who served their masters in life and, apparently, in death. Ubelaker et al. (1995) analyzed these skeletal remains for age at death, sex, and stable isotopes of carbon and nitrogen. The stable isotope of carbon, ^{13}C, can determine if foods in the diet were based on plants using the C_3 or the C_4 photosynthetic pathway. The more ^{13}C in a skeleton the more C_4 plants in the diet. Included among C_4 plants are the domesticated grains maize, millet, and sugarcane, while C_3 plants include virtually all those growing wild in temperate regions. The only C_4 plant that ancient people of highland Ecuador consumed in quantity was maize. The amount of stable nitrogen isotope, ^{15}N, in human skeletons is lowest when the diet is mostly plant food and higher as more animal protein is included in the diet.

Ubelaker and colleagues found that the skeletons ranged in age from 5 to 50 years at the time of death, with children and adolescents in both the elite and the low-status samples. Age at death had no effect on the levels of stable isotopes in these skeletons, but there is a statistically significant difference in the ^{13}C levels between the two groups. The elites have higher levels, indicating they consumed more maize than the low-status individuals. There was no difference between the two groups for ^{15}N levels, indicating equal amounts of animal protein in the diet. Ubelaker et al. point out that these findings contradict the conventional wisdom that elites always ate more animal protein while low-status people ate mostly vegetable-based foods. The authors explain that the extra maize consumed by the elites was in the form of an expensive and politically restricted food called beer. Elites controlled the production and consumption of beer. Maize beer was produced by the chief's household and was doled out to the commoners at feasts in return for their labor. Chiefs also paid tribute to each other in the form of beer and offered copious amounts of beer at royal funerals. Chiefs were buried with many ceramic vessels, and at La Florida 70.5 percent of these were devoted to the brewing and serving of maize beer.

The Sr/Ca trace element analysis was used by Schoeninger (1982) to analyze fossil remains of archaic and modern *H. sapiens* from sites in Israel dating between 70,000 and 10,000 years ago. The purpose of the study was to see if a change in diet, from relatively more meat to relatively more plant food consumption, correlated to the change in human form from archaic to modern (e.g., modern people have more gracile skeletal features than archaic forms). Care was taken to control for differences in the amount of calcium and strontium in the soils of different fossil sites and other confounding geological variables. It was found that Sr/Ca ratios in bone increased with time, suggesting more plant food in the diet, but the increase occurred 20,000 years after the modern human form appears in the fossil record. Schoeninger concludes that the morphological transition from archaic to modern *H. sapiens* was not due to the utilization of new foods, rather it was due to "alterations in the means of procuring or processing the same kinds of foods that had been utilized earlier in time" (p. 37). In other words, behavioral and cultural changes were more important than diet change per se in bringing about the biological form of modern humans. This along with the other examples of trace element and stable isotope analysis clearly shows the biocultural nature of people and food.

STUDIES OF LIVING HUNTERS AND GATHERERS

Today, 99.9 percent of people derive their food from some form of agriculture. However, from the time of the *Australopithecus* until about 10,000 years ago, a time period that covers 99 percent of human evolution, all hominids lived by foraging—the gathering, scavenging, and, more recently, hunting of wild foods. Most human physical traits, and perhaps many behavioral propensities, evolved during the time that hominids lived as hunters and gatherers. That biobehavioral evolution includes current human dietary requirements, adaptations for food acquisition and processing, and biocultural responses to food intake. Studies of the few remaining cultures of hunting and gathering peoples offer an indirect view of that style of life, now nearly extinct. These ethnographic and ecological studies complement the information derived from paleontological and archaeological sources.

Foragers are a diverse group geographically and culturally, ranging from the arctic Inuit and Eskimo, to the tropical forest Ache (Paraguay), to the dry scrub San (Africa) and the desert Australian Aborigines. Yet research shows some consistencies in behavior and diet. The diversity of food resources utilized is high among gathering and hunting peoples compared with agriculturalists. The !Kung San of southern Africa, for instance, eat 105 species of plants and 144 species of animals (Lee 1984). The Australian North Queensland Aborigines exploit 240 species of plants and 120 species of animals (Gould 1981). The Ache forage on fewer species, about 90 types of plants and animals (Hill and Hurtado 1989). Even the Dogrib, residing in the subarctic of Canada, gather 10 species of plants and 33 species of animals (Hayden 1981). That is a small food base for hunters and gathers, but still a large number relative to agriculturalists who, on a worldwide basis, subsist largely on four species of plants and two species of animals. Of nine species of staple plant foods, wheat, rice, potatoes, and maize together account for

Table 6.3
Demographic Characteristics of Forager Groups

Group (location)	Group size	Population density/100 mi²	Frequency of moves
Nootka (Canada)	1,500	200	180 days
Andamanese (Asia)	45	200	60 - 180 days
Paliyans (India)	24	200	as needed, ≈45 days?
!Kung San (Africa)	20	41	14 - 21 days
Hazda (Africa)	9	40	14 days
G/wi San (Africa)	55	16	21 days
Ache (S. America)	48	8	daily, .143 days
Guayaki (S. America)	16	7	3 days
Western Desert Australians	20	3	7 - 14 days
Mistassini (Canada)	15	1	180 days

Source: Hayden 1981. Ache data from Hill and Hurtada 1989.

1,680 of the 2,284 million metric tons consumed (sorghum, sweet potatoes, barley, millet, and cassava are the other five staples, [Garine 1994]). Of the animal foods, cattle and hogs account for 80 out of every 100 metric tons of domesticated animal meat. Poultry, lamb, goat, buffalo, and horse make up the bulk of the remaining 20 metric tons (Bogin 1985).

A second common feature is that gathered foods (plants, insects, birds' eggs, turtles, etc.) are the primary subsistence base in most foraging societies. Lee (1968) compared 58 forager groups and found that the primary subsistence source was gathering for 29, fishing for 18, and hunting for 11. Ten of the hunting groups and 16 of the fishing groups lived north or south of the 40-degree parallel. Thus, not only is gathering the most common subsistence pattern, it is correlated with tropical, subtropical, and low-temperate habitats. Such habitats were the home for all species of hominids until the middle to late paleolithic period.

Often the use of many species for subsistence is correlated with the high diversity, low density, or seasonality of food items in the environment. In habitats where low density is combined with the wide dispersal of foods, foragers must be mobile and live in small groups. Thus a small, mobile social group is a third typical feature of forager societies, but, as shown in Table 6.3, it is not a universal feature. Leaving aside the Nootka, average group size ranges from 9 to 55 and average densities range from 1 to 200 people per 100 square miles. Mobility ranges from daily movement from camp to camp in the case of the Ache to seasonal sedentariness at one camp (e.g., a winter lodge) in the case of the Mistassini (hunters of the Canadian boreal forests).

The Ache are unusual in their daily movement, but contemporary Ache live at agricultural mission settlements and only travel on foraging trips 25 to 35 percent of the year (Hill and Hurtado 1989). Based on foods consumed, the purpose of these trips appears to be hunting, with up to 66 percent of calories consumed while traveling coming from mammalian meat. Thus their daily movement may be the result of intense hunting over a short period rather than a typical pattern of mobility. The Nootka are also unusual due to both large group size and density. The Nootka lived on the Pacific coast of Canada. Oceanic conditions, high rainfall, and varied terrestrial topography make this region extremely abundant in plants and animals. The Nootka had available a nearly inexhaustible supply of food, so much food that of 16 forager groups studied by Hayden (1981), the Nootka had the longest list of edible plants and animals that were, in fact, avoided. Their diverse and reliable food base allowed the Nootka to form large camps to exploit seasonal foods (such as salmon and whales) and maintain permanent villages.

The high density of the Andamanese and Paliyans is due to their being restricted to relatively small areas. The Andamanese live on an island rich in food resources from both land and sea. The Paliyans (of southern India) live in a rich habitat capable of supporting high densities and are surrounded by agriculturists—which means they live, effectively, within an ecological island. All of the other groups have much lower population densities. Even with all this culture to culture variability there are some general trends in this small sample of foragers; larger groups tend to be more densely populated, and the larger, or more densely populated groups tend to move less often. For the statistically minded reader, the Pearson correlation coefficients between the three variables—size, density, moves—vary from 0.51 to 0.58, indicating a moderate association among the variables.

A fourth common feature is that all foragers depend on technology to procure, process, and store food. Technology ranges from simple to complex, both in its amount and its sophistication. Savanna and desert foragers, such as the !Kung and Australians, use a digging stick to get at roots and tubers that are hidden from view or not possible to extract using the hands alone. The digging stick seems simple, but that tool more than doubles the calories available to the people who use it as compared to nonhuman primates living in similar habitats (Washburn and Moore 1980). The !Kung also use bow and arrow to hunt large game. The bow is lightweight and not, by itself, capable of delivering a lethal blow to prey. Rather, the shaft of the arrow carries a dose of a neurotoxin that paralyzes the animal without spoiling the meat. The toxin is derived from the larva of a beetle, which must be specially processed to be effective. The simplicity of the material culture of the !Kung belies the effectiveness and sophistication of their system of hunting. At the other extreme of material culture are the Inuit and Eskimo, who possess dozens of pieces of equipment for hunting or fishing, including hooks, spears, sleds, knives, and specialized clothing. The relative complexity of Inuit and Eskimo material culture is required to extract food from a harsh environment.

Food preparation techniques include cooking (e.g., boiling, steaming, roasting, frying), soaking, grinding and grating, pounding, drying, fermenting, and putrefying (as in "aged" meat). Many human foods are poisonous prior to preparation by one or more of these techniques. Acorns and horse chestnuts, eaten by many North American Indian foragers, are toxic when raw. Manioc, a root crop and dietary staple of many African societies, is poisonous until it is processed. The toxins in all of these foods are removed by leaching, that is, by boiling them in water and then allowing the food to dry prior to consumption. Rhubarb and cashews, eaten by some people in modern industrial societies, are also toxic until cooked by boiling or roasting. Finally, food storage by drying, caching, and, where possible, freezing or salting is common to many forager groups. It is essential to remember that dependence on technology for food procurement, the processing of food, and food storage are all behaviors unique to the human species and found universally in all known human cultures.

Sharing and the division of labor compose a fifth characteristic of foragers. Much has been made of both food sharing and division of labor because these two behaviors were considered necessary consequences of the "hunting hypothesis" for human evolution (Washburn and Lancaster 1968; Issac 1978). The basic premise is that male hominids ranged widely to hunt large game while female hominids, encumbered by pregnancy and dependent children, gathered plant food within a smaller area. Both sexes returned to a home base and shared the fruits (and ribs) of their labor with each other and the children. That hypothesis is out of favor currently, because there is no fossil evidence for the type of big game hunting that requires sharing and division of labor to be effective prior to the appearance of *Homo sapiens*. Nevertheless, the fact that all known living hunters and gatherers share some food, even small game and vegetables in many cultures, and have some division of labor indicates that this is a universal human nutritional adaptation.

Although universal, the degree to which sharing occurs is not constant in all cultures. Some forager groups share food regularly and have cultural rules to encourage food exchange. The !Kung and Ache, for example, prohibit hunters from keeping their own kills, rather the meat must be given to others, often a respected elder, for distribution to all members of the band. Ache women who share plant food are given praise by others, and "children are taught that stinginess is the worst trait a person can have" (Hill and Hurtado 1989:439). In contrast, several Australian groups and the Paliyans share less regularly. Hayden's (1981) review of these cultures shows that Australian men usually ate all the game they hunted in the bush, rarely bringing meat back to camp for their wives and daughters. Women and children might eat more than 50 percent of their total food intake while foraging (Hayden calls this "snacking"), and would bring back to camp only those foods needing processing. The Paliyans also practiced snacking while foraging and brought back little food to be shared at the camp.

Sharing and division of labor may best be viewed as behaviors that: (1) reduce the effects of unpredictability and variance in food supply, and (2) increase reproductive fitness. By dividing the social band into working groups based on sex and age, more of the necessary subsistence tasks can be accomplished in a shorter period of time. Adults can gather plant foods, honey, insects, and other small animal foods and hunt larger animal prey. Children can remain at the camp in age-graded play groups, with older children caring for younger children, or can accompany their parents to learn foraging techniques (Bogin 1988a). Or, children may provide significant amounts of foraged food, as they do in Hadza society (Blurton-Jones 1993). Men often range over larger areas in search of food and hunt larger prey than do women, and this serves to further increase the total supply and diversity of food. Using statistical analysis and mathematical models of food behavior among the Ache, Hill and Hurtado (1989) find that division of labor and sharing results in an 80 percent increase in nutritional status and nearly a threefold increase in the predictability and regularity of daily food intake.

Reproductive fitness, measured by the number of offspring that survive to reproductive age, is increased by division of labor and sharing. Most animals must acquire all of their own food. A few primates, including baboons and chimpanzees, are known to share some food, but only in a limited way compared to people. Chimpanzees are more like people in terms of reproductive biology, that is, both species take a relatively long time to reach sexual maturity and typically bear one offspring at a time. This places a tremendous reproductive constraint upon the chimpanzee. Chimpanzee females in the wild reach menarche (the first menstruation) at 10 to 11 years of age (Goodall 1983). The average period between successful births in the wild is 5.6 years, and young chimpanzees are dependent on their mothers, which precludes a subsequent pregnancy, for about 4.5 years (Teleki et al. 1976; Goodall 1983). Just to reproduce herself and one of her mates, a female must live to be about 25 years old. This is a long time for the animal to struggle for its own existence, find food, avoid predators, and compete with conspecifics. It is longer than most chimpanzees live. Teleki et al. (1976) and Goodall (1983) estimate that in one African game reserve only about 35 percent of all live-born chimpanzees survive to their mid-twenties. Even so, it is a significantly greater rate of survival than most other species of mammals. Lions, another social mammalian species, successfully rear about 14 to 16 percent of their offspring to adulthood (Lancaster and Lancaster 1983). The female chimpanzee's parental investment of time and energy is efficient when viewed in this context.

People living in traditional hunting and gathering societies delay reproductive age even longer than chimpanzees, but do not wait as long between successful births. The best documented example are the !Kung of southern Africa. A woman's age at her first birth averages 19 years, and subsequent births follow about every 3.6 years for an average of 5.1 births per woman (Howell 1976, 1979; Short 1976). As with all human children, the !Kung child is dependent on its parents, or other adults, for at least seven years (Bogin 1995). The traditional !Kung lived under relatively austere ecological conditions, including moderate malnutrition during childhood (Tobias 1975). Thus it may be safe to assume that for earlier hominids living under better conditions, the average amount of time between successful births was no longer than for the !Kung. Indeed the Ache, foragers of a tropical rainforest and living part-time on mission settlements, average only 3.1 years between births and 7.2 births per woman (Hill and Hurtado 1989). This presents a paradox; human birth spacing is shorter than that of chimpanzees, but human childhood dependency is longer and development slower. How can hunting and gathering people have it both ways, when for all other primates dependent young preclude another birth?

To have it both ways requires some assurance that the birth of a new infant will not result in the death of an earlier-born child (or children) still receiving basic care. Human parents "solve" this problem in two ways: (1) weaning infants by about age three and (2) by provisioning all their children with food. By weaning infants from breast milk to other foods the mother can reproduce again and be free to nurse her new infant. The weaned child may eat special weaning foods or some version of the adult diet. In either case, older individuals must prepare these foods, since children lack the skill and knowledge to do so for themselves (Bogin 1995). Lancaster and Lancaster (1983) call the provisioning of children with food "the hominid adaptation," for no other primate provides this type of investment. Some female nonhuman primates will share food items with their young, although complete provisioning is extremely rare. Male nonhuman primates do not share vegetable food with their mates or with their young; male chimpanzees will share meat with other adult males and estrus females. Human parents, male and female, regularly share food with their offspring, and this may be viewed ecologically as both a feeding and reproductive strategy. "Human hunter-gatherers, even without benefit of modern medicine, successfully raise to adulthood about one out of every two children born to them" (Lancaster 1985).

Thus adults may be able to increase their net reproductive output during a relatively short period of time. In this way sharing leads to greater reliability and predictability of food intake, better nutritional status, and increased reproduction and survival of the young. It is easy to see how these behaviors would have evolved by natural selection during the course of human history.

Table 6.4

The Nine Universal Features of Human Nutrition and Food Behavior and
the Sources of Evidence Used to Study Their Evolution

Universal features	Sources of evidence
1. Large number of essential nutrients	Primate studies, biomedical research
2. Each culture has a cuisine	Archaeology, ethnography
3. Extreme omnivory	Primate studies, hunters & gatherers
4. Transport of foods	Archaeology, ethnography
5. Storage of foods	Archaeology, ethnography
6. Complex technology for acquisition and preparation	Archaeology, ethnography
7. Sharing and division of labor	Primate studies, hunters & gatherers
8. Food taboos	Ethnography
9. Non-nutritional use of potential foods	Archaeology, ethnography

SUMMARY OF EVIDENCE FOR THE EVOLUTION OF HUMAN NUTRITION

Table 6.4 lists the nine universal features of human nutrition and food behavior. Also listed in the table are the sources of evidence that allow an understanding of the origin and function of these universals. The human place in nature as primates explains our broad requirements of essential nutrients. Fossil and archaeological evidence accounts for the development of cuisines and the technology for food acquisition, preparation, and storage. The study of living hunting and gathering peoples complements and supports these other sources of evidence. Five features of food and behavior are typically found in hunting and gathering societies: (1) a high diversity of food types; (2) greater dependence on gathering over hunting; (3) small, mobile social groups; (4) dependence on technology for acquiring and processing foods; (5) and division of labor and sharing. Additionally, forager studies detail the nature of human food transport for exchange and sharing and provide some information on the origin of food taboos and nonnutritional uses of foods.

"CAVEMAN CUISINE"

Using the methods of research described here, archaeological and paleontological evidence, ethnographic studies of living hunting and gathering people, and the nutritional analysis of wild plant and animal food, Eaton and Konner (1985) reconstructed the diet of paleolithic people living during

Table 6.5
The Paleolithic Diet of 15,000 Years B.P., the Current American Diet, and
One Set of Dietary Recommendations for the United States

Daily Intake	Paleolithic	American[1] M	American[1] W	Recommended[2]
Total dietary energy (%)				
Protein	34	15	15	12
Carbohydrate	45	48	50	58
Fat	21	34	34	30
Alcohol	trace	4	2	--
P:S ratio[3]	1.41	0.56	.61	1.00
Daily intakes				
Cholesterol (mg)	591	395	244	300
Fiber (g)	46	19	13	30-60
Sodium (mg)	690	4659	3002	2000
Calcium (mg)	1580	1075	778	1200
Ascorbic acid (mg)	392	121	87	60
Simple sugars (g)	trace	≈154		≈50

[1]American diet for adults 20–29 years old surveyed between 1988 and 1991, published by the
Centers for Disease Control, 1994; M = men, W = women. Based on a diet of 3,025 calories per day for men and 1,957 calories per day for women.
[2]Recommendations of U.S. Senate Select Committee and Food and Nutrition Board, National
Academy of Sciences. Values for adults, sexes combined.
[3]Ratio of polyunsaturated to saturated fats from all foods.
Source: Paleolithic diet: Eaton and Konner 1985; American diet: Guthrie and Picciano 1995,
appendix K.

the last glacial period in western Europe, about 15,000 years ago. Garn and
Leonard (1989) point out that this diet was not typical of the majority of
people alive at that time. The majority lived at tropical or subtropical latitudes and consumed more wild grains and less animal meat—recall Schoeninger's (1982) analysis of paleolithic diets from Israel. Garn and Leonard
state that "many of our ancestors ate poorly, . . . and they were often at risk
for vitamin deficiencies, food-borne diseases, and neurotoxins" (1989: 337).
Despite these caveats, the paleolithic diet reconstructed by Eaton and Konner offers some useful data, especially when compared with the modern
American diet.

Table 6.5 compares this paleolithic diet with that of modern Americans
and U.S. government recommendations for a safe and healthy diet. These
glacial people ate more protein and less fat than we do. Eaton and Konner's
analysis of living foragers indicates that the average diet consists of 35 percent of calories from meat and 65 percent of calories from vegetable foods.
Although plants contribute protein to the diet, Eaton and Konner estimate
that most of the protein was from animals, including fish, insects, and other
invertebrates. Fat intake was lower in the paleolithic due to the low content

of fat in wild game. The average carcass fat content of 15 species of wild herbivore surveyed by Eaton and Konner is 3.9 percent compared to an average of 25 to 30 percent in domesticated carcasses (cattle, hogs, etc.). Moreover, compared with domesticated meat, the fat of wild game is about five times higher in the polyunsaturated form. Along with plant foods rich in polyunsaturated fats, the paleolithic diet has a high ratio in polyunsaturated to saturated fats. Cholesterol intakes appear to have been higher in the ancient diet. In the early 1980s, however, the ancient and modern diets contained similar amounts of cholesterol, and fat intake of the American diet was about 42 percent of total calories. It seems that Americans have learned to eat foods with less fat and cholesterol. Unfortunately, Americans are also eating more total food (i.e., calories) than in 1980. So, despite a decrease in fat consumption there has been an increase in body weight, mostly due to fatness, for both average and obese children and adults (Yip and Scanlon 1995).

The modern ethnographic data and the archaeological data indicate that paleolithic people would have gathered a wide assortment of wild plant foods and many species of animals, ensuring variety in both vitamin and mineral content and in taste and appearance. In contrast, the many people living in agricultural and industrial societies eat from an extremely narrow range of food options. Modern people eat more wheat, rice, potatoes, and maize than the next 26 most often consumed plants combined (when did you last eat a turnip?). There are many reasons for this. For most of the world the reasons are associated with economics. Wheat, rice, potatoes, and maize are grown on a large scale to make profits for national or multinational agribusiness corporations. The intensive production of these and a few other crops is very efficient in terms of business practices and profits. These crops may be produced relatively cheaply, making them more affordable to the 80 percent of the world population who live in less-developed nations and who are at or near the poverty level. The more affluent 20 percent of the world's people, living mostly in the more-developed nations of Europe, Japan, Australia, and North America, can eat a much wider variety of foods. They can afford to buy more expensive foods that are produced in limited quantities and often shipped long distances. The Japanese and French, for example, eat dozens of species of animals, including many mammals (rabbits, sheep, horses) and ocean species (shell fish, sea urchins, fish) as part of their regular diet. The modern American diet, on the other hand, is much more restricted in food choice. A survey of most supermarkets will reveal a limited variety of animal protein sources (when did you last eat horse, rabbit, or even fish?). Americans eat more ground beef, usually in the form of hamburgers, than any other animal protein food. It is estimated that 12,000 hamburgers are consumed each minute in the United States—a rate of 200 per second (Lieberman 1991). The consumption of ground beef also accounts for about one-half of the total fat and three-fourths of the saturated fat in the American diet. Surveys of food consumption generally find that the uniformity and limited variety of offerings available at fast-food restaurants depicts the current American diet very well.

The Eaton and Konner reconstruction also indicates that our ancestors ate much more fiber, calcium, and vitamin C, but far less sodium. Our ancestors ate simple sugars only in natural forms, for instance from fruits, but today we each eat about 124 pounds of simple sugar (mostly sucrose and corn syrup) a year. Paleolithic foragers consumed no dairy products, except for mother's milk during infancy, and little alcohol. Consumption of dairy foods is a by-product of animal domestication, and thus less than 12,000 years old. Even today, dairy products are staple foods in only a few societies. Most adults lack the enzyme lactase needed to digest the milk sugar lactose (Kretchmer 1972). Some societies do eat cheeses or yogurt, for these foods have their lactase digested by bacteria, but these foods are often too expensive for most of the world's people. The wealth of the developed nations allows their populations to consume large quantities of dairy products. In the United States, 20 percent of protein, and most calcium, comes from milk and cheeses. These foods, unfortunately, also contain high amounts of fat and sodium, which also typify the American diet. Alcohol is, basically, also a product of domestication—the domestication of grains such as maize and barley. Some alcoholic beverages (beer, mead, wine) contains some nutrients, but alcohol itself provides no essential nutrients. Even so, alcohol contains energy—seven calories per gram—and contributes a measurable percent of calories to the American diet.

High intakes of fat, especially saturated fat, simple sugars, sodium, and alcohol are linked with health problems, such as obesity, heart disease, and liver disease. Apparently, Americans are aware of a problem, for example, millions of dollars are spent annually for weight loss programs. The weight loss programs usually have little long-term success, indeed the average weight and fatness of Americans has increased in the last few decades. A narrow diet is also a risk for nutrient deficiencies, such as the low calcium intake of many Americans. The response of the people is to purchase nutritional supplements and special "health foods." The U.S. Food and Drug Administration (note that food and drugs are lumped together by American culture) estimates that 40 percent of adults regularly take at least one vitamin and mineral product (Moss et al. 1989). Taking vitamin pills to compensate for a narrow diet was not the nutritional behavior followed by our ancestors. Consumption of vitamins via pills is not bad, or harmful, in and of itself. Our bodies make no distinction between the vitamins in food and those synthesized by chemists. Eating food, however, provides the physical and emotional satisfaction of taste, aroma, and a full stomach, along with other nutritional factors that are linked with good health, such as fiber. Of course, one can also buy and consume "fiber pills." Indeed, there are pills to reduce high serum cholesterol levels, induced by all those hamburgers, and to lower blood pressure, induced, in part, from our sodium overload. Perhaps it is best to view American nutritional habits as part of a biocultural system with its own internal logic. The system works, in the sense that there are fewer nutritional deficiency diseases in the United States today than ever before.

Nutritional oversufficiency is the single biggest dietary problem in the United States. In this regard, it is important to mention one other major difference between Paleolithic people and contemporary Americans. The former were required to perform high levels of both aerobic and anaerobic exercise, while the latter are sedentary ("couch potatoes" in the vernacular). Foraging people of the past and of today have the physique and cardiovascular conditioning of athletes. No amount of diet change or pill consumption for Americans and people of the other developed nations will improve health without a simultaneous increase in physical activity.

AGRICULTURE AND THE DECLINE OF HUMAN NUTRITION AND HEALTH

Some of the nutritional problems of modern world societies are: (1) a narrow food base, leading to deficiencies for some essential nutrients, (2) an inadequate supply of energy (i.e., undernutrition of total calories from all food sources) for about 60 percent of the world's population, especially the poor in the least-developed countries, and (3) an oversupply of energy, leading to obesity and related diseases in the developed nations and, increasingly, among the more affluent in the developing nations. The immediate causes of these problems include a host of social problems, such as poverty and other economic inequalities, political unrest (such as civil and ethnic wars), inadequate water management, and unregulated population growth. Although these are significant proximate causes for the world's current nutritional crisis, there is a more fundamental explanation that had its origin at the end of the Paleolithic period.

The major culprit of the nutritional dilemma is agriculture. More recently, industrialization and urbanization have compounded the effects of agriculture on the nutritional status and health of human populations. Agriculture, industrialization, and urbanization are often stated to be the hallmarks of "progress" of the human species. Although progressive in a technological sense, each of these achievements has had negative consequences for human nutrition and health.

There is much evidence from the developing nations of the world that the food production systems of rural people correlate strongly to their nutritional status. The classic study of Indonesian peoples by Geertz (1963) shows that simple horticulturalists have the most abundant variety and amount of foods, while food shortages and frank malnutrition are most common in areas of intensive rice agriculture. Whyte (1974) extended these findings to much of tropical Asia. Whyte's analysis shows that foragers, hor-

ticulturalists, and fishing societies have diversified diets, but often inadequate calorie intakes. These societies are better nourished, however, than
peoples practicing mixed agriculture-pastoralism and intensive irrigation agriculture, especially of rice. The agriculturalists suffer marginal to serious
malnutrition for total calories and many vitamins, minerals, and protein.

The dilemma of modern agricultural societies has deep historical roots.
Studies of archaeological populations show that several indicators of biological stress increase with the transition from foraging to horticulture and agriculture (Cohen and Armelagos 1984). These stress indicators include bone
lesions due to anemia (called porotic hyperostosis), deficits in enamel formation in teeth (hypoplasias), loss of bone tissue from the skeleton, bone
lesions due to infectious disease, such as tuberculosis (called periosteal reaction), and reduced skeletal growth in children and adults (Goodman et al.
1988). The Dickson Mounds site of the Illinois River Valley provides a
classic example. From A.D. 950 to 1300 the human population of that area
changed from mobile foragers to sedentary intensive agriculturalists. During
this short time period, "the shift in subsistence led to a fourfold increase in
iron deficiency anemia (porotic hyperostosis) and a threefold increase in infectious disease (periosteal reaction). The frequency of individuals with both
iron deficiency and infectious lesions increased from 6% to 40%" (Goodman
et al. 1988:180).

The incidence of enamel hypoplasias (malformations of the tooth crown
that include pitting, linear furrowing, or complete lack of enamel) also increases from the forager to agricultural period. These dental deficiencies
occur when malnutrition or disease disrupt the secretion of enamel-forming
material. For the permanent teeth that process takes place during infancy
and childhood. Thus enamel hypoplasias leave a permanent record in the
teeth of nutritional or disease stress that people experienced in early life. In
the Dickson Mound skeletal material the prevalence of hypoplasia increases
with time, going from 45 to 80 percent of individuals affected. Furthermore,
the number of hypoplasias correlates to mortality. Individuals with one hypoplasia died, on average, five years earlier than people with no hypoplasias.
With two or more hypoplasias age at death was reduced by nine years (Goodman et al. 1988:180). Since peoples' teeth form in a fixed pattern that is
virtually the same in all human beings, it is possible to correlate the frequency of hypoplasias found on different teeth to the age of the individual
when the disease stress occurred. At Dickson Mound that correlation indicates that infants and young children were especially subject to health stress
at the age of weaning (about two to four years of age). Deficiencies in the
weaning diet, combined with increased exposure to infections and other
diseases at the time of weaning, were very likely the cause of the hypoplasias
(Goodman et al. 1988).

With the development of agriculture the Dickson Mound people shifted
from a diverse food base to one dependent on maize. The emphasis on

monoculture reduced the supply of essential nutrients, especially amino acids and vitamins not found in maize, and this compromised the health of the people. Compounding these nutritional problems was rapid population growth. Despite a lowering in the average age at death at the Dickson mound site, population sizes increased due to a shorter interval between births (about two years as compared with four years in forager populations). Larger populations and sedentarism gave rise to the conditions favorable for the spread of infectious disease, and the poor nutritional state of the people made them more susceptible to these diseases.

POLITICAL ECONOMY, FOOD, AND HEALTH

There are other archaeological examples of decline in human health with the spread of agriculture, including sites in Africa, the Middle East, Latin America, and Asia. But, not all people living in agricultural societies suffered health problems. The social organization and political economy of each society played a major role in the distribution of resources, especially food and health care. One example comes from nearly three decades of research on ancient and medieval Nubia (Van Gerven et al. 1995). Nubia is region of the Nile River valley from southern Egypt to northern Sudan, bounded by the First Cataract at Asswan to about the Fourth Cataract in modern Sudan. For the past 5,000 years the people of Nubia lived by the agricultural production of "sorghum, millet (locally known as *dura*), barely, beans, lentils, peas, dates, and wheat. In addition, a few cattle, sheep, and pigs were kept, but animal products appear to have been a minor part of the Nubian diet" (ibid: 469). While the dietary base remained stable for millennia, the political base of Nubia changed many times. From about 350 B.C. to A.D. 350, called the Meroitic period, there was political unification of all Nubia under a centralized, militaristic state society. The Meroitic state had great wealth, great urban centers, but also great social stratification. The following Ballana period (ca. A.D. 350–550) was politically decentralized, with people living in smaller but more self-sufficient settlements. Overall, health status, as revealed from skeletal and dental indicators, was better in the Ballana period than in Meroitic times. People also lived longer during the Ballana period.

By the end of sixth century A.D. Nubia was again unified under a series of Christian kingdoms. The Christian period ended in A.D. 1365, following the ascension of a Moslem prince to the throne in A.D. 1323. Van Gerven and colleagues analyzed skeletons from a Christian period cemetery located in the town of Kulubnarti, near the Dal Cataract. The early Christian period was highly centralized and socially stratified, and the people of Kulubnarti "were but a small and contributing satellite to a centralized and distant authority" (Van Gerren et al. 478). The people contributed taxes in the form of food surplus and labor. By the late Christian period, the central state authority was in decline and satellite communities like Kulubnarti were essentially ignored and independent. The populous of Kulubnarti reverted to subsistence agriculture, local political control, and were free of taxation. The skeletons from the cemetery show that infant and child mortality was greatest during the early Christian period. Enamel hypoplasias occurred at earlier ages and were more frequent, and there was more evidence of anemia during early Christian times. Late Christian–period people suffered from all of these indicators of poor health too, but less so. All of this shows, again, that the political economy of a society interacts with the food base to shape the pattern of health of the people.

CONQUEST, FOOD, AND HEALTH

Colonization of the New World, Africa, and Asia by the Spanish and other Europeans introduced new plants, animals, foods, and diseases. Europeans also introduced a new political economy. Generally, the diet and health of native people suffered. A book edited by Larsen and Milner (1994) provides up-to-date reviews of the biological effects of New World conquest. The colonizers, however, also suffered from the introduction of new foods to their diets. Pellagra is a nutritional disease caused by a lack of niacin (vitamin B_3). The word pellagra is Italian, meaning rough or painful skin, and was used to describe the disease when it first appeared in the eighteenth century in that country. In Spain the same disease also appeared at that time, but it was called *mal del sol* ("sun disease"). Pellagra's classic symptoms are the four D's—dermatitis, diarrhea, depression, and dementia. The early symptom of light-sensitive dermatitis gave the condition its Spanish name. However, sunlight only aggravated the real cause, a diet based on the consumption of highly refined maize. Maize was domesticated in the New World and exported to Europe after contact with native American people. Maize grew well in Europe and quickly became an abundant and inexpensive food that replaced many traditional grains. This was true especially in the diet of the poor of southern Europe which, by the 1700s, was predominantly based on maize, molasses (derived from sugarcane, which is of Asian origin), and salt pork.

Maize is naturally low in the amino acids lysine, tryptophan, and cystine, and in the vitamin niacin. Molasses and salt pork are also deficient in these same nutrients. Milling the maize removes the husk and germ, further reducing the niacin content, from 2.4 mg per cup to 1.4 mg per cup. The minimum daily need for niacin in adults is set at 13 mg per day by the World Health Organization. For cultural reason, Europeans preferred the bleached white appearance of the highly milled maize, as it imitated the more expensive wheat flour consumed by the wealthy. For the poor, who followed a monotonous diet based on maize flour, pellagra was the result. Pellagra spread to the United States as Europeans and their diets became the dominant cultural force. It was confined to cotton producing and cotton milling areas in the southern states where the maize, molasses, and salt pork diet was common. Even as late as 1918 an estimated 10,000 deaths from pellagra occurred in the United States, and 100,000 cases were reported. Hospitals and mental institutions treated the disease as an endemic condition (endemic diseases are particular to a people or a region). At that time the cause of pellagra was blamed on heredity, unsanitary living conditions, or an infectious agent in spoiled maize (Guthrie and Picciano 1995).

In an experiment conducted in 1917, inmates in a United States prison were asked to switch from the normal prison diet to the maize, molasses, and salt pork diet in exchange for reprieve. After five months the prisoners developed pellagra, and the nutritional cause of the disease was established. Not until 1937, however, was the specific cause, niacin deficiency, discovered.

In the Americas, where maize was first domesticated, some populations received 80 percent of their total caloric intake from maize. The living Maya, the people of corn, still consume this amount of maize. Yet pellagra was unknown in the New World prior to European contact. The reason for this is that New World people used the whole grain of the maize, including the germ, and prepared the maize in a manner that enhanced the tryptophan content and the available niacin. Throughout Central America, Mexico, and those regions of the United States where maize was (or is) the dietary staple, the following method of preparation is commonly used. Ears of maize are dried and the kernels removed from the cob. The kernels are ground by hand (minimal milling, see Figure 6.1) and placed in a pot of water. Ground limestone (calcium carbonate) is added to the pot and the contents are boiled. The mixture is removed and dried until it forms a malleable dough (called *masa* in Latin American Spanish) that can be shaped into foods such as tortillas and tamales. The limestone is an alkali and reacts chemically with the maize and the water to increase the tryptophan content of the maize by hydrolysis (Katz et al. 1974). Tryptophan, in turn, is a precursor to niacin, that is, in the human body tryptophan can be converted into niacin by metabolic processes. The rate of conversion is about 60 mg of tryptophan for 1.0 mg of niacin (Guthrie and Picciano 1995). The limestone used to make *masa* also adds calcium to the diet. A cup of dry cornmeal (unenriched) provides 1.4 mg of niacin and 8.0 mg of calcium, while a cup of dry *masa* flour contains 4.8 mg of niacin and 211.6 mg of calcium. Thus a diet in which 80 percent of the calories are derived from *masa*-based foods provides sufficient niacin and calcium.

INDUSTRIALIZATION, URBANIZATION, AND THE FURTHER DECLINE OF NUTRITION AND HEALTH

Industrialization, and its concomitant urbanization, compounded the problems started with the introduction of agriculture. Industrial peoples are removed yet another step from their food sources, and often become more dependent on a limited variety and quality of food. Industries and cities divert vast amounts of water from agriculture and food production, to be used instead for power generation and more recently for materials processing and cooling. Industrial processes cause pollution of the environment, that is, they concentrate naturally occurring but widely dispersed substances that are toxic to people, such as lead, coal dust, and hydrocarbons, into small areas. Industrial process also create new substances that are toxic to people, such as polychlorinated biphenals (PCBs) and dioxin. Industrialization further concentrates people in smaller areas, increasing the opportunity for contact with pollutants and the transmission of infectious disease. Industrialization increases sedentarism, restricts outdoor activity, breaks up traditional kinship-based societies, and increases socioeconomic stratification. The sharing of food and other goods and services decreases. Finally, patterns of food consumption are regimented in industrial societies. Foragers and subsistence farmers tend to eat smaller amounts more frequently throughout the day (snacking). Industrial workers tend to eat fewer meals, for example "three meals per day," rather than snacking. Each of these changes in behavior and social organization has the potential to impact negatively on human nutrition and health.

Historical records for the population of the Connecticut River Valley during the eighteenth and nineteenth centuries show that as the market economy and industrialization increased so did the incidence of tuberculosis and diarrheal infections (Meindl and Swedlund 1977; Swedlund et al. 1980). Infectious disease can impair nutritional status by curtailing appetite and food intake and impairing the absorption of nutrients by the digestive system while at the same time increasing the body's need for nutrients, especially protein (Scrimshaw and Young 1976). Poor nutrition may make a person more susceptible to disease by suppressing the body's immune responses (Chandra 1990). This synergism between malnutrition and infection shows up clearly in records of physical growth in height and weight of individuals or populations. Since growth is dependent on an adequate supply of all essential nutrients, both malnutrition and infection work against optimal growth. Public health workers, epidemiologists, anthropologists, economists, and historians use records of physical growth to measure the health and well-being of human populations (Schell 1986).

During the years 1750 to 1900, the time of the industrial revolution in the Western world, the growth in height of people living in industrialized areas was less than that of people living in agricultural areas (Bogin 1988b). In a historical study of eighteenth-century British military recruits, Steegmann (1985) found that men from rural areas averaged 168.6 cm while the average height of men born in urban areas was 167.5 cm, a small but statistically significant difference. Steegmann noted that during the eighteenth century Britain was a developing nation. Industrializing urban regions were becoming increasingly dependent on food supply from rural areas. Crop fail-

Figure 6.3
Eighteenth-Century Military Stature

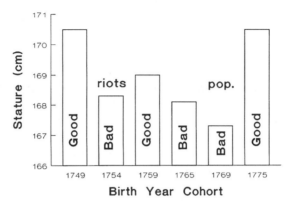

Birth Year Cohort

The dates of each birth year cohort begin with the year indicated and continue until the next
  birth cohort; that is, the earliest cohort was born between 1749 and 1753, the next cohort
  was born between 1754 to 1758, and so on. "Good" and "Bad" are relative terms which
  refer to historical estimates of food availability in England. "Riots" refers to years of food
  shortages so severe as to cause riots, and "pop." indicates a period of rapid population
  growth (after Steegmann 1985).

ures, unreliable transportation, lack of food storage and preservation techniques, and demand from higher-paying external markets resulted in
periodic food shortages in cities. Figure 6.3 illustrates the relationship between food availability and the stature of military recruits based on the year
of birth of those men for all of England and Ireland between 1750 and 1778.
The average height of men born in "bad" (food shortages) years are significantly less than those of men born in "good" (food adequacy) years. Industrializing areas were particularly hard pressed in bad years, and in 1753
and 1757 there were food riots in some cities. Research with modern populations shows that severe malnutrition during infancy and childhood has a
permanent stunting effect on human growth in height (Bogin 1988b). Steegmann's British data for the 1700s concurs with undernutrition as the cause
for the reduced height of men born during periods of food shortages.

    A recent example of the effects of industrialization and pollution on hu-
man growth and well-being is the work of Paigen and colleagues (1987) at
Love Canal. The site of the research was a residential neighborhood in
Niagara Falls, New York, that was constructed above a 3,000 meter long
unfinished canal. Prior to building homes and a school at the site in the
1950s, the canal "was used as a burial site for 19,000 metric tons of organic
solvents, chlorinated hydrocarbons, acids, and other hazardous waste during
the 1940's" (Paigen et al. 1987: 490). By 1977, the presence of unsafe levels
of chemicals in the ground water, the soil of the school playground, and the

indoor air of homes was established. In 1978, due to an excess of miscarriages by women from Love Canal, the state of New York evacuated 235 families. In 1980 the Federal government of the United States evacuated the remaining 800 families.

Prior to the 1980 evacuation, Paigen and colleagues measured the height and weight of 921 children between the ages of 1.5 and 16.99 years from 424 households of Love Canal. A second control sample of 428 children from Niagara Falls was also measured. The children of the control sample were from homes in noncontaminated neighborhoods but similar to the Love Canal sample in terms of socioeconomic and ethnic background. No difference in weight was found between the Love Canal and control samples. However, children born and residing in Love Canal for at least 75 percent of their lives were significantly shorter than the children from Niagara Falls. That difference could not be accounted for by statistically controlling the effect of parental height, socioeconomic status, nutritional status, birth weight, or history of chronic illness. The authors of the report conclude that chronic exposure to the toxic industrial wastes is a likely cause of the growth retardation of Love Canal residents.

One does not have to live on top of a toxic waste dump to suffer the effects of industrial pollutants. Lead dust in the air, water, and soil of industrialized countries affects virtually all of the population (Schell 1992). Toxic levels of lead causes neurological disease in both children and adults. The lead dust comes from a variety of sources, especially leaded gasolines and water pipes joined with lead solder. The nutritional impact of lead is that food grown in areas with high levels of automobile traffic may be contaminated with lead from the soil. Even worse, anyone living in an older home is at risk for lead in drinking water. Even though lead was virtually removed from gasolines in the 1980s and banned from plumbing solder in the United States in 1986, the accumulation of lead in water and soils is so great that all Americans have measurable lead accumulations in their bodies.

DIET AND THE DISEASES OF MODERN LIFE

After the year 1900, the affluent people of industrial areas in Britain and other Western nations begin to achieve adult heights greater than those of people in rural areas. The technology of Western nations, including efficient transport of regional and nonnative foods, refrigeration, nutritional supplementation, treated water, and public sanitation, allowed their people to overcome some of the nutritional and health deficits of agriculture, industrialization, and urbanization (Bogin 1988b). Other evidence for the improving conditions of life in developed nations comes from mortality statistics. Prior to 1850, deaths from epidemic diseases were a leading cause of mortality in the cities of Europe and North America. Death rates were so high that urban populations required massive migration from rural areas just to maintain constant numbers (McNeill 1979). Between 1850 and 1900 death rates in urban and rural areas began to equalize, and since 1900, urban mortality rates, for all ages, have been lower, generally, than rural mortality rates. The process of modernization in developed counties that resulted in better physical growth and lower rates of mortality for urban populations is now taking place in developing nations. Conditions for life in many Third World cities are still abominable for the poor underclass. However, current trends in some Third World countries indicate that these nations may follow the historical path toward modernization that occurred in Western nations (Bogin 1988a).

Improved physical growth and longer life do not mean that modern urban populations are free of the specter of malnutrition and disease. Rather, as the threat of undernutrition and infectious disease relaxed, a suite of new diseases related to the diet and life-style of industrialized/urbanized people developed to burden modern affluent people. Data from 1990 show that cardiovascular disease and cancer are the two leading causes of death in the United States. They are followed by cerebrovascular disease (e.g., stokes), accidents (mostly motor vehicle and firearm accidents), pulmonary diseases, and diabetes. The literature on the relationship of diet to heart disease, cancer, and diabetes is abundant and controversial. Alcohol, a dietary component as well as a drug, contributes substantially to accidents and many of the other leading causes of death.

The increase of cardiovascular disease in developed nations in this century can be linked to diet in several ways. An intriguing hypothesis to account for the epidemic of heart disease that occurred after World War II is proposed by Barker (1992). Using both geographical analysis and the health history of thousands of individual people, Barker and his colleagues show that babies with some indication of growth retardation (low birth weight, small but normal size, or small head circumference) have a higher risk of cardiovascular disease as adults. Growth retardation at birth is very often a nutritional problem. Either the mother is poorly nourished, or, despite adequate maternal nutrition, not enough nutrients cross the placenta to the fetus.

Poor nutrition during childhood may add to the risk of heart disease. Fellague-Ariouat and Barker (1993) interviewed women from England and Wales aged 80 years or older about their food habits when they were 10 to 15 years old (spanning the years 1899 to 1924). All of the women grew up in families of lower economic status. The women who lived in areas that today have low cardiovascular mortality tended to be rural, "to eat four meals a day rather than three, to live in households which had gardens, kept hens or livestock, and to go into domestic service, where diets were generally good. Those who grew up in areas which have high cardiovascular mortality tended to eat less red meat, live in houses without gardens, to enter industrial occupations and have higher fertility rates" (p. 15). The high mortality areas were more industrialized—mainly cotton mills—when the women were young. These industrial regions seem to have decreased the quality of diet and frequency of food consumption of young people, leading to poorer health in adulthood.

Other research links heart disease to adult behaviors that included high calorie intakes and a sedentary life-style, which lead to obesity. Long-term studies find that since World War II, as industrialization, sedentary life-styles, and sugar and fat consumption increased in Japan, Israel, many African countries, Polynesia, Micronesia, and among Native Americans and Eskimos, so did the incidence of obesity and cardiovascular disease (Weiss et al. 1984; Hamilton et al. 1988). Of course these associations are only correlations and do not prove that sugar or fat are among the causes of heart diseases. Indeed, other populations have not responded to increased sugar and fat consumption in the same manner. What seems clear, however, is that in susceptible populations there is a synergistic interaction among industrial/urban life-styles, diet, and metabolic diseases (Weiss et al. 1984).

Dental decay and gum disease are linked with a high consumption of sugar. As shown in Table 6.5, the average American consumes 154 grams of sugar per day, or about 124 pounds per year. At the turn of this century the average sugar intake was about 20 pounds per year, mostly from whole-food sources. About half of the sugar in the modern diet comes from refined white sugar (sucrose) and the other half from corn syrup (fructose), both of which are added to virtually all processed foods as sweeteners and preservatives.

Other disease risks of obesity are type II diabetes, a disease of glucose regulation, and certain cancers. Glucose is one of the major sources of energy used by the body to maintain metabolism. Normally, the amount of glucose in the bloodstream and in body cells is regulated by food intake and insulin. The carbohydrates in food are converted by the body into glucose, and insulin, secreted by cells in the pancreas, triggers body cells to absorb the glucose. Type I diabetes, which occurs in about 20 percent of people with the disease, is due to the lack of insulin production. In type II diabetes, the type found in about 80 percent of diabetes suffers, the body cells become resistant to insulin and blood levels of glucose stay too high. This leads to hypertension, kidney disease, general circulatory disease, blindness, and death. Sugar does not cause diabetes, but obesity and lack of exercise play an important role. Most type II diabetes cases can be controlled or cured with a diet lower in fats and sugars and an increase in exercise—behaviors that are more in line with our forager ancestors.

A relationship between diet and cancer is well founded, but as with diabetes and heart disease, the exact causes are unclear. What is clear is that evidence of cancer is rare in prehistoric times and the historic period prior to the industrial revolution. Less than 200 cases of cancer are known from all of the skeletons so far examined by paleopathologists (E. Strouhal, personal communication). No tumors have been found in any Egyptian or

Nubian mummy (D. Moerman, personal communication). A carcinogen (cancer-causing substance) is usually needed to provoke a cancer. Many carcinogens are industrial products, but some are found naturally in foods. Cancer rates for modern people change as food preferences change. Takasaki and colleagues (1987) studied the rates for different types of digestive system cancer in the Japanese population during the period 1950 to 1983. The researchers argue that between 40 to 60 percent of the incidence of cancer may be attributable to diet, especially in those cases in which carcinogens come into direct contact with the gastrointestinal tract. In the earlier years, the typical Japanese cuisine was based on rice seasoned with highly salted condiments, some green and yellow vegetables, and very little milk or diary products. Takasaki et al. report that this type of diet is linked with stomach cancer, and stomach cancer is the most frequent type of digestive system cancer in Japan. During the 1960s, the postwar industrialization and economic recovery of Japan proceeded rapidly. One of the consequences of that expansion was a shift from the traditional cuisine to one that included significantly more dairy products and fat. Between 1965 and 1983 rice consumption dropped from about 300 gm per person per day to about 200 gm/person/day. Milk and dairy products increased from about 75 to 150 gm/person/day. Diets high in fats are associated with cancers of the intestine and colon. In Japan, mortality rates (age adjusted) per 100,000 population for stomach cancers dropped from about 37 to 22, while the same rates for intestinal cancer increased from about 2 to 4.5.

Epidemiological studies such as Takasaki and colleagues' Japanese research show many links between cancer and specific foods or cuisines. The same holds true for heart disease, diabetes, and the other diseases of modern life. This research negates the belief that these diseases are the natural consequence of aging. Rather, these diseases are potential indicators of the environmental quality of life and the well-being of human populations. The fact that heart disease, cancers, and diabetes are the major causes of death in developed nations belies the notion of "progress" that is a central belief of European and American culture. While it is true that the average age at death has increased steadily in developed nations in this century, most of the increase is due to the control of infant and child mortality from infectious disease. Adults suffer as much, or more, disease than 100 years ago, and may suffer these diseases from an earlier age.

Food is safer today than 100 years ago in that processing, refrigeration, and other technologies prevent spoilage and food poisoning. However, the processing that increases short-term safety also adds salt, sugar or artificial sweeteners, and, often, fats (both natural and artificial) to our diet that may lead to long-term health risks. Advances in food technology also permit producers and consumers to eat more preferred foods. Preferred foods may be "good" or "bad" for people depending on the scientific, philosophical, and moral code of a society. Many Americans, for example, abhor horse meat

Table 6.6
Energy Inputs for Processing Common Food Items of Industrial Societies,
the Energy Provided by Eating These Same Foods, and the Energy Cost to
Produce the Container for These Foods

Processed food	Energy input (kcal/kg)	Energy return (kcal/kg)	Container (kcal)
Instant coffee	18,948	2,645	2,213
Chocolate	18,591	5,104	722
Breakfast cereal (corn flakes)	15,675	3,877	722
Beet sugar (≈17% sugar in beets)	5,660	4,000	≈400
Cane sugar (≈20% sugar in cane)	3,380	4,000	≈400
Fruits and vegetables (frozen)	1,815	≈500	722
Fish (frozen)	1,815	1,058	≈400
Baked goods (white bread)	1,485	2,680	559
Meat (hamburger)	1,206	2,714	≈400
Ice cream (vanilla)	880	2,015	722
Fruit and vegetables (canned)	575	≈500	2,213
Flour (enriched, sifted)	484	3,643	≈400
Milk (3.7% fat)	354	643	2,159

Source: Energy inputs and containers: Harris 1993; energy returns: Guthrie and Picciano 1995, appendix K.

both for reasons of food safety and morality—horses are "pets" not "food." The French, in contrast, insist that horse meat is best for making the dish steak tartar, prepared from ground meat, which is seasoned with many spices and flavorings and then eaten uncooked. The French state that horse meat is safer to eat, as it is "free of parasites" (D. Moerman, personal communication).

The ability to produce virtually unlimited quantities of preferred foods may be one reason that people in the developed nations, especially the United States, tend to eat more food than ever before. In addition to the technological advances in food production, there are social and ideological reasons for this. In the more developed nations, food production and consumption have become part of the industrial and commercial social structure of the society (Lieberman 1991). Food is part of "big business," that is, the economic, social, and political organizations that structure social organization in industrial nations. Consider the social impact of the fast-food industry, McDonald's Corporation for example. In the United States, the industrialization of food production has reached the point where far more energy is expended by the machines that harvest, process, and transport food than is returned as food calories. Listed in Table 6.6 are several processed foods, the amount of energy it takes to manufacture them, the energy return from the foods themselves, and the energy cost of the container used to package the food. To manufacture one kilogram of instant coffee, for example, requires 18,948 kilocalories. Drinking all that as coffee, slightly more than 529 six-ounce cups, provides 2,645 kilocalories. The metal and plastic container that the coffee is packaged in costs an additional 2,213 kilocalories to manufacture. Chocolate, breakfast cereals, table sugar from beets and sugar cane, frozen fruits and vegetables, and frozen fish also require more, or as much, energy to produce and package than they return as food energy. Hamburgers, the bread they are sandwiched into, and ice cream provide relatively high-energy returns for the cost to processing these foods. But people do not live by hamburgers and ice cream alone, not even Americans. Less-processed foods such as fruits, vegetables, flour and milk provide as much or more energy than they cost to process. This energy profit is countered by relatively high-energy losses for manufacturing the container that holds these foods. The figures in Table 6.6 do not include the costs to grow, harvest, and transport the foods, nor the cost of operating factories and stores that process and sell the foods. From an ecological perspective, one that measures energy flow through a society, industrial food production systems operate at an energy loss. Every other species of living things would go extinct under these conditions. People living in industrial societies manage to survive because industrial and business activities are able to generate substantial financial profits, which can be used to offset food production costs. Unfortunately, these financial profits often come at the expense of the biologically evolved nutrition needs of the people.

Evidence of the commercialism of food and diet is easy to find. Print and electronic media bombard people with the message that food promotes pleasure. This is especially true of foods that are high in fats and sugars. Igor de Garine (1987), a French anthropologist of food, observes that the style of food consumption today in wealthy nations reflects more a quest for pleasure and increased social status than a desire to fulfill human biological necessity. Of course this has been the case since at least the time of the ancient Maya and Romans. Only recently, however, are people able to eat any food, in any quantity, as often as they wish, if they can afford the price. This may make people happier, and even more productive, in some sense, but there are biological consequences of this sensual and socioeconomic pursuit of satisfaction. There is an increasing body of research that shows that in addition to the body fat that accumulates from overeating, the chemical by-products of excessive food digestion are themselves harmful. This includes the digestion of any food, including low fat foods, sugar-free foods, and any other so-called health food. These digestive by-products may cause cellular damage that induces metabolic disease, such as diabetes, and accelerate aging (Weindruch 1996). Maybe today is a good time to go on that diet that you have been thinking about.

CONCLUSION

This chapter offers one perspective on the evolution of human nutrition. The mammalian and primate background for human nutrition, the hominid fossil and archaeological evidence, the behavior and diet of human foraging societies, and the development of modern foods and life-styles are treated in some depth. Other aspects of human evolution related to food and nutrition are neglected here, such as a detailed discussion of food taboos, ritual and profane foods, and the effect of seasonal periods of food shortage and abundance on human biology and behavior. Also neglected are connections between food production systems and diseases that are not directly caused by food or diet. Malaria, for example, spread to human populations following the introduction of agriculture in Africa (Livingstone 1958). Malaria kills more people, even today, than any other inofectious disease, and, consequently, is a potent agent of natural selection and human evolution. There is evidence that some African societies have developed biocultural systems to produce and consume food, especially cassava, that reduce the threat of malaria (Jackson 1990).

The most pressing nutrition problem of the twentieth century is also barely mentioned. This is the undernutrition and starvation that afflicts three-fourths of the world's children—nearly two billion people. The toll that this takes on human health, productivity, and happiness is virtually unmeasurable. The cause of this suffering lies in the social economic, and political inequalities between rich and poor; inequalities that the affluent populations are unwilling to change (Foster 1992; Shields 1995). These and other topics dealing with human nutritional biochemistry, genetics, history, ethnology, and psychology relating to food may be pursued in other sources of reference, including other chapters in this book. The primary message of all of these sources, and this chapter, is that food is central to human life. From a biological perspective food is central because of the essential nutrients needed for growth, repair, and maintenance of the body. From a sociocultural perspective food is central because of the behaviors and beliefs that have evolved around foods and their use. From a medical perspective food is central because of the consequences of diet and food behavior for human health. Combining these discrete perspectives into a single holistic framework leads to the conclusion that human nutrition is a biocultural phenomenon.

ACKNOWLEDGMENTS

Professor Daniel Moerman and Dr. Alan Goodman read earlier versions of this chapter, offering many suggestions to improve the presentation and correct errors of fact. Their help and friendship is much appreciated.

REFERENCES

Barker, D. J. P., ed. 1992. *The Fetal and Infant Origins of Adult Disease.* London: British Medical Journal Books.

Binford, L. R. 1984. *Faunal Remains from the Klasies River Mouth.* New York: Academic Press.

———. 1987. "American Association of Physical Anthropologists Annual Luncheon Address, April 1986: The Hunting Hypothesis, Archaeological Methods, and the Past." *Yearbook of Physical Anthropology* 30:1–9.

Blakely, M. 1989. "Bone Strontium in Pregnant and Lactating Females from Archaeological Samples. *American Journal of Physical Anthropology* 80:173–85.

Blumenschine, R. J., and J. A. Cavallo. 1992. "Scavenging and Human Evolution." *Scientific American* 267(10):90–96.

Blurton-Jones, N. G. 1993. "The Lives of Hunter-Gather Children: Effects of Parental Behavior and Parental Reproductive Strategy." In *Juvenile Primates.* M. E. Pereira and L. A. Fairbanks, eds. Oxford: Oxford University Press, 309–26.

Bogin, B. 1985. "The Extinction of *Homo Sapiens.*" *Michigan Quarterly Review* 24:329–43.

———. 1988a. "Rural-to-Migration." In *Biological Aspects of Human Migration.* G. W. Lasker and C. G. Mascie-Taylor, eds. Cambridge: Cambridge University Press, 90–129.

———. 1988b. *Patterns of Human Growth.* Cambridge and New York: Cambridge University Press.

———. 1995. "Growth and Development: Recent Evolutionary and Biocultural Research." In *Biological Anthropology: The State of the Science.* N. T. Boaz and L. D. Wolfe, eds. Bend, Oregon: International Institute for Human Evolutionary Research, 49–70.

Brain, C. K. 1981. *The Hunters or the Hunted? An Introduction to African Cave Taphonomy.* Chicago: Chicago University Press.

Bryant, V. M., Jr. 1974. "Prehistoric Diet in Southwest Texas: The Coprolite Evidence." *American Antiquity* 39:407–20.

Bryant, V. M., Jr., and G. Williams-Dean. 1975. "The Coprolites of Man." *Scientific American* 232:100–109.

Burghardt, R. 1990. "The Cultural Context of Diet, Disease and the Body." In *Diet and Disease in Traditional and Developing Societies.* G. A. Harrison and J. C. Waterlow, eds. Cambridge: Cambridge University Press, 307–25.

Caraway, C. 1981. *The Mayan Design Book.* Owing Mills, Maryland: Stemmer House.

Cartmill, M. 1974. "Rethinking Primate Origins." *Science* 184:436–43.

Cavallo, J. A. 1990. "Cat in the Human Cradle."*Natural History* (2):52–60.

Chagnon, N. A. 1983. *Yanomamo-The Fierce People.* New York: Holt, Rinehart and Winston.

Chandra, R. K. 1990. "McCollum Award Lecture: Nutrition and Immunity: Lessons from the Past and New Insights into the Future." *American Journal of Clinical Nutrition* 53:1087–1101.

Cohen, M. N. and G. J. Armelagos, eds. 1984. *Paleopathology at the Origins of Agriculture.* London: Academic Press.

Conroy, G. C. 1990. *Primate Evolution*. New York: W. W. Norton

Dart, R. A. 1957. *The Osteodontokeratic Culture of Australopithecus Prometheus*. Pretoria: Transvaal Museum Memoirs, No. 10.

Darwin, C. 1871. *The Descent of Man, and Selection in Relation to Sex*. Reprint, Princeton, N.J.: Princeton University Press, 1981.

Eaton, S. B. and M. Konner. 1985. "Paleolithic Nutrition." *The New England Journal of Medicine* 312:283–89.

Ezzo, J. A., C. S., Larsen, and J. H. Burton. 1995. "Elemental Signatures of Human Diets from the Georgia Bight." *American Journal of Physical Anthropology* 98: 471–81.

Fellague-Ariouat, J., and D. J. P. Barker. 1993. "The Diet of Girls and Young Women at the Beginning of the Century." *Nutrition and Health* 9:15–23.

Figueroa, R. 1986. *Leyenda de la formación de los hombres de maíz* (summary). In *Cocina Guatemalteca*. C. Figueroa, ed. Guatemala City: Editorial Piedra Santa, xiii–xiv.

Foster, P. 1992. *The World Food Problem*. Boulder, Colo.: Lynne Rienner.

Franken, R. E. 1988. *Human Motivation*. 2nd ed. Pacific Grove, Calif.: Brooks/Cole.

Garine, I. de. 1994. "The Diet and Nutrition of Human Populations." In T. Ingold (ed.), *Companion Encyclopedia of Anthropology*. London: Routledge, 226–64.

Garn, S. M., and W. R. Leonard. 1989. "What Did Our Ancestors Eat?" *Nutrition Reviews* 47:337–45.

Geertz, C. 1963. *Agricultural Involution*. Berkeley: University of California Press.

Glander, K. E. 1982. "The Impact of Plant Secondary Compounds on Primate Feeding Behavior." *Yearbook of Physical Anthropology* 25:1–18.

Goodall, J. 1983. "Population Dynamics During a 15-Year Period in One Community of Free-Living Chimpanzees in the Gombe National Park, Tanzania." *Zietschrift fur Tierpsychologie* 61:1–60.

Goodman, A. H., R. B., Thomas, A. C. Swedlund, and G. J. Armelagos. 1988. "Biocultural Perspectives on Stress in Prehistoric, Historical, and Contemporary Population Research." *Yearbook of Physical Anthropology* 31:169–202.

Gould, R. A. 1981. "Comparative Ecology of Food-Sharing in Australia and Northwest California." In *Omnivorous Primates*. R. S. O. Harding and G. Teleki, eds. New York: Columbia University Press, 422–54.

Guthrie, H., and M. F. Picciano. 1995. *Human Nutrition*. St. Louis Mo.: Mosby.

Hladik, C. 1981. "Diet and the Evolution of Feeding Strategies among Forest Primates." In *Omnivorous Primates*. R. S. O. Harding and G. Teleki, eds. New York: Columbia University Press, 215–54.

Hamilton, E. M. N., E. N. Whitney, and F. S. Sizer, 1988. *Nutrition: Concepts and Controversies*. 4th ed. St. Paul, Minn.: West.

Harding, R. S. O. 1981. "An Order of Omnivores: Nonhuman Primate Diets in the Wild." In *Omnivorous Primates*. R. S. O. Harding and G. Teleki, eds. New York: Columbia University Press, 191–214.

Harris, M. 1993. *Culture, People, Nature*. 6th ed. New York: Addison-Wesley

Hayden, B. 1981. "Subsistence and Ecological Adaptations of Modern Hunter/Gatherers." In *Omnivorous Primates*. R. S. O. Harding and G. Teleki, eds. New York: Columbia University Press, 344–421.

Hill, K., and A. M. Hurtado. 1989. "Hunter-Gathers of the New World." *American Scientist* 77:436–43.

Howell, N. 1976. "The Population of the Dobe Area !Kung." In *Kalahari Hunter-Gatherers*. R. B. Lee and I. DeVore, eds. Cambridge: Cambridge University Press, 137–57.

———. 1979. *Demography of the Dobe !Kung*. New York: Academic Press.

Issac, G. L. 1978. "The Food Sharing Behavior of Proto-human Hominids." *Scientific American* 238(4):90–108

Jackson, F. L. 1990. "Two Evolutionary Models for the Interactions of Dietary Organic Cyanogens, Hemoglobins, and Falciparum Malaria." *American Journal of Human Biology* 2:521–32.

Katz, S. H., M. L. Heideger, and L. A. Valleroy. 1974. "Traditional Maize Processing Techniques in the New World. *Science* 184:765–73.

Kay, R. F. 1985. "Dental Evidence for the Diet of *Australopithecus*." *Annual Review of Anthropology* 14:315–41.

Kinzey, W. G., and M. A. Norconk. 1990. "Hardness as a Basis of Fruit Choice in Two Sympatric Primates." *American Journal of Physical Anthropology* 81:5–15.

Kretchmer, N. 1972. "Lactose and Lactase." In *Human Nutrition*. N. Kretchmer and W. van B. Robertson, eds. San Francisco: W. H. Freeman, 130–38.

Lancaster, J. B. 1985. "Evolutionary Perspectives on Sex Differences in the Higher Primates." In *Gender and the Life Course*. A. S. Rossi, ed. New York: Aldine.

Lancaster, J. B. and C. S. Lancaster. 1983. "Parental Investment: The Hominid Adaptation." In *How Humans Adapt*. D. J. Ortner, ed. Washington, D.C.: Smithsonian Institution Press, 33–65.

Larsen, C. S., and G. R. Milner, eds. 1994. *In the Wake of Contact: Biological Responses to Conquest*. New York: Wiley-Liss.

Lee, R. B. 1968. "What Hunters Do for a Living, or, How to Make Out on Scarce Resources." In *Man the Hunter*. R. B. Lee and I. DeVore, eds. Cambridge, Mass.: Harvard University Press.

———. 1984. *The Dobe !Kung*. New York: Holt, Rinehart and Winston.

Lee R. B., and I. DeVore, eds. 1968. *Man the Hunter*. Cambridge, Mass.: Harvard University Press.

Leonard, W. R. and M. L. Robertson. 1994. "Evolutionary Perspectives on Human Nutrition: The Influence of Brain and Body Size on Diet and Metabolism." *American Journal of Human Biology* 6:77–88.

Lieberman, L. S. 1991. "The Biocultural Consequences of Contemporary and Future Diets in Developed Countries." *Collegium Antropologicum* 15:73–85.

Livingstone, F. B. 1958. "Anthropological Implications of Sickle Cell Gene Distribution in West Africa." *American Anthropologist* 60:533–62.

Martin, R. D. 1983. *Human Brain Evolution in an Ecological Context*. Fifty-second James Arthur Lecture. New York: American Museum of Natural History.

McNeill, W. H. 1979. "Historical Patterns of Migration." *Current Anthropology* 20:95–102.

Meindl, R. S. and A. C. Swedlund. 1977. "Secular Trends in Mortality in the Connecticut Valley, 1700–1850." *Human Biology* 49:389–414.

Moerman, D. E. 1986. *Medicinal Plants of Native America*. 2 vols. Ann Arbor: University of Michigan Museum of Anthropology.

———. 1989. "Poisoned Apples and Honeysuckle: The Medicinal Plants of Native America." *Medical Anthropology Quarterly* 3:52–61.

Moss, A. J., A. S. Levy, I. Kim, and Y. K Pak. 1989. "Use of Vitamin and Mineral

Supplements in the United States." *Advance Data from Vital and Health Statistics* 174. Hyattsville, Md.: National Center for Health Statistics.

Oates, J. F. 1987. "Food Distribution and Foraging Behavior." In *Primate Societies.* B. B. Smuts, D. L. Cheney, R. M. Seyfarth, R. W. Wrangham, and T. T. Struhsaker, eds. Chicago: University of Chicago Press, 197–209.

Paigen, B., L. R. Goldman, M. M. Magnant, J. H. Highland, and A. T. Steegmann, Jr. 1987. "Growth of Children Living Near the Hazardous Waste Site, Love Canal." *Human Biology* 59:489–508.

Pelto, J. P. and G. H. Pelto. 1983. "Culture, Nutrition, and Health." In *The Anthropology of Medicine.* L. Romanucci, D. Moerman, and L. R. Tancredi, eds. New York: Praeger, 173–200.

Potts, R. B., and P. Shipman. 1981. "Cutmarks Made by Stone Tools on Bones from Olduvai Gorge, Tanzania." *Nature* 291:577–80.

Reinhard, K. J. 1989. "Coprolite Evidence of Medicinal Plants." Paper presented at the annual meetings of the Paleopathology Association, San Diego, California.

Saenz de Tejada, E. 1988. "Analytical Description of the Food Patterns in Mesoamerica since Prehistoric Times to the Present, with Special Attention to the *Triada.* (Translated from the Spanish title.) Thesis, Universidad del Valle de Guatemala, Guatemala City.

Schaller, G. B. and G. R. Lowther. 1969. "The Relevance of Carnivore Behavior to the Study of Early Hominids." *Southwest Journal of Anthropology* 25:307–41.

Schell, L. M. 1986. "Community Health Assessment through Physical Anthropology: Auxological Epidemiology." *Human Organization* 45:321–27.

———. 1992. "Risk Focusing: An Example of Biocultural Interaction." In *Health and Lifestyle Change: MASCA Research Papers in Science and Archaeology.* R. Huss-Ashmore et al., eds. 9:137–44.

Schoeninger, M. J. 1979. "Diet and Status at Chalcatzingo: Some Empirical and Technical Aspects of Strontium Analysis." *American Journal of Physical Anthropology* 51:295–310.

———. 1982. "Diet and the Evolution of Modern Human Form in the Middle East." *American Journal of Physical Anthropology* 58:37–52

Scrimshaw, N. S. and V. R. Young. 1976. "The Requirements of Human Nutrition." In *Human Nutrition.* N. Kretchmer and W. van B. Robertson, eds. San Francisco: W. H. Freeman, 156–70.

Shields, D. L. L. 1995. *The Color of Hunger.* London: Rowman and Littlefield.

Short, R. V. 1976. "The Evolution of Human Reproduction." *Proceedings, Royal Society,* Series B 195:3–24.

Sillen A., and M. Kavanagh. 1982. "Strontium and Paleodietary Research: A Review." *Yearbook of Physical Anthropology* 25:67–90.

Steegmann, A. T., Jr. 1985. "18th Century British Military Stature: Growth Cessation, Selective Recruiting, Secular Trends, Nutrition at Birth, Cold and Occupation." *Human Biology* 57:77–95.

Strum, S. 1981. "Processes and Products of Change: Baboon Predatory Behavior at Gilgil, Kenya." In *Omnivorous Primates.* R. S. O. Harding and G. Teleki, eds. New York: Columbia University Press, 255–302.

Sussman R. W. and W. G. Kinzey. 1984. "The Ecological Role of the Callitrichidae: A Review." *American Journal of Physical Anthropology* 64:419–49.

Swedlund, A. C., R. S. Meindl, and M. I. Gradie. 1980. "Family Reconstitution in the Connecticut Valley: Progress on Record Linkage and the Mortality Survey." In *Genealogical Demography*. B. Dyke and W. Morril, eds. New York: Academic Press, 139–55.

Takasaki, Y., C. Pieddeloup, and S. Anzai. 1987. "Trends in Food Intake and Digestive Cancer Mortalities in Japan." *Human Biology* 59:951–57.

Tedlock, D., trans. 1985. *Popol Vuh*. New York: Simon and Schuster.

Teleki, G. 1981. "The Omnivorous Diet and Eclectic Feeding Habits of Chimpanzees in Gombe National Park, Tanzania." In *Omnivorous Primates*. R. S. O. Harding and G. Teleki, eds. New York: Columbia University Press, 303–43.

Teleki, G., E. Hunt, and J. H. Pfifferling. 1976. "Demographic Observations (1963–1973) on the Chimpanzees of the Gombe National Park, Tanzania." *Journal of Human Evolution* 5:559–98.

Tobias, P. V. 1975. "Anthropometry among Disadvantaged Peoples: Studies in Southern Africa." In *Biosocial Interrelations in Population adaptation*. E. S Watts, F. E. Johnston, and G. W. Lasker, eds. The Hague: Mouton, 287–305.

Ubelaker, D. H., M. A. Katzenberg, and L. G. Doyon. 1995. "Status and Diet in Precontact Highland Ecuador." *American Journal of Physical Anthropology* 97: 403–11.

Van Gerven, D. P., S. G. Sheridan, and W. Y. Adams 1995. "The Health and Nutrition of a Medieval Nubian Population." *American Anthropologist* 97:468–80.

Walker, A. C. 1981. "Dietary Hypotheses and Human Evolution." *Philosophical Transactions of the Royal Society* B292:58–64.

Walker, A., M. R. Zimmerman, and R. E. F. Leakey. 1982. "A Possible Case of Hypervitaminosis A in *Homo Erectus*." *Nature* 296:248–50.

Washburn, S. L., and C. H. Lancaster. 1968. "The Evolution of Hunting." In *Man the Hunter*. R. B. Lee and I. DeVore, eds. Cambridge, Mass.: Harvard University Press.

Washburn, S. L. and R. Moore. 1980. *Ape into Human: A Study of Human Evolution*. 2nd ed. Boston: Little, Brown.

Weindruch, R. 1996. "Caloric Restriction and Aging." *Scientific American* 274(1):46–52.

Weiss, K. M., R. E. Ferrell, and C. L. Hanis. 1984. "A New World Syndrome of Metabolic Diseases with a Genetic and Evolutionary Basis." *Yearbook of Physical Anthropology* 27:153–78.

Whyte, R. O. 1974. *Rural Nutrition in Monsoon Asia*. Kuala Lampur: Oxford University Press.

Yip, R., and K. Scanlon. 1995. "The Changing Body Mass of US Children: Implications for Future Growth Curves." Paper presented at the Human Growth Workshop, Emory University, October 2–3.

Zihlman, A. L. 1981. "Women as Shapers of Human Adaptation." In *Women the Gatherer*. F. Dahlberg, ed. New Haven, Conn.: Yale University Press, 75–120.

7

Zoonoses and the Origins of Old and New World Viral Diseases: New Perspectives

LINDA M. VAN BLERKOM

Disease affects culture, and culture in turn affects disease. Epidemic diseases provoke social and medical response, while cultural behaviors influence the transmission and evolution of infectious diseases. Acquired immune deficiency syndrome (AIDS) illustrates this well. Medical procedures and sexual behavior have changed as a result of the AIDS epidemic, while cultural responses such as screening blood and using condoms have slowed its spread. Changing human behavior probably contributed to the origins of the AIDS pandemic (Feldman 1990; Ewald 1994), and the AIDS virus has continued to evolve since then (Yokoyama and Gojobori 1987; Li et al. 1988; Gao et al. 1992; Sternberg 1992). HIV and other emerging viruses are powerful reminders that we do not control our environment and cannot prevent threats to human health posed by new infectious diseases.

The appearance of new human infections is dependent on a number of factors that favor transmission and endemicity. Demographic factors such as population size, density, and interaction with other populations are important because causative agents need a minimum host population size in order to continually find new susceptibles. This size varies with the requirements and characteristics of each disease. *Varicella zoster* virus (chicken pox) remains latent throughout its host's life, often causing painful eruptions of shingles in old age. This virus requires only a few thousand people in contact for its persistence, while measles, with its short, virulent infection resulting in lifelong immunity or death, must have a host population of at least half a million (Black 1966). More densely settled societies suffer more frequent epidemics, as do those with extensive trade and communication networks that include other large societies. The presence of several civilized centers in the Old World and their increased interaction contributed to the many epidemics that have plagued Europeans since the Roman era (McNeill 1976).

The presence of pathogens in the environment, and climatic and cultural factors that affect their survival, virulence, and transmission, also affect infectious disease evolution. Many infections require arthropod vectors for transmission. Mosquitos and other arthropods are sensitive to temperature, humidity, and altitude, and they must have suitable breeding places (often unwittingly supplied by humans). Especially important sources of human disease are the infections of other animals and cultural practices that put humans in infectious foci or in contact with infected animals or vectors. Unlike human epidemic infections such as influenza or AIDS, which are widely distributed and somewhat independent of environment (like their host), most wild animal diseases are localized in more or less defined niches, called foci or nidi (Pavlovsky 1966). Human contact with such foci may result in the interspecific transmission of infection. For example, sylvatic yellow fever in South America is usually found only in the upper canopy inhabited by the monkeys and mosquitos it infects. People can acquire the infection by felling trees, which brings the mosquitos temporarily to ground level (Fiennes 1964:55). Clearing new land for agriculture is notorious for its association with zoonotic disease. Other human cultural activities, such as trapping and skinning infected animals or living with domesticated and commensal species, also contribute to the potential for infection with zoonoses, animal infections that can also affect humans.

Once a person is infected with a zoonosis, the potential exists for adaptation to human hosts and person-to-person transmission. The more frequently human infection occurs, the greater the likelihood of the zoonosis evolving into a new, specifically human disease. Most of our infectious diseases came to us recently in our evolution, and from other animals (Table 7.1). Some infections (e.g., herpes, colds, malaria, poxvirus infections) evolved along with us, with related strains in other primates. But entirely new human diseases are most likely to be either new strains of existing human pathogens (by mutation or infection of bacteria such as staph or strep by toxin-producing bacteriophages) or microorganisms acquired from an animal population. Therefore cultural practices that favor the transmission of zoonoses should also favor the evolution of new human infections. The Old World's greater reliance on domesticated animals and higher tolerance of large commensal rodent and primate populations in human settlements contributed to the large number of epidemic diseases native to that hemisphere (Table 7.2; Van Blerkom 1985).

These are the same diseases that killed a major portion of the population of the Americas in the first century after contact. Estimates range as high as 95 percent for some areas (Dobyns 1966). While the extent of depopulation is disputed, most agree that Native Americans were unfamiliar with most of the infections from Europe and Africa. For the paleoepidemiologist or med-

Table 7.1
Common Diseases of Probable Zoonotic Origin

Human Diseases	Related Animal Diseases
Measles*	Canine distemper, bovine rinderpest
Influenza*	Swine, equine, or wild bird influenza
Smallpox*	Poxvirus infections in many primates and domesticates
Dengue fever* and urban yellow fever*	Sylvatic yellow fever
AIDS*	Retrovirus infections of other primates
Plague	Rat plague
Tuberculosis	Bovine and avian TB
Relapsing fever (louse-borne)	Sylvatic relapsing fever (tick-borne)
Typhus (louse-borne)	Murine typhus (flea-borne)
Trypanosomiasis (African sleeping sickness, Chagas' disease in New World)	Trypanosomiasis in wild herd animals in Africa; American reservoir still unknown

*Human viral infections.

ical historian, this is no surprise, because the two hemispheres had had no substantial contact for at least twelve thousand years, and most epidemic diseases appeared after the development of large sedentary populations in the Neolithic (Armelagos and McArdle 1975; Armelagos and Dewey 1978). The surprise is that Native Americans appear to have had so few epidemics of their own with which to ravage their conquerors. This is especially hard to explain in Mesoamerica, where population densities were comparable to those in the Old World and should have been sufficient to sustain a chain of infection (Van Blerkom 1985).

The epidemic diseases that killed so many Native Americans after European contact probably had zoonotic origins. The biggest killers appear to have been smallpox, measles, typhus, and influenza (Ashburn 1947). Native Americans may have had their own strains of influenza A, as this virus is carried by migrating wild birds of both hemispheres. New and unfamiliar strains coming from other populations can still have severe consequences, however—for example in the 1918 influenza pandemic.

Cultural differences can help explain why fewer infectious diseases evolved in the New World. Different styles of interaction with animals led to unequal numbers of infectious diseases in the pre-Columbian Old and New Worlds. A lesser degree of dependence on domesticated animals, especially herd animals that are milked and stalled in human habitations, and

Table 7.2
Pre-Columbian Distribution of Major Human Infections

	Old World	Both	New World
Viral diseases	Dengue fever Measles Mumps Rubella Smallpox Yellow fever	Chickenpox Colds Hepatitis Herpes Influenza Polio	Changuinola fever
Bacterial	Diphtheria Gonorrhea Leprosy Relapsing fever Scarlet fever Typhoid fever Yaws	Pertussis Salmonellosis Shigellosis Staph infections Strep infections Trachoma Tuberculosis	Bartonellosis Pinta Syphilis
Rickettsial	Typhus		
Protozoal	Amoebiasis Malaria African trypanosomiasis	Giardiasis	Chagas' disease
Fungal		Candidiasis Piedra Ringworm	
Helminths	Guinea worm Filariasis Loiasis Onchocerciasis Schistosomiasis	Hookworm Pinworm Roundworm Tapeworm Trichinosis Trichuriasis	

the hunting of rodents and primates attracted to human structures and activities (which kept these animals' populations below epizootic levels) are among the factors that decreased Native Americans' potential for acquiring new infections. But this supposedly more "healthy" state of affairs had tragic consequences during contact with Europeans and Africans.

Three of the four major killers of Native Americans are viral diseases. Table 7.2 shows that the distribution of viral infections was particularly skewed toward the Old World before contact. The only human virus to evolve in the pre-Columbian New World is the Changuinola fever virus of humans and sand flies *(Phlebotomus)* in Central America. This arbovirus, which produces a three- to four-day fever and malaise, probably infected Spanish invaders, but as death from this infection is unknown (Benenson 1990:44), it had little effect on the conquest. Most viruses are host-specific, so their zoonotic sources can be determined. For these reasons, and to keep

Table 7.3
Viral Zoonoses with Pre-Columbian Worldwide Distribution

Infection	Reservoir	Transmission
Encephalomyocarditis	Commensal rats (Old World *Rattus* and New World *Sigmodon*) and other rodents	Ingestion of infected meat, urine, or feces
Influenza type A	Migratory waterfowl; also turkeys, ducks, chickens, swine	Direct contact or inhalation of airborne droplets
Kemerovo virus infection	Many animals and birds	Tick
Phlebotomus fever	Gerbils (Old World); arboreal rodents and monkeys (New World)	Sandfly
Psittacosis (Ornithosis)	Parakeets, parrots, pigeons, turkeys, ducks, and other birds	Inhalation of desiccated droppings
Rabies	Dogs, cats, wild carnivores (esp. Eur. foxes, Asian wolves), bats, N. Am. raccoons and skunks	Bite

the scale of this study manageable, it is limited to analysis of viral zoonoses and the evolution of human viral diseases. The study suggests that the New World contained no important indigenous human viruses because its inhabitants were less likely to acquire zoonotic viral infections.

METHOD OF ANALYSIS

Tables 7.3 to 7.5 include all zoonoses listed in the volumes on viral zoonoses in *Handbook Series on Zoonoses* (Beran 1981). The infections are organized by hemispheric distribution before contact, along with their reservoirs and most frequent sources of human disease. This information came primarily from the *Handbook Series*, with help from other sources (Benenson 1990 especially; also Bisseru 1967; Fiennes 1967; Hubbert et al. 1975; Schwabe 1984).

Some zoonoses, especially those with wide host ranges or carried by migrating birds, were probably found in both hemispheres before contact (Table 7.3). They are few, however, compared to the longer lists of viral zoonoses found in each hemisphere alone (Tables 7.4 and 7.5). Inhabitants of the New World were more likely to acquire zoonotic infections from the bites of arthropod vectors (arboviral infections) or while hunting, while Old World people suffered from many more diseases requiring proximity to infected animals.

Tables 7.3–7.5 are summarized in Table 7.6, which shows there was little difference in the pattern of animal involvement for vector-borne zoonoses in the two hemispheres. Transmission of these infections does not require

Table 7.4
Viral Zoonoses Indigenous to the Western Hemisphere

Infection	Reservoir	Transmission
Arenaviral hemorrhagic fevers (Junin and Machupo)	Field rodents (*Calomys*) of Argentina & Bolivia	Ingestion or inhalation of dust contaminated by rodent urine or feces
Bussuquara fever	Rodents (*Proechimys*) of Panama, Columbia, and Brazil	Mosquito
California encephalitis	Squirrels and chipmunks, U. S. and Canada	Mosquito
Colorado tick fever	N. Am. ground squirrels (*Citellus*), chipmunks (*Eutamias*), deer mice (*Peromyscus*), porcupines	Tick
Eastern equine encephalitis	Wild passerine birds, esp. pheasants; amplifying host, horses, since conquest	Mosquito
Group C bunyaviral fevers	Central and South American rodents	Mosquito
Mayaro fever (Uruma)	New World monkeys and marmosets	Mosquito
Mucambo fever	South American rodents (*Oryzomys*)	Mosquito
Oropouche fever	Monkeys (*Alouatta and Cebus*) of Trinidad and Brazil	Midge (*Culicoides*)
Piry fever	Amazon opossums or other wild animals	Mosquito
Powasson encephalitis	Canadian and U. S. squirrels and groundhogs	Tick
Rocio encephalitis	Wild birds of coastal Brazil	Mosquito
St. Louis encephalitis	Wild birds	Mosquito
Venezuelan equine fever	Wild rodents; amplifying hosts: dogs; horses, and other domesticates since conquest	Mosquito
Vesicular stomatitis	Arboreal & semi-arboreal mammals in tropics; horses, cattle, and swine since conquest	Sandfly
Western equine encephalitis	Wild birds, esp. blackbirds, swallows, U. S. and Canada	Mosquito

Table 7.5
Viral Zoonoses Indigenous to the Eastern Hemisphere

Infection	Reservoir	Transmission
Banzi fever	Unknown (Africa)	Mosquito
Bunyamwera fever	Unknown (Africa)	Mosquito
Bwamba fever	Unknown (Africa)	Mosquito
Central European tick-borne encephalitis	Wild vertebrates (hedgehogs, shrews, voles, etc.); amplifying hosts: cattle, sheep, goats	Tick or infected goat's milk
Chikungunya fever	Old World canopy monkeys; amplifying host: baboon (*Papio*)	Mosquito
Crimean-Congo hemorrhagic fever	Hares (*Lepus*) and other small Eurasian mammals; amplifying hosts: sheep, goats, horses, cattle	Tick or nosocomial; migrating birds carry infected ticks to Africa
Dengue fever	Canopy primates of W. Malaysia and W. Africa	Mosquito
Dugbe viral fever	West African cattle	Tick
Ebola-Marburg virus disease	Unknown (Africa)	Nosocomial (contact with infected blood, semen, secretions, or organs)
Far Eastern tick-borne encephalitis	Eurasian rodents	Tick
Foot and mouth disease	Cloven-footed animals, incl. cattle, sheep, goats, swine, camels	Inhalation of aerosol droplets or contact with discharges
Germiston fever	Unknown (Africa)	Mosquito
Getah virus infection	Domestic mammals and fowl, Malaysia and Australia	Mosquito
Japanese encephalitis	Herons, egrets in Asia & Pacific; amplifying hosts: swine	Mosquito
Keterah virus infection	Asian bats	Tick

Table 7.5 (Continued)

Infection	Reservoir	Transmission
Korean hemorrhagic fever	Eurasian field mice (*Apodemus*) and voles (*Clethrionomys*); urban rats and mice (*Rattus* and *Mus*)	Aerosol transmission from rodent excreta
Kunjin fever	Unknown (Australia and Malaysia)	Mosquito
Kyasanur Forest disease	Indian rats, shrews (*Suncus*), cattle	Tick
Langat virus infection	W. Malaysian wild rats	Tick
Lassa fever	African multimammate mouse (*Mastomys*)	Ingestion or inhalation of infected urine
Louping ill	Ticks, sheep, red grouse (*Lagopus*) and deer in the U. K.	Tick
Lymphocytic choriomeningitis	House mouse (*Mus*); also found in hamsters (*Mesocricetus*)	Ingestion or inhalation of infected urine, or bite
Murray Valley encephalitis	Water birds of N. Australia, New Guinea	Mosquito
Newcastle disease	Chickens, other birds	Contact with infected carcasses
Omsk hemorrhagic fever	Siberian muskrats and other rodents	Tick
O'nyongnyong	Unknown (Africa)	Mosquito
Orf virus disease	Sheep, goats, reindeer, and musk oxen	Contact with infected animals
Poxvirus infections: Cowpox Horsepox Monkeypox Pseudocowpox Tanapox Yabapox	Cattle Horses W. African monkeys Cattle African primates W. African monkeys	Contact with respiratory discharges or skin lesions
Quaranfil	African herons	Tick

Table 7.5 (Continued)

Infection	Reservoir	Transmission
Rift Valley fever	Wild res. unknown; amplifying hosts sheep and cattle, Africa	Mosquito, or handling infected carcasses
Ross River fever	Australian rodents and marsupials	Mosquito
Scrapie	Sheep and goats	Ingestion or contact with infected brains
Semliki Forest viral fever	Wide variety of African birds and animals	Mosquito
Sendai virus infection	Mice (*Mus*)	Droplet spread or contact with respiratory secretions
Simian B virus disease	Old World monkeys	Bite or contact with infected saliva or tissue cultures
Simian parainfluenza virus infection	African green (*Cercopithecus*) and rhesus monkeys (*Macacus*)	Droplet spread or contact with respiratory secretions
Sindbis fever	Wild birds	Mosquito
Spondweni fever	Unknown (Africa)	Mosquito
Tahyna virus infection	Small mammals of Europe and Africa	Mosquito
Tanjong Rabok viral infection	W. Malaysian arboreal mammals	Unknown arthropod vector
Wesselsbron fever	Unknown (Africa); amplifying host sheep	Mosquito or handling infected carcasses
West Nile fever	Birds of Africa, Europe, and Asia	Mosquito
Yellow fever	African primates; New World primates since conquest	Mosquito
Zika Forest fever	Old World monkeys	Mosquito
Zinga fever	Large wild mammals and monkeys of Central Africa	Mosquito

Table 7.6
Animals Most Frequently Involved in Viral Zoonoses

	Old World	Both	New World
Vector-borne viral diseases:			
Reservoir: wild animals (includes primates)	29*	2	15
Reservoir: domesticates (cattle, sheep, goats)	4 (3)**	0	0
Amplifying hosts: domesticates (cattle, sheep, goats)	5 (4)	0	3 (2)
Amplifying host: baboon	1		
Total Zoonoses	33	2	15
Nonvector-borne diseases:			
Reservoir: domesticates (cattle, sheep, goats)	7 (6)	3	0
Reservoir: commensal rodents	4	1	1
Reservoir: primates	5	0	0
Reservoir unknown	1		
Total Zoonoses	17	4	1
Grand Total	50	6	16

*Reservoirs of nine unknown, presumably in nondomesticated animals.
**Numbers in () equal zoonoses of domesticates involving cattle, sheep, and goats.

direct contact with their reservoir hosts, so most of these diseases are maintained in wild animals. While activities that take people into the foci of these diseases are still a factor, these diseases are more independent of culture and custom concerning the uses and treatment of animals. Domesticated animals are involved in 4 of the Old World's 33 arboviral infections and are amplifying hosts for 5 others (and 3 New World arboviruses since European contact). An amplifying host is a species that, while not the usual reservoir, can support a chain of infection and propagate the causative agent such that the probability of human infection is greatly increased.

Diseases requiring contact with an infected vertebrate or its discharges were more frequent in the Old World (Table 7.6) probably because of closer relationships between humans and other species in that hemisphere. Domesticates and commensal rodents (rats and mice attracted to human settlements and dependent on human activities) contribute to all the New World diseases of this type and almost all in the Old World, where primates are also a disease risk. Domesticates involved in the Americas were mostly turkeys and dogs, while cattle, sheep, and goats are implicated in most Old World zoonoses of domesticated animals. Today these three important multipurpose animals act as amplifying hosts in the western hemisphere as well.

The frequency of Old World contact infections acquired from domesticates, commensal rodents, and primates suggests that the difference in infectious disease load carried by inhabitants of the two hemispheres can be explained at least in part by differences in types and frequency of interactions with animals.

DISCUSSION

New and dangerous human viruses continue to appear, in spite of modern medicine and public health surveillance. Novel strains of influenza virus cause local epidemics almost every year and pandemics approximately every decade (Benenson 1990:225). Agents such as Ebola, Machupo, hanta, Lassa, and new varieties of dengue virus can cause fatal infection in humans. An as yet unnamed morbillivirus (a relative of measles and canine distemper) killed 13 horses and a human trainer in Australia in September 1994 (Nowak 1995). The study of these emerging viruses is an important focus in virology today (Morse 1993, 1994), and their evolution is now better understood.

Perhaps the most famous emerging virus of recent times is human immunodeficiency virus (HIV), the causative agent of AIDS (although dissenting voices exist on this point—see Cohen 1994; Duesberg 1994). Where did HIV come from, and how and why did it evolve? Efforts to understand this virus and its origins have been strenuous and nearly as prolific as the virus itself. Researchers have discovered a complex picture of rapid viral change that illustrates the potential of RNA viruses to evolve into new epidemic threats.

Most of our pathogenic viruses, and virtually all zoonotic and emerging viruses, are RNA-based (see Table 7.7). RNA viruses evolve very rapidly for a variety of reasons (Holland et al. 1982), including error-prone replication processes that lack proofreading enzymes (leading to error rates in the order of a million times those of DNA-based organisms; Domingo and Holland 1994); astronomical numbers of replication events during diseases outbreaks that multiply further the chance of mutation; and high frequencies of recombination (Chao 1994). These all facilitate rapid evolution of expanded host range and enhanced virulence. Retroviruses such as HIV are now known to share these capabilities (Doolittle et al. 1989).

Table 7.7
Human Viruses and Related Strains in Animals

Viral Family	Viruses of Humans	Animal Viruses
RNA Viruses		
Arenaviridae	Zoonotic only	Rodent arboviruses of Lassa fever, lymphocytic choriomeningitis, arenaviral hemorrhagic fevers, and others
Bunyaviridae	Human phlebotomus fever virus	Arboviruses such as California encephalitis Crimean-Congo hemorrhagic fever Hantaviruses Phlebotomus fever Rift Valley fever Bunyamwera fever Nairobi sheep disease, and more than 200 others
Coronaviridae	Respiratory viruses (colds)	Respiratory viruses of many species
Filoviridae	Ebola and Marburg viruses (zoonotic?)	Ebola, Marburg (presumed but as yet unknown animal reservoirs)
Orthomyxoviridae	Influenza types A, B, and C (many strains of each)	Influenza type A of horses, swine, birds, and fowl Other arborviruses of Africa and Europe
Paramyxoviridae	Parainfluenza viruses Mumps	Simian parainfluenza Newcastle and other parainfluenza viruses of birds Sendai (mice and pigs)
	Measles	Canine distemper Bovine rinderpest Australian equine morbillivirus Peste de petits ruminants (rodents)
	Human respiratory syncytial virus	Bovine respiratory syncytial virus Mouse pneumovirus

Table 7.7 (Continued)

Viral Family	Viruses of Humans	Animal Viruses
Picornaviridae	70 enterovirus such as Polioviruses	Enteroviruses of cattle, pigs, and other animals
	Coxsackie A and B viruses	Swine coxsackie Foot-and-mouth disease
	Echoviruses	Primate echoviruses
	Hepatitis A	Duck hepatitis
	Human cardioviruses	Encephalomyocarditis in rodents and birds
	More than 100 rhinoviruses (colds)	Rhinoviruses in chimps and gibbons Perhaps also caliciviruses of sea lions, swine, and cats; bacterial ribophages
Reoviridae	Human rotavirus (infantile diarrhea)	Rotaviruses of cattle, swine, mice, monkeys
	Reoviruses of enteric tract	Reoviruses in many animals
	Changuinola virus	Colorado tick fever and some arboviruses of Europe and Africa Sheep blue tongue African horse sickness
Retroviridae	Human AIDS viruses (HIV-1 and 2)	SIV and AIDS viruses of other animals Equine infectious anemia virus Caprine arthritis encephalitis virus Visna virus of sheep
	Human T-cell leukemia (HTLV-1 and 2) and possibly other oncogenic human viruses	Simian AIDS ("D-type") viruses Oncogenic and leukemia viruses of many animals and birds
	Foamy agents, perhaps Hepatitis C	Simian foamy agents
Rhabdoviridae	Humans are now a reservoir for Piry virus	Rabies viruses Piry virus of opossums Lagos bat virus Some viruses of fish, insects, and plants Vesicular stomatitis

Table 7.7 (Continued)

Viral Family	Viruses of Humans	Animal Viruses
Togaviridae	Rubella virus	Group A arboviruses (Alphaviruses) such as Venezuelan, Eastern, and Western equine encephalitis viruses
	Dengue virus	Group B arboviruses (Flaviviruses) including yellow fever and dengue in primates Tick-borne encephalitis viruses (rodents) Louping ill of sheep Bat salivary gland virus Japanese and St. Louis encephalitis viruses and many others, especially in bats and rodents Hog cholera and other pestiviruses of cattle and swine
DNA Viruses		
Adenoviridae	33 human respiratory viruses, some oncogenic	Adenoviruses of primates, other mammals, and birds
Herpesviridae	Human herpesviruses: Types 1 and 2 (*Herpes simplex*) Type 3 (*Varicella zoster*)	Simian B virus and other alphaherpesviruses of Old and New World primates, cattle, horses, dogs, cats, fowl Pseudorabies of swine and cattle
	Type 4 (Epstein-Barr virus)	Gammaherpesviruses of primates Lymphoproliferative viruses of turkeys and rabbits Betaherpesviruses in primates,
	Type 5 (Cytomegalovirus)	mice, and swine
Iridoviridae	No human forms at present	Insect iridescent viruses African swine fever Viruses in frogs and fish

Table 7.7 (Continued)

Viral Family	Viruses of Humans	Animal Viruses
Papovaviridae	Human SV40 virus, a polyomavirus (tumorigenic viruses)	Polyomaviruses of monkeys, mice, rabbits
	At least 24 human papillomaviruses (warts)	Papillomaviruses of rabbits, cattle, dogs, sheep, goats, horses, hamsters, deer, and many other species
Parvoviridae	Adeno helper viruses	Adeno-associated viruses in primates, dogs, cattle, horses, and birds Insect densoviruses
	Norwalk and other gastroenteritis viruses Erythema infectiosum, and perhaps, Hepatitis B	Parvoviruses of many species worldwide
Poxviridae	Smallpox Vaccinia	Poxviruses of monkeys and cattle are most closely related; poxviruses also found in sheep, goats, birds, water buffalo, camels, swine, and most other animals, including insects
	Molluscum contagiosum	Milker's nodule virus Orf virus Myxomatosis in New World hares

Most emerging viruses are also zoonoses, with human cases arising from the same domestic and wild animals that were important role-players in the past (e.g., primates: Ebola, Marburg, probably HIV as well; rodents: hanta, Lassa, Machupo; and domesticates: pandemic influenza, Australian morbillivirus). Domesticated animals are probably less important today because of the relative constancy of our interaction with them, that is, we are not entering into new contacts or relationships with these familiar animals as we are with rodents and primates. New viruses tend to emerge after human activities take people (and their domesticates) into new environments or change the landscape in some fashion, thus bringing them into closer contact with wild species and vectors.

The existence of animal viruses related to viruses causing disease in humans suggests several conclusions about the evolution of human infections. First, human and other viruses in the same family may be derived from a fairly recent common ancestor. This is probably true for most of the RNA viruses, given their brisk mutation rates. Other viruses have coevolved with their hosts at the slower rate of DNA evolution. Herpes viruses illustrate this model, as each primate species has its own (Yokoyama and Gojobori 1987).

Another implication of the viral relationships shown in Table 7.7 is the potential for interspecific recombination when two strains coinfect the same individual. This can lead to greatly changed infectious agents with serious consequences for human health. Influenza pandemics have been traced to recombination between duck and pig viruses replicating simultaneously in pigs (Webster 1993). Host cell DNA and viral genomes can also recombine.

In spite of the small size of viral genomes and our ability to sequence them, identifying ancestral viruses and their hosts is still difficult unless, as in the case of hanta virus, a virus is caught in the act of emerging and the reservoir host can be identified. Yet after several serious outbreaks of Ebola in Africa, researchers still haven't discovered its reservoir. Human cases can follow contact with monkeys, but the disease is also fatal in these animals, indicating some other usual host.

Furthermore, estimating the time depth of phylogenetic relationships based on viral RNA sequences is nearly impossible. First of all, RNA virus evolution violates the assumption of rate uniformity necessary for molecular clocks. Viral mutation rates are higher during active outbreaks than during periods of latent infection in small populations. Rates of sequence change depend on whether viral genomes are being replicated by error prone processes using RNA polymerases or reverse transcriptases during active infection or by DNA polymerases after integration into host DNA during latent infection. Under these conditions, mutation/evolution rates are much slower and similar to those of the host (Doolittle 1989; Doolittle et al. 1989).

Second, RNA viruses can change fast enough to accumulate multiple forward and backward mutations at any position relatively quickly. This means genetic distance (i.e., sequence divergence) is linearly related to time for only the last 30 years or so (Eigen and Nieselt-Struwe 1990).

Third, populations of these viruses, even in a single infected cell, are not uniform strains of a single genotype, but rather "quasispecies"—collections of highly variable genetic sequences (Domingo et al. 1985; Eigen 1993). Sequencing them, even with the use of polymerase chain reaction (PCR), produces a snapshot of a statistical average of base sequences in this population rather than that of a discrete strain or species.

Finally, viral recombination produces base sequence shifts that totally confound a tree based on the assumption of point mutations. All of this spells difficulties in interpreting phylogenetic trees for RNA viruses, and not surprisingly there is a good deal of uncertainty and debate over the origins of HIV as a result.

An older view (Van Blerkom 1991) is that HIV-1 (the family of strains found in central Africa, Europe, Asia, and the United States) originated from a simian immunodeficiency virus of African green monkeys, SIV_{AGM}, more than a century ago (Fukasawa et al. 1988). HIV-2 (a less virulent group of strains found primarily in West Africa) (Clavel et al. 1987) was thought to have arisen from a similar virus of sooty mangabeys, SIV_{SMM}, as did a number of SIV's causing AIDS-like disease in captive macaques (Chakrabarti et al. 1987). All of these primate viruses were thought to be ultimately derived from a common ancestor 300 to 500 years ago, thus producing a simple picture of primate retrovirus phylogeny.

Today's view is considerably different. Retrovirus molecular biology and evolution are better understood. Some primate retroviruses are believed to be much older than 500 years (Allan et al. 1991). Many more strains of both HIV and SIV have been discovered and sequenced, leading to the *approximate* phylogenetic tree shown in Figure 7.1 (Eigen and Nieselt-Struwe 1990; Myers et al. 1992, 1993; Mindell et al. 1995). The closest simian relative of HIV-1 is now believed to be SIV_{CPZ}, discovered in two wild chimpanzees captured in Gabon (Peeters et al. 1989; Huet et al. 1990). Like other naturally infected nonhuman primates in Africa, chimpanzee SIV infections are asymptomatic. SIV strains have been discovered in many other species of African primate, but have been omitted from Figure 7.1 for simplicity. Note also that all these retroviral strains are themselves quite variable.

Based on this tree, some researchers believe HIV is not a new human virus but instead one that only recently, as a result of changes in human behavior, became more virulent (Ewald 1994; Mindell et al. 1995). According to this view, some SIVs may have evolved from HIVs, instead of the other way around. Evidence for this perspective includes the phylogenetic tree, which appears to show SIV_{SMM} and SIV_{MAC} evolving from HIV-2, and SIV_{CPZ} evolving from HIV-1. Also, this diagram shows that if HIV-1 and HIV-2 have a common human ancestor, that virus may also be ancestral to other SIVs, depending on how the area of uncertainty in Figure 7.1 is drawn. Those who hold this view argue that it requires fewer interspecies transmissions and better explains how HIV-1 and 2 can cause nearly identical diseases. They also present evidence of correlation between increased HIV virulence and higher frequency of sexual intercourse in selected African villages. Therefore they conclude that HIV has been present, but latent, in small isolated human populations for a long time and only recently increased in virulence with increased sexual promiscuity.

This is a compelling hypothesis. However, it treats the viral phylogenetic tree with a degree of precision that is probably unwise. There are too many ambiguities concerning order of branching points and genetic distances involved (Eigen and Nieselt-Struwe 1990). No two sets of researchers agree on how to draw this tree, and because of rapid rates of change and the quasispecies nature of viral populations, the separate strains shown in most diagrams (and mostly left out of Figure 7.1) may be illusions. Also, HIV readily recombines with other HIV strains (Howell et al. 1991; Robertson et al. 1995), with retroviruses of other animals (Lusso et al. 1990), and perhaps even with host cell genes (Doolittle et al. 1989).

As is the case for other RNA viruses, rate heterogeneity complicates the interpretation of these phylogenies. Does a large sequence difference (as,

Figure 7.1
Molecular Phylogeny of Primate Retroviruses

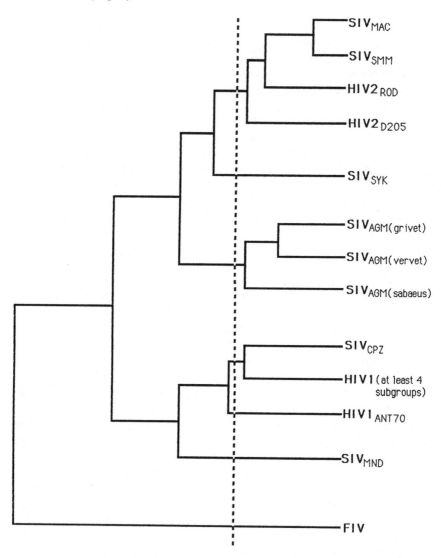

Shows approximate sequence relationships of immunodeficiency viruses of humans (HIV-1 and HIV-2, both highly variable); African green monkeys (SIV_{AGM}, with different strains in vervet, grivet, and sabaeus populations); chimpanzee (SIV_{CPZ}); macaques (SIV_{MAC}, a number of strains in different species); mandril (SIV_{MND}); sooty mangabey (SIV_{SMM}); Sykes monkey (SIV_{SYK}); and, for comparison, domestic cats (FIV). Note that all relationships shown to the left of the dotted line are uncertain. (Composite and simplification of figures in Eigen and Nieselt-Struwe 1990; Myers et al. 1992, 1993; Mindell et al. 1995).

for example, between HIV and SIV$_{AGM}$ [Fukasawa et al. 1988]) reflect millions of years of evolution as part of host genomes or rapid evolutionary rates operating over two centuries or less? Does sequence similarity (as in HIV-1 and SIV$_{CPZ}$ [Peeters et al. 1989; Huet et al. 1990]) indicate recent interspecies transmission or the close evolutionary relationship of the hosts?

Note also that phylogenies indicate sister relationships of extant viruses but cannot identify ancestors. Must the scenario with the fewest interspecies transmissions necessarily be correct? The incidence of modern zoonotic infections plus the frequency of interspecies transmission of primate retroviruses argues otherwise.

The SIV$_{AGM}$-African green monkey connection seems to be an ancient one and is the easiest to resolve. Of all monkeys caught in the wild, 30 to 50 percent are seropositive for this virus (Mulder 1988). There are three major strains of SIV$_{AGM}$ whose phylogenetic relationships reflect those of their hosts—vervet, grivet, and sabaeus monkeys (Allen et al. 1991)—and these infections are all subclinical, implying a long period of coevolution (at least 10,000 years, since the three species of monkey diverged). While infectious disease evolution does not invariably lead toward attenuation (as, for example, in the case of infections in which virulence enhances transmission [Ewald 1994]), SIV$_{AGM}$ doesn't require virulence for its transmission and survival, so here the assumption that attenuation implies a long-standing host-parasite relationship is probably a good one. Consistent with this is that SIV$_{MAC}$ (recently derived from SIV$_{SMM}$, which is asymptomatic in its natural host) induces AIDS-like disease in macaques.

So what, if anything, can one conclude about the evolution of the AIDS virus? Clearly, interspecies transmission was at some point involved. Some retroviruses have transferred between primate species (Novembre et al. 1992), and some have remained latent for long periods in the same hosts (Allen et al. 1991). Unfortunately, at the moment we can't tell whether HIV-1, HIV-2, or both are ancient human viruses or recently emerged from zoonotic origins. We can't determine ancestral viruses from relationships between modern quasispecies. And we can't treat RNA virus phylogenies like the phylogenies of their hosts for the purpose of estimating the rate of a molecular clock. Therefore we don't know when HIV evolved. All we do know is when the AIDS pandemic began. And this makes an important point—the evolution of a disease is not necessarily the same as the evolution of its infectious agent. Human behavior and culture also affect the expression and symptomology of disease, which brings us back to the opening point of this chapter: disease affects culture, and culture affects disease.

Culture affects the potential for interspecies transmission of infectious agents. If zoonotic in origin, HIV may have originated with changes in human behaviors affecting interaction with primates as, for example, in hunting, laboratories, or vaccine research. Activities that favor outbreaks of viral zoonoses include forest work (yellow fever and other arboviral infections),

clearing new agricultural areas (Eastern equine encephalitis), field work, especially during harvest season (hemorrhagic fevers, Lassa fever), crowding
animals and people together in barns and peasant huts (influenza and other
respiratory infections, cowpox), milking or drinking milk (milker's nodules,
cowpox, Central European encephalitis), storing water in uncovered vessels
(yellow and dengue fevers and other mosquito-borne arboviruses), medical
work (Ebola/Marburg infections), laboratory use of monkeys (simian B virus
infection, simian AIDS), irrigating rice paddies (Japanese encephalitis),
butchering (Newcastle disease, Rift Valley fever, Wesselsbron fever), and
eating sheep brains (scrapie). These are just some viral infections; cultural
styles promote or protect from many bacterial, rickettsial, protozoal, fungal,
and helminthic zoonoses as well.

Comparison of disease burdens and cultures of Old and New World civilizations suggests that differences in practices relating to animals contributed to the relative lack of epidemic disease in the Americas. Greater
reliance on domesticated herd animals in the Old World, and more intensive
contact with them (milking, stalling—often in the same structure as humans,
riding, harnessing to vehicles and plows, etc.), provided many opportunities
for communication of infection. Compare this with the Andean style of using
camelids, in which llamas and alpacas are herded but never fed by humans
or milked, only occasionally ridden, and eaten only after their useful lives
as pack or fleece-bearing animals are over (Gade 1969). Furthermore, the
relative lack of domesticated meat sources in the New World contributed to
overhunting in some areas, which reduced the density and diversity of fauna
near large settlements.

Cultural attitudes in Old World civilizations, such as the Hindu doctrine
of *ahimsa*, or reverence for life, and a general reluctance to eat rodents,
contributed to the buildup of commensal rats and mice, first in Asia, where
many of our epidemic diseases were born, and eventually throughout the
Old World (Zinsser 1934). Both *Rattus* and *Mus*, as well as these attitudes,
were transplanted to cities of the New World. But indigenous reactions to
rats and other rodents were to hunt, trap, and eat them, especially the large
species of South America (Gilmore 1950; Linares 1976). Garden trapping
resulted in lower commensal populations, and hunting may have contributed
to the extinction of several species (Gilmore 1950). Diminished rodent populations not only reduce the likelihood of contacting a diseased one but also
lessen the probability of rodent epidemics in the first place. It's interesting
that domesticated guinea pigs did not contribute any viruses to the human
disease pool. Being kept within Indian huts probably insulated them from
most wild rodent diseases. They have recently been implicated in zoonoses
of Old World commensal rodents, such as plague (Hubbert et al. 1975).

Ahimsa protects cattle and monkeys in India as well as rats. Cattle, like
other milked domesticates, can carry many important zoonoses. People of
India consider rhesus macaques and langurs sacred and tolerate a certain

amount of mingling in Indian urban areas. This contrasts with tropical America, where monkeys are almost completely arboreal in their habits, and so in less intimate contact with humans. This even inhibits sharing of insect vectors, which are adapted to different heights in the canopy. Native Americans also hunt monkeys, which reduces the chance of infection for the same reasons their hunting of rodents does.

So humans in the eastern hemisphere were surrounded by animals with which they interacted closely at times, because of cultural differences more than environmental ones. Large populations of humans and their commensal and domesticated species, especially in southern Asia where tropical latitudes provided high biodiversity, provided the perfect conditions for the evolution of viral epidemics. People in the New World hunted rather than domesticated most of the animals of their environments. This kept animal densities low and afforded fewer opportunities for zoonotic infection and subsequent adaptation to a human host.

CONCLUSION

For a new human viral disease to arise, there must be a suitable virus available in the environment, humans must come into contact with it in a fashion conducive to transmission, and there must be enough new susceptibles in the human population to sustain a chain of infection. The virus also must adapt to human hosts, but since most viruses evolve rapidly and because viral infections produce astronomical numbers of virus particles, this is easily accomplished.

Zoonoses are a frequent source of new human infections. Therefore anything that increases animal population size, density, disease load, or contact with humans increases the chance of human disease, as veterinarians have been pointing out for a long time (Schwabe 1984). Differences in the disease burdens of the Old and New Worlds before contact are at least partly the result of differences in coresident animal populations and in attitudes and practices concerning them.

We must be aware of the continuing evolution of new human diseases in a global environment we cannot totally control. Just as AIDS seemed to come from nowhere, with terrible loss of life in Africa and in several risk groups in the United States, other infections will surface, especially those we can least control. The use of antibiotics sets up perfect laboratory conditions for the selection of drug-resistant strains. Our ability to influence so many aspects of our environment means that future plagues will be even harder to stop, as their epidemiology will increasingly involve factors we control the least (like human sexual and addictive behavior).

We are ourselves animals, part of natural ecosystems, in spite of culture and our ability to mold our environments (our technology may be our biggest threat, for it now poisons nature and selects for those diseases we can least control). Infectious epidemics like AIDS still remind us of our species' vulnerability in evolution's cosmic game of chance.

APPENDIX: SHORT DESCRIPTIONS OF ANIMAL VIRUS FAMILIES

Viruses are classified according to morphology and serology rather than by mode of transmission, target organ, or type of disease.

Adenoviridae. Nonenveloped, icosahedral double-strand DNA viruses that replicate in cell nuclei. Associated with respiratory infections with prolonged latency in many mammals (Genus *Mastadenovirus*) and birds *(Aviadenovirus)*. Some produce tumors.

Arenaviridae. Genus *Arenavirus*: Spherical enveloped viruses with segmented single-strand RNA genomes that replicate in the cytoplasm and mature by budding from the plasma membrane. Associated with chronic inapparent infections in rodents.

Bunyaviridae. Over 200 roughly spherical, enveloped arboviruses, with tubular nucleocapsids, single-strand RNA in three circular segments that replicate in the cytoplasm and mature by budding from intracytoplasmic membranes. Consists of the genus *Bunyavirus* and others as yet unclassified. All multiply in and are transmitted by arthropods.

Coronaviridae. Genus *Coronavirus*: Spherical enveloped single-strand RNA viruses with tubular nucleocapsids that replicate in the cytoplasm, bud from intracytoplasmic membranes, and cause respiratory disease in a variety of animals.

Herpesviridae. Enveloped, icosahedral, double-strand DNA viruses that replicate in the nucleus and bud from the nuclear membrane. Associated with latent or persistent infections in many animals and often cause a vesicular rash; some are oncogenic.

Iridoviridae. Genus *Iridovirus*: Large, nonenveloped, icosahedral, double-strand DNA viruses that replicate in the cytoplasm. Include insect iridescent viruses and viruses of fish, amphibians, and African swine fever. Vertebrate iridoviruses are enveloped.

Orthomyxoviridae. Genus *Influenzavirus*: Spherical enveloped viruses with segmented single-strand RNA and tubular capsids that multiply in the cytoplasm and mature by budding from the plasma membrane. Important cause of respiratory disease in animals and human beings.

Papovaviridae. Nonenveloped, icosahedral viruses with circular, double-strand DNA that multiply relatively slowly in the nucleus. Cause latent and chronic infections and tumors, mostly benign, in a variety of animals if the viral genome becomes integrated into host cell DNA. Genera *Papillomavirus* (causative agents of warts) and *Polyomavirus* (oncogenic viruses of primates, mice, rabbits).

Paramyxoviridae. Genera *Paramyxovirus*, *Pneumovirus*, and *Morbillivirus*: Viruses similar to the Orthomyxoviridae, except the RNA genome is in one piece and does not recombine. Associated with respiratory disease and skin rashes.

Parvoviridae. Small, icosahedral, single-strand DNA viruses that multiply in the nucleus. Genera *Parvovirus* (many rodent and other viruses), *Densovirus* (in insects), and the adeno-associated virus group that replicates only in the presence of an adeno-virus.

Picornaviridae. A large group of small, single-strand RNA viruses with no envelopes and icosohedral nucleocapsids that replicate in the cytoplasm and generally cause inapparent infection. Genera include *Enterovirus*, in the intestines of many animals; *Rhinovirus*, causing mild respiratory infections; *Calicivirus*, in swine, sea lions, and cats; *Cardiovirus*, mostly in rodents; and *Aphthovirus*, foot-and-mouth and equine rhi-noviruses.

Poxviridae. Largest animal viruses. Brick-shaped, double-strand DNA viruses with a DNA-containing core surrounded by several envelopes of viral origin. They replicate in the cytoplasm and mature within cytoplasmic foci. Recombination can occur within genera. Involved in many diseases of mammals, birds, and humans, often with ves-iculo-pustular rash. Subfamilies Chordopoxviridae, in vertebrates, and Entomopox-viridae, in insects.

Reoviridae. Nonenveloped viruses with segmented double-strand RNA and icosa-hedral double capsids that replicate in the cytoplasm. Genera *Reovirus* and *Rotavirus*, found in human and animal enteric tracts, and *Orbivirus*, a group of arboviruses.

Retroviridae. Spherical, enveloped viruses with icosahedral inner shells, tubular nu-cleocapsids, and single-strand RNA that is transcribed by viral reverse transcriptase into DNA proviruses capable of integration into the cellular genome. Subfamilies Lentiviridae, slow viruses of sheep plus human AIDS and related viruses (all with long incubation periods before the onset of clinical symptoms); Oncoviridae, onco-genic and leukemia viruses of many species, including integrated genomes occurring naturally in normal cells; and Spumaviridae, or "foamy agents" causing inapparent infections in cats, monkeys, and cattle.

Rhabdoviridae. Enveloped single-strand RNA viruses with double-helical nucleocap-sid inside a bullet-shaped shell. Replicates in the cytoplasm and buds from the plasma membrane. Genera *Lyssavirus*, rabies and related viruses with wide distri-bution in nature, including insects and plants; *Vesiculovirus*, vesicular stomatitis, re-lated arboviruses, and some viruses of fish; and *Sigmavirus*, found in *Drosophila*.

Togaviridae. Spherical, enveloped, single-strand RNA viruses with icosahedral nu-cleocapsids that replicate in the cytoplasm. *Alphavirus* (Group A arboviruses, all mos-quito-borne) and *Rubivirus* (rubella) mature by budding from the plasma membrane, while *Pestivirus* (found in cattle, pigs, horses) and *Flavivirus* (Group B arboviruses, mosquito- and tick-borne) bud from intracytoplasmic membranes. Purified RNA of this family is infectious.

REFERENCES

Allan, Jonathan S., Mary Short, Maria E. Taylor, Shiawhwa Su, Vanessa M. Hirsch, Philip R. Johnson, George M. Shaw, and Beatrice H. Hahn. 1991. "Species-Specific Diversity among Simian Immunodeficiency Viruses from African Green Monkeys." *Journal of Virology* 65:2816–28.

Armelagos, George J., and John R. Dewey. 1978. "Evolutionary Response to Human Infectious Diseases." In *Health and the Human Condition: Perspectives on Medical*

Anthropology. Michael H. Logan and Edward E. Hunt, Jr. eds. Belmont, Calif.: Wadsworth, 101–7.

Armelagos, George J., and Alan McArdle. 1975. "Population, Disease, and Evolution." In *Population Studies in Archaeology and Biological Anthropology: A Symposium.* Alan C. Swedlund, ed. Memoirs of the Society for American Archaeology, No. 30 (American Antiquity 40, No. 2 Part 2):1–10.

Ashburn, P. M. 1947. *The Ranks of Death: A Medical History of the Conquest of America.* Frank D. Ashburn, ed. New York: Coward-McCann.

Benenson, Abram S., ed. 1990. *Control of Communicable Diseases in Man.* 15th ed. Washington, D.C.: American Public Health Association.

Beran, George W. 1981. *Viral Zoonoses.* Vols. 1 and 2. In *Handbook Series in Zoonoses.* James H. Steele, editor-in-chief. Boca Raton, Fla.: Chemical Rubber Company Press.

Bisseru, B. 1967. *Diseases of Man Acquired from His Pets.* Philadelphia: J. B. Lippincott.

Black, Francis L. 1966. "Measle Endemicity in Insular Populations." *Journal of Theoretical Biology* 11:207–11.

Chakrabarti, L., M. Guyader, M. Alizon, M. D. Daniel, R. C. Desrosiers, P. Tiollais, and P. Sonigo. 1987. "Sequence of Simian Immunodeficiency Virus from Macaque and its Relationship to other Human and Simian Retroviruses." *Nature* 328:543–47.

Chao, Lin. 1994. "Evolution of Genetic Exchange in RNA Viruses." In *The Evolutionary Biology of Viruses.* Stephen S. Morse, ed. New York: Raven Press, 233–50.

Clavel, François, Kamal Mansinho, Sophie Chamaret, Denise Guetard, Veronique Favier, Jaime Nina, Marie-Odette Santos-Ferreira, Jose-Luis Champalimaud, and Luc Montagnier. 1987. "Human Immunodeficiency Virus Type 2 Infection Associated with AIDS in West Africa." *New England Journal of Medicine* 316:1180–85.

Cohen, Jon. 1994. "The Duesberg Phenomenon." *Science* 266:1642–49.

Dobyns, Henry F. 1966. "Estimating Aboriginal American Population, I: An Appraisal of Techniques with a New Hemispheric Estimate." *Current Anthropology* 7:395–416.

Domingo, Esteban, and John J. Holland. 1994. "Mutation Rates and Rapid Evolution of RNA Viruses." In *The Evolutionary Biology of Viruses.* Stephen S. Morse, ed. New York: Raven Press, 161–84.

Domingo, Esteban, E. Martinez-Salas, F. Sobrino, J. C. de la Torre, A. Portela, J. Ortin, C. López-Galindez, P. Pérez-Breña, N. Villanueva, R. Nájera, S. VandePol, D. Steinhauer, N. DePolo, and J. Holland. 1985. "The Quasispecies (Extremely Heterogeneous) Nature of Viral RNA Genome Populations: Biological Relevance—A Review." *Gene* 40:1–8.

Doolittle, Russell F. 1989. "The Simian-Human Connection." *Nature* 339:338–39.

Doolittle, Russell F., D. -F. Feng, M. S. Johnson, and M. A. McClure. 1989. "Origins and Evolutionary Relationships of Retroviruses." *Quarterly Review of Biology* 64:1–30.

Duesberg, Peter H. 1994. Letter to the Editor. *Science* 267:313–14.

Eigen, Manfred. 1993. "Viral Quasispecies." *Scientific American* 269(1):42–49.

Eigen, Manfred, and Katja Nieselt-Struwe. 1990. "How Old is the Immunodeficiency Virus?" *AIDS* 4 (suppl 1):S85–S93.

Ewald, Paul W. 1994. *Evolution of Infectious Disease*. New York: Oxford University Press.

Feldman, Douglas A. 1990. *Culture and AIDS*. New York: Praeger.

Fiennes, Richard. 1964. *Man, Nature, and Disease*. London: Weidenfeld and Nicolson.

———1967. *Zoonoses of Primates: The Epidemiology and Ecology of Simian Diseases in Relation to Man*. Ithaca, N.Y.: Cornell University Press.

Fukasawa, Masashi, Tomiyuki Miura, Akira Hasegawa, Shigeru Morikawa, Hajime Tsujimoto, Keizaburo Miki, Takashi Kitamura, and Masanori Hayami. 1988. "Sequence of Simian Immunodeficiency Virus from African Green Monkey: A New Member of the HIV/SIV Group." *Nature* 333:457–61.

Gade, Daniel W. 1969. "The Llama, Alpaca, and Vicuña: Fact vs. Fiction." *Journal of Geography* 68:339–43.

Gao, F., L. Yue, A. T. White, P. G. Pappas, J. Barchue, A. P. Hanson, B. M. Greene, P. M. Sharp, G. M. Shaw, and B. H. Hahn. 1992. "Human Infection by Genetically Diverse SIV_{SM}-related HIV-2 in West Africa." *Nature* 358:495–99.

Gilmore, Raymond M. 1950. "Fauna and Ethnozoology of South America." *Handbook of South American Indians*, 6:345–464. Bureau of American Ethnology Bulletin 143. Washington, D.C.: American Ethnology Society.

Holland, John, Katherine Spindler, Frank Horodyski, Elizabeth Grabau, Stuart Nichol, and Scott VandePol. 1982. "Rapid Evolution of RNA Genomes." *Science* 215:1577–85.

Howell, R. M., J. E. Fitzgibbon, M. Noe, Z. Ren, D. J. Gocke, T. A. Schwartzer, and D. T. Dubin. 1991. "In Vivo Sequence Variation of the Human Immunodeficiency Virus Type 1 *env* Gene: Evidence for Recombination Among Variants Found in a Single Individual." *AIDS Research and Human Retroviruses* 7: 869–76.

Hubbert, William T., William F. McCulloch, and Paul R. Schnurrenberger, eds. 1975. *Diseases Transmitted from Animals to Man*. 6th ed. Springfield, Ill.: Charles C. Thomas.

Huet, Thierry, Rémi Cheynier, Andreas Meyerhans, George Roelants, and Simon Wain-Hobson. 1990. "Genetic Organization of a Chimpanzee Lentivirus Related to HIV-1." *Nature* 345:356–59.

Li, Wen-Hsiung, Masako Tanimura, and Paul M. Sharp. 1988. "Rates and Dates of Divergence between AIDS Virus Nucleotide Sequences." *Molecular Biology of Evolution* 5:313–30.

Linares, Olga F. 1976. "Garden Hunting in the American Tropics." *Human Ecology* 4:331–49.

Lusso, P., F. di Marzo Veronese, B. Ensoli, G. Franchini, C. Jemma, S. E. DeRocco, V. S. Kalyanaraman, and R. C. Gallo. 1990. "Expanded HIV-1 Cellular Tropism by Phenotypic Mixing with Murine Endogenous Retroviruses." *Science* 247:848–52.

NcNeill, William H. 1976. *Plagues and Peoples*. Garden City, N.Y.: Anchor Books.

Mindell, David P., Jeffrey W. Shultz, and Paul W. Ewald. 1995. "The AIDS Pandemic Is New, but Is HIV New?" *Systematic Biology* 44:77–92.

Morse, Stephen S. 1993. *Emerging Viruses*. New York: Oxford University Press.

———1994. *The Evolutionary Biology of Viruses*. New York: Raven Press.

Mulder, Carel. 1988. "Human AIDS Virus Not from Monkeys." *Nature* 333:396.

Myers, Gerald, Kersti MacInnes, and Bette Korber. 1992. "The Emergence of Simian/Human Immunodeficiency Viruses." *AIDS Research and Human Retroviruses* 8:373–86.

Myers, Gerald, Kersti MacInnes, and Lynda Myers. 1993. "Phylogenetic Moments in the AIDS Epidemic." In *Emerging Viruses*. Stephen S. Morse, ed. New York: Oxford University Press, 120–37.

Novembre, Francis J., Vanessa M. Hirsch, Harold M. McClure, Patricia N. Fultz, and Philip R. Johnson. 1992. "SIV from Stump-Tailed Macaques: Molecular Characterization of a Highly Transmissible Primate Lentivirus." *Virology* 186: 783–87.

Nowak, Rachel. 1995. "Cause of Fatal Outbreak in Horses and Humans Traced." *Science* 268:32.

Pavlovsky, Eugeny N. 1966. *Natural Nidality of Transmissible Diseases*. Trans. Frederick K. Plous, Jr. N. D. Levine, ed. Urbana: University of Illinois Press.

Peeters, M., C. Honoré, T. Huet, L. Bedjabaga, S. Ossari, P. Bussi, R. W. Cooper, and E. Delaporte. 1989. "Isolation and Partial Characterization of an HIV-Related Virus Occurring Naturally in Chimpanzees in Gabon." *AIDS* 3:625–30.

Robertson, David L., Paul M. Sharp, Francine E. McCutchan, and Beatrice H. Hahn. 1995. "Recombination in HIV-1." *Nature* 374:124–26.

Schwabe, Calvin W. 1984. *Veterinary Medicine and Human Health*. 3rd ed. Baltimore, Md.: Williams and Wilkins.

Sternberg, Steve. 1992. "HIV Comes in Five Family Groups." *Science* 256:966.

Van Blerkom, Linda M. 1985. "The Evolution of Human Infectious Disease in the Eastern and Western Hemispheres." Ph.D. dissertation, University of Colorado, Boulder.

———. 1991. "Zoonoses and the Origins of Old and New World Viral Diseases." In *The Anthropology of Medicine: From Culture to Method*. 2nd ed. Lola Romanucci-Ross, Daniel E. Moerman, and Laurence R. Tancredi, eds. New York: Bergin & Garvey.

Webster, Robert G. 1993. Influenza. In *Emerging Viruses*. Stephen S. Morse, ed. New York: Oxford University Press, 37–45.

Yokoyama, Shozo, and Takashi Gojobori. 1987. "Molecular Evolution and Phylogeny of the Human AIDS Viruses LAV, HTLV-III, and ARV." *Journal of Molecular Evolution* 24:330–36.

Zinsser, Hans. 1934. *Rats, Lice and History*. Boston: Little, Brown.

8

MALARIA, MEDICINE, AND MEALS: A BIOBEHAVIORAL PERSPECTIVE

NINA L. ETKIN AND PAUL J. ROSS

The study of indigenous medicines commands a prominent position in medical anthropological study that seeks to comprehend, from multicultural and crosscultural perspectives, how people manage health and illness. Intellectually, such inquiry is most meaningfully cast in the theoretical idioms of a human ecology that explores not only the cultural and social construction of therapeutics but also the physiologic outcomes of health-seeking behaviors. Since the publication of pioneering research that revealed the extent to which the category "medicine" overlaps that of "food" (Etkin 1986b; Etkin and Ross 1982, 1991; Johns 1990), studies of indigenous medicine increasingly include dietary and other contexts of plant use in order to assess the extent to which people are exposed to pharmacologically active plant constituents. Such investigations embody the biobehavioral perspective of medical anthropological inquiry (Etkin 1986a, 1988, 1990, 1994a; Browner et al. 1988; Armelagos et al. 1992; Franquemont et al. 1990).

Working in more narrow intellectual frameworks, phytochemists and pharmacologists are optimistic that the study of indigenous medicines will expand the biomedical pharmacopoeia, at the same time—ironically—that biological and cultural diversity are conserved (Abbink 1995; Anyinam 1995; Chadwick and Marsh 1994; Kinghorn and Balandrin 1993; see also the *Journal of Ethnopharmacology*, *Planta Medica*, *Economic Botany*). For their part, ministries of health in developing nations have formalized policies that champion indigenous medicine, both to accommodate the limited availability of biomedical resources and to serve political ends through the reaffirmation of traditional institutions. Compelled by a more applied agenda, international agencies such as the World Health Organization (WHO) have made explicit recommendations to study indigenous medicines (Akerele

1987; Chunhuei 1994; Last 1990). At present, more than 20 centers around the globe collaborate in the WHO Traditional Medicine Program, the primary objective of which is to conduct systematic investigations of efficacy and risk and to integrate local medicine into the provision of state health care.

All of those concerns are resonated in this chapter through a revised version of our contributions to earlier editions of this volume. We present data on Hausa medicine and diet, which are then interpreted through a unique model of disease adaptation. For the present version, we review findings from our research on plants used in both diet and medicine: the findings of two principal field sessions, 1975–1976 and 1987–1988, are compared and amplified by the results of continuing data analysis, including the laboratory investigation of plants used in the prevention and treatment of malaria.[1] Additional observations/data that inform these analyses are regularly conveyed to us by the Nigerian member of our research team, Ibrahim Muazzamu of the Department of Medicinal Plants, National Institute for Pharmaceutical Research and Development, Abuja, Nigeria.

Comparing results of the two field studies suggests the temporal applicability of our model of disease adaptation: the seasonal fluctuation in consumption of certain plant foods/medicines that we invoked to explain low rates of malaria infection during the 1975–1976 period was no longer apparent during 1987–1988. This shifting perspective underscores the dynamic nature of the interrelationships among medicines, foods, and illness, emphasizing that knowledge and understanding are emergent, that in science the "facts" and their configurations constantly undergo change. Longitudinal research such as described here offers the opportunity to retest and refine explanatory models to accommodate changing conditions as the physical and cultural landscapes are transformed over time.

STUDY SITE AND DATA COLLECTION

Our research was conducted among an agricultural Hausa-Fulani community located 50 kilometers southeast of the urban center Kano, in northern Nigeria. The village core of Hurumi (a pseudonym) is a nucleated settlement of 400 residents, with dispersed compounds in the outlying hamlets raising the population total to approximately 4,000. The size of compounds in this rural settlement ranges from 2 to close to 40 occupants. These living units customarily include a compound head, his wife (or wives), his sons and their wives, and children. Not atypically, compounds are constituted by more than one "household"—people who "eat from the same pot." This creates the potential for intracompound variability in access to resources, including, in the present context, knowledge of plants and composition of diet.

Hurumi's economy centers on intensive agriculture supplemented by the raising of livestock (primarily sheep, goat, and fowl, with some cattle) and trade in locally produced and imported commodities. Although clearly less remote today than during our initial investigation, the village still is not served by paved roads and has neither electricity nor piped water. The greater part of subsistence labor—from planting through harvest, supplemented by gathering in the "wild"—is neither mechanized nor assisted by draft animals.[2]

Hausa Medicine

Data on Hausa medicine, diet, and health were first collected in the course of a 22-month investigation during 1975 and 1976, a time when Hurumi residents relied almost exclusively on an extensive botanical pharmacopoeia for all therapeutic and preventive measures. Information was collected regarding Hausa understandings of disease etiology and nosology in order to describe the most commonly perceived symptoms and their appropriate treatments. Extensive interviews were conducted with individuals who were identified by others, and who perceived themselves, as most conversant in matters related to health. Five women and nine men constituted a core of principal respondents and included among them a woman whose knowledge of plant medicines, especially for spirit-caused illness, earned her district-wide recognition and clientele. Other respondents represented more narrow foci of medically related knowledge: a barber-surgeon, three midwives, and authorities in such specific areas as venereal diseases, jaundice, weaning medicines, witchcraft, and sorcery (predominantly ascribed to malfeasance among co-wives, and jealousy). Other interviews and observations throughout the village revealed that most adults are familiar with at least several medicines for a variety of common disorders, including gastrointestinal complaints, fevers, children's illnesses, and skin conditions.

Open-ended interviews were organized around the following: a catalogue of 637 plants, for which individuals described the physical attributes, availability, and medicinal and other uses of each; and an inventory of 808 diseases, symptoms, and related terms for which respondents described commonly used medicines, including source, preparation, additional constituents, approximate dose and schedule of administration, therapeutic objectives, and alternatives for circumstances in which that medicine is not available or does not produce the expected results. Our data are more or less consonant with observations in other parts of Hausaland; differences are of a magnitude one would expect given temporal and ecologic variability and compounded by the varying methodologies (especially ethnographic depth) of other reporters—for example, Adam et al. (1972), Busson et al. (1965), Dalziel (1937), Darrah (1980), Oliver (1986), Prietze (1913–1914), Stock (1980), and Wall (1988).

For the year-long follow-up study (1987–1988), we employed a more rigorous methodology in order to extend the depth of our inquiry, to understand better the antecedents and sequelae of plant use by Hausa, and to collect additional antimalarial plants for further laboratory investigation. Plants still were the predominant medicines for prevention and therapy— this despite the dramatic incursion of biomedicine over the last decade and the marked increase in availability and widespread use of pharmaceuticals (Etkin et al. 1990). Using the same plant and disease/symptom inventories, extensive interviews combined with observations of therapeutic and preventive events elicited the details of plant selection, preparation, application, and desired outcome. Two nonspecialists—a man and a woman—participated in the study as principal respondents; villagewide consensus identified them as most generally conversant regarding therapeutic and preventive objectives and plant identification. A representative, villagewide interview schedule (including 50 respondents) supplemented practitioner- and specialist-focused studies to provide a broader (exoteric rather than esoteric) base for compiling the knowledge that more accurately represents preventive and therapeutic modalities that affect the majority of villagers on a day-to-day basis. These data were supplemented by field and market surveys to assess plant availability, cost, and so forth. The medical investigation was amplified by a monthly village health survey that recorded all disease episodes for all households. In addition, we conducted a two-month investigation at the recently opened biomedical facility located eight kilometers from Hurumi. Patients and staff participated in entry and exit interviews that explored, among other factors, reasons for clinic attendance and prior treatments, patient-physician encounters, and "compliance" with prescriptive and other instruction—topics that have potential influence on the continued viability and form of "local medicines."

During 1987 and 1988, villagewide interviews yielded nearly 5,000 medicinal preparations. Excluding replications, the number of remedies is 3,165. (A distinct remedy is defined by a unique combination of constituents, or each time that combination is used for another illness category.) Table 8.1 lists the more common of the 211 categories for which these preparations are administered. Of those medicines, 89 percent (2,801) include a total of 374 plants. Three hundred forty-five of all plants are used for diseases that we have termed "overtly physiologic" (in application and in therapeutic objectives) (Table 8.2). These are illnesses whose etiology Hausa attribute to naturalistic phenomena such as dirt or disharmony along such axes as dry-wet, cold-hot, sweet-salty, bitter-sweet, and permutations thereof, and whose prevention and treatment include dislodgement or externalization of disease substance, palliation of pain or discomfort, and, finally, symptom resolution.

Heeding the very inclusive Hausa definition of medicine—*magani*, literally, anything that improves or repairs something—necessitates attention also to plants used in the management of disorders attributed to human malfeasance or the intervention of extrahuman agency. Two hundred sixty-

Table 8.1
Most Common Categories for Hausa Medicinal Preparations

Hausa Nosology	General Analogue	n medicinal preparations
ISKA	Spirit caused illness	104
SAMMU	Sorcery	103
CIWON CIKI	General GI disorders	94
CIWON CIKIN KABA	Acute GI disorders	90
SHAWARA	Hepatitis, malaria	72
KYANDA	Measles	70
MAYE	Witch caused illness	66
ZAZZABI	Febrile disorders	64
DANSHI	Pediatric malaria	59
MAYANKWANIYA	"Wasting," anemias	59

Source: Adapted from Etkin and Ross 1994.

six of all plants are used for the mediation of sorcery, spirits, and witches; this is accomplished largely through preventive measures but can be treated after the fact as well. To the extent that these intercessions include ingestion, topical application, fumigation, inhalation, and other close contact with plant constituents, these contexts of use also have physiologic implications. We do not propose that the management of spirits, witches, and sorcery entails a unique constellation of plants, for it does not. We draw attention to the issue here precisely because most researchers have not concerned themselves with plant applications whose rationale and objectives fall outside the context of disorders of naturalistic origin. Further, Hausa exposure to constituents of these plants increases dramatically because they actively engage these imperceptible threats to well-being on at least a daily basis and not just when the fact of illness is established.[3,4]

Hausa Diet

For the 1975–1976 study, a dietary survey of eight households was conducted to understand the sources, distribution, and preparation of foods and to document consumption. This was implemented for 24-hour periods, randomly selected twice per week per household, for 48 consecutive weeks to coincide with the end of one harvest and the beginning of the next, these being the most meaningful delineators of the annual agricultural cycle. Pre-

Table 8.2
Plant Medicines

Intended Use:	"Semi-Wild" Plants		All Plants	
	n plants	n remedies	n plants	n remedies
Physiologic	254	1854	345	2275
Other	215	452	266	526
TOTALS	272[a]	2306	374[a]	2801[b]

[a]Totals are less than the sums due to multiple plant uses.
[b]Excluded are five remedies that specify plant location or situation rather than a particular
    genus or species.
Source: Adapted from Etkin and Ross 1994.

cise weight measures of unprocessed foods were augmented with extensive interviews and observations. The participating households contained a mean of 46 residents and were selected as a reasonable cross section of the larger hamlet, representing the relatively narrow range of economic, social, and demographic variability in Hurumi.

For each of the three daily meals, all foods were weighed prior to cooking and other preparation. For all food preparers in the study, independent and repeated assessments of all food types and preparations included weight and volume measures for all ingredients, tabulated sequentially through all stages of preparation to final cooked (or otherwise modified) consumable form. This permitted extrapolation from the unprocessed weight measures for each household to quantified approximations of nutrient values (for calories, protein, etc.) based on published food composition values (e.g., Duke and Atchley 1986; Longhurst 1984; Simmons 1976; Wu Leung 1968). All foods, including snacks, consumed by adults and obtained from extrahousehold sources—such as vendor, market, or gift—were recorded in the same way, assessing step-by-step preparation and using collateral data such as cost per unit of prepared food, fluctuating market prices, and so on.[5] Thus, the full food consumption cycle is accounted for, including seasonal variation, deviations related to illness or idiosyncratic disposition, celebratory meals ("feasting"), and fasting (during Ramadan).

The dietary survey conducted during our follow-up study helped us to further understand the multicontextual use of plants. Building on the earlier investigation, the more recent survey replicated the methodology outlined above: the same eight households (54 residents) were monitored for a full 48-week harvest-to-harvest cycle. The range of items contributing to diet had expanded over the 12-year period as a result of increased interregional and international communication and trade. In both medicine and diet, more subtle changes were suggested by shifting environmental circumstances that affected the availability of medicinal and food plants. The changes in Hausa diet are discussed in greater detail elsewhere (Ross et al. 1996). For this chapter, we review only the yearly fluctuations in relative quantities of different food types, particularly with reference to grain-based foods (porridges and gruels, the mainstay of morning and evening meals) and foods that include "vegetables" (leafy and other herbaceous plants).

HOW DOES ONE SELECT PLANTS FOR STUDY?

Conventionally, investigations of indigenous medicines evaluate therapeutic efficacy on the basis of treatment for simple, discrete symptoms. Antimicrobial activity has been tested in plants used in the treatment of wounds (Macfoy and Cline 1990), tooth and gum disease (Elvin-Lewis 1986; Etkin 1981; Kaufmann and Elvin-Lewis 1995), dermatoses (Apisariyakul et al. 1995; Palanichamy and Nagarajan 1990; Paranjpe and Kulkarni 1995), and gastrointestinal disorders (Caceres et al. 1990; Etkin and Ross 1982). Antipyresis and analgesia are targets for medicines used in the treatment of fevers (Agwu and Akah 1990; Iauk et al. 1993; Lanhers et al. 1991). Effects on platelet and phagocyte function (Hammerschmidt 1986; Teng et al. 1994; Kagawa et al. 1993) and systemic arterial pressure (Fitzpatrick et al. 1995; Mao et al. 1995; Stevenson 1986) generate most interest for plants used in the treatment of cardiovascular disorders. Studies of fertility-regulating plants deal principally with estrogen-modulating actions (Benie et al. 1990; Desta 1994) but also with effects on male fertility (Zhang et al. 1995) and abortifacient actions (Goonasekera et al. 1995).

By contrast, our model for the empirical evaluation of plant medicines directs attention to the potential efficacy of therapies used in the treatment of disorders characterized by interrelated and superficially indiscernible symptom complexes. As we have discussed elsewhere (Etkin 1979, 1981), investigation of indigenous treatments of symptom-complex disorders such as malaria is particularly important in view of the associated high morbidity and mortality, and because it is in the prevention and treatment of those complex diseases that one confronts the most tension between biomedical and indigenous explanatory models (Bastien 1995; Counts and Counts 1989; Etkin 1992, 1994b; Etkin et al. 1990; Green 1988).

Pharmacologic investigations of indigenous antimalarials tend to consider only those plants described specifically for the treatment of the malaria symptom complex in its entirety, a biomedical construct that not all medical paradigms recognize. Studies of antimalarials of which we are aware do not acknowledge the potential lack of concordance between biomedical and other nosologies and, so, do not include plants used only for one or some of the symptoms or for emically nonmedical purposes such as food, hygiene, and cosmetics. (We do not count here wholesale screening of plants and compounds for antimalarial activity, since those studies tend to be informed by the paradigms of botany and phytochemistry and have virtually no bearing on *ethno*medicine.)

The plants that we selected for laboratory investigation following the 1975–1976 research are among the more common Hausa medicines used in the treatment of one or more components of what biomedicine understands to be the malaria symptom complex. These include the intermittent fevers that are the signature of malaria infection as well as more equivocal markers such as anemia, hemoglobinuria, spleno/hepatomegaly, and jaundice. In this way, our analysis incorporates medicines used to treat the full range of symptoms, singly or in some combination.

LABORATORY AND PHARMACOLOGIC STUDIES OF HAUSA PLANTS

Investigations of Antimalarial Activity: Series 1

Rationale: Our first laboratory investigations drew conceptually on indirect measures of efficacy in malaria therapy, specifically perturbations of red blood cell oxidation-reduction (redox) equilibrium. That approach was an important departure from conventional pharmacologic studies of antimalarial activity, which until that time had been primarily constituent analyses probing for quininelike alkaloids or for compounds that approximate the structure, and presumably the activity, of known synthetic antimalarials (Gilles and Warrell 1993; Peters and Richards 1984).

The significance of redox fluctuations in the course of malaria infection has been amply demonstrated over the last two decades (e.g., Clark et al. 1989; Eaton et al. 1976; Etkin 1995a, 1995b; Etkin and Eaton 1975; Golenser et al. 1991; Vennerstrom and Eaton 1988). Recently other researchers also include redox phenomena in their investigations of antimalarial plants (e.g., Borris and Schaeffer 1992; Chawla and Kumar 1991; Pollack et al. 1990).[6] The most salient point for the present discussion is that increased oxidation compromises host red cell integrity and interferes with *Plasmodium* metabolism to the extent that parasite maturation is impaired, resulting in the interruption of what would ordinarily be the regular, serial infection of new blood cells.

Red blood cell integrity is dependent upon suppression of chemical equilibrium with molecular oxygen. That equilibrium is offset in normal cells by redox reactions that are part of or integrally linked to the pentose phosphate shunt (PPS). This secondary pathway for glucose catabolism uses glucose to produce carbon dioxide (CO_2) and NADPH, a source of reducing (antioxidant) capacity and potential energy. This can link at three points with the primary, Embden-Meyerhof pathway, which metabolizes glucose to lactate and produces potential energy (ATP) (Figure 8.1). Whereas ordinarily about 11 percent of red cell glucose passes through the PPS, that amount increases

Figure 8.1
Glucose Catabolism through the Pentose Phosphate Shunt

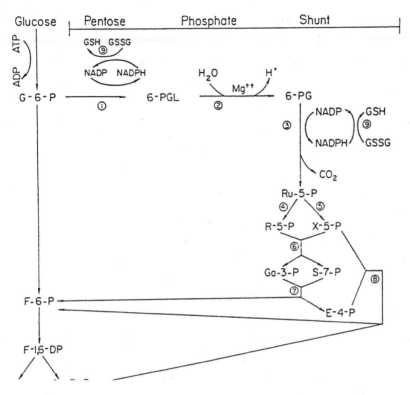

Abbreviations relevant to the text discussion: NADP/NADPH and NAD/NADH = oxidized/
reduced forms of the enzyme cofactors nicotinamide adenine dinucleotide phosphate and
nicotinamide adenine dinucleotide. GSSG/GSH = oxidized/reduced forms of glutathione.
Circled numbers correspond to enzymes. For the present discussion, note that 1 = glucose-
6-phosphate dehydrogenase. Adapted from Eaton and Brewer 1974. Reprinted with permission from J.W. Eaton and G.W. Brewer, "Pentose Phosphate Metabolism," in *The Red
Blood Cell*, Vol. I, D.M. Surgenor, ed., pp. 435–471. New York: Academic Press, 1974.

when levels of intracellular oxidation are elevated. Such elevations occur in
the course of normal metabolic fluctuations, in certain genetic anomalies, in
the presence of infectious and other pathologies, and as a reaction to some
foods, drugs, and other xenobiotics. The most salient point for the present
discussion is that increased oxidation compromises the integrity of host red
cells. This interrupts plasmodial development and leaves immature parasite
forms that cannot transfer the infection to new red cells.

Evidence of oxidation during plasmodial infection includes elevated methemoglobin (metHb), coenzymes NAD and NADP, and glutathione (GSSG)
relative to their reduced counterparts (hemoglobin, NADH and NADPH,

GSH); inhibition of catalase by aminotriazole (which requires the presence of the oxidant hydrogen peroxide, H_2O_2); lipid peroxidation; spontaneous generation of radical oxygen species; and parasite incorporation of host superoxide dismutase. These observations are understood to reflect both intraerythrocytic oxidation (of plasmodial origin and red cell response) and activation of leukocyte defense, including the release of reactive oxygen species among the immunomodulators (reviewed by Etkin 1995a, 1995b).

The summary point is that *elevated intracellular oxidation, some of plasmodial origin, selectively renders infected cells more susceptible to hemolysis* through peroxidation of membrane lipids and decomposition of sulfhydryl-containing enzymes, hemoglobin, and other key cellular constituents. Red cell destruction interrupts maturation of the plasmodium, which cannot survive extracellularly as an immature blood form. A range of circumstances that protect humans against fulminant malaria infection are thus explained: oxidant sensitivity in G6PD deficiencies (including "favism," a severe hemolytic reaction to the ingestion of the fava bean), some hemoglobinopathies (α- and-ß-thalassemias, hemoglobins S and E), vitamin E deficiency, free-radical intermediates in the metabolism of certain pharmaceuticals, and naturally occurring endoperoxides (Docampo and Moreno 1984; Eaton et al. 1976; Etkin and Eaton 1975; Friedman 1981; Hebbel et al. 1982; Kitayaporn et al. 1992; Meshnick et al. 1989; Vennerstrom and Eaton 1988).

In view of that evidence, we investigated the oxidizing potential of Hausa plant medicines used to treat one or more symptoms of malaria. We hypothesized that the combined effects of plant- and parasite-generated intraerythrocytic oxidation would overwhelm host cell oxidant defenses, resulting in lysis of infected red cells and release of immature parasites.

Conversion of Hemoglobin to Methemoglobin: Methemoglobin generation is a sensitive indicator of erythrocyte oxidant damage and is determined through standardized assays (see Etkin and Eaton 1975 for details). Extracts were prepared from macerated plant materials in solutions of isotonic saline and neutralized to physiologic pH. Normal red call hemolysates in dilute hemoglobin suspensions were incubated at 37°C in equivolume ratios with plant extracts, and metHb levels were determined after two hours' incubation. Control samples were identically prepared, sans plant extract. Data are summarized in Table 8.3, with two-hour metHb concentrations expressed as percentages of original Hb that was converted to the oxidized metHb. In this study, *Guiera senegalensis* leaves appear to be the most potent oxidant generators, with 100 percent conversion of Hb $\rightarrow$ metHb.

Glutathione Oxidation: Our second measure of oxidizing potential evaluated plant extracts for the ability to convert reduced glutathione (GSH) to its oxidized counterpart (GSSG). Extracts, hemolysates, and controls were prepared as for the metHb studies, with starting GSH concentrations at 2.0 millimoles (mM). Samples were incubated for two hours at 37°C and residual GSH measured at 30-minute intervals (methods as reported in Etkin and

Table 8.3
Methemoglobin Generation by Plant Extracts

Genus and Species	Hausa Name	Plant Part	% Hb ---> MetHb
Acacia nilotica Del. Fabaceae	Gabaruwa	Root	56%
Azadirachta indica A. Juss. Meliaceae	Darbejiya	Leaf	42%
		Bark	9%
		Root	7%
Cassia occidentalis L. Fabaceae	Majamfari	Root	78%
		Leaf	68%
Cassia tora L. Fabaceae	Tafasa	Leaf	35%
		Root	29%
Cochlospermum tinctorium Rich., Cochlospermaceae	Rawaya	Root	51%
Guiera senegalensis JF Gmel.,Combretaceae	Sabara	Root	47%
		Leaf	100%
Securidaca longipedunculata Fres., Polygalaceae	Sanya	Root	29%
Controls			0.5%

Eaton 1975). Results are summarized in Table 8.4, in which both relative rates of GSH depletion and glutathione residua for all samples are displayed. Highest oxidant activity is indicated for leaf extracts of *Guiera senegalensis*, *Azadirachta indica*, and *Cassia tora*, which had the lowest final GSH concentrations.

The results of these preliminary investigations of methemoglobin generation and GSH depletion suggest that some Hausa plant medicines have oxidizing activity, indirectly recommending their efficacy in the therapy of malaria infection. On this basis we selected the best candidates for inclusion in direct in vivo tests of efficacy against an analogue of human malaria, murine *Plasmodium berghei*, studies of which represent most of the basic experimental work in human malaria therapy (Peters and Richards 1984).

In vivo Studies: Malaria infection is maintained in laboratory animals by

Table 8.4
Gluthatione Oxidation by Plant Extracts

Genus and Species	Hausa Name	Plant Part	0 min.	30 min	60 min	120 min
Acacia nilotica Del. Fabaceae	Gabaruwa	Root	2.0mM	1.3mM	0.9mM	0.2mM
Azadirachta indica A. Juss. Meliaceae	Darbejiya	Leaf	2.0	1.2	0.7	0.1
		Bark	2.0	1.7	1.6	1.4
		Root	2.0	1.8	1.8	1.7
Cassia occidentalis L. Fabaceae	Majamfari	Root	2.0	1.9	1.7	1.5
		Leaf	2.0	1.9	1.6	1.0
Cassia tora L. Fabaceae	Tafasa	Leaf	2.0	0.4	0.4	0.1
		Root	2.0	1.5	1.3	0.9
Cochlospermum tinctorium Rich., Cochlospermaceae	Rawaya	Root	2.0	1.8	1.7	1.2
Guiera senegalensis J.F. Gmel., Combretaceae	Sabara	Root	2.0	1.8	1.5	1.5
		Leaf	2.0	0.5	0.1	0.1
Securidaca longipedunculata Fres., Polygalaceae	Sanya	Root	2.0	1.8	1.7	1.5
Controls			2.0	1.9	1.9	1.9

intraperitoneal (IP) injection of healthy subjects with plasmodium-infected red blood cells drawn from heavily parasitized animals. We interrupted this process with an incubation phase in order to expose parasites to extracts of the medicinals *Acacia nilotica* root, and leaves of *Azadirachta indica*, *Cassia tora*, and *Guiera senegalensis*. After two hours' incubation, infected blood was injected into healthy subjects. We monitored time elapsed before the infection reached patency and the duration of infection prior to death, two standard evaluations used in the testing of antimalarial drugs (Peters and Richards 1984). The toxicity of plant extracts was ruled out by a parallel series of investigations in which neutralized extracts were injected IP over a course of seven days. Results are summarized in Table 8.5. Exposure to extracts of *Acacia nilotica*, *Azadirachta indica*, and *Guiera senegalensis* clearly suppressed infection, while *Cassia tora* extended survival only insignificantly.

Table 8.5
Effects of Plant Extracts on Plasmodial Infection

Genus and Species	Hausa Name	Plant Part	Parasitemia Day 7
Acacia nilotica Del. Fabaceae	Gabaruwa	Root	0%
Azadirachta indica A. Juss. Meliaceae	Darbejiya	Leaf	0%
Cassia tora L. Fabaceae	Tafasa	Leaf	83%
Guiera senegalensis JF Gmel., Combretaceae	Sabara	Leaf	1%
Controls			87%

The findings of these preliminary investigations of Hausa antimalarial plants could be clarified by more rigorous laboratory protocols to fractionate the specific constituents responsible for in vitro oxidant activity, establish whether ingestion of these oxidizing plants raises intraerythrocytic oxidation to levels that disrupt malaria parasite development, and determine whether the apparent in vivo effects against *Plasmodium berghei* can be attributed to those other constituents. Our preliminary findings were sufficiently promising as a prototype study to sustain our investigatory energy. We reported those results in the first edition of this volume principally to highlight a unique methodology for the evaluation of antimalarial plants.

Investigations of Antimalarial Activity: Series 2

Rationale: In view of the growing body of literature confirming the role that oxidant sensitivity plays in protection against malaria (discussed above), the argument is still compelling that this feature should be explored in the continuing search for new antimalarial drugs. Other methodological advances need to be embraced as well, including two important advances that were developed since the late 1970s, when we began our antimalarial studies. Refinement of a continuous culture technique for *Plasmodium falciparum* (Trager and Jensen 1976) has made possible the propagation and ever more intricate manipulation of human malaria parasites, and long-term maintenance of cell cultures provides a system for the direct and quantifiable measurement of in vitro antimalarial activity.

We took advantage of this elaborated protocol to further assess the antimalarial potential of Hausa plants. Having expanded our original data base through the extensive follow-up study in 1987–1988, we tested 309 specimens representing 134 species for activity against *P. falciparum* cell cultures. This time, we further specified the sample by invoking the criterion of multicontextual use (see discussion that follows) and selected from among 126 Hausa antipyretics 82 plants that are used in diet as well, thereby increasing people's exposure to any pharmacologic (and other) action. Primary aqueous/ethanol extractions (I) of 23 specimens (22 species, 27%) demonstrated in vitro activity against *P. falciparum*. Differential extraction with saline (II NaCI) and chloroform (II Chlor), and finally extraction of the remaining insoluble residue with ethanol (III) revealed antimalarial activity in additional fractions (Table 8.6).[7] It is important to distinguish between this direct test for antiplasmodial action and the earlier, indirect assessment that probed for oxidant action. The two series of laboratory investigations employed different methodologies, but results are not mutually exclusive: failure to demonstrate oxidizing potential in some plants does not confirm lack of antiplasmodial action—they may be effective through another mechanism of action; and efficacy demonstrated by plants in the later series may or may not be linked to their ability to increase intracellular oxidation. The methodological advances of the later series no doubt account in some measure for the disparity between the lists of "positives" that distilled from the two series of investigations; further testing will reconcile these differences.

A second strategic advance for research on antimalarial plants is access to NAPRALERT (NAtural PRoducts ALERT), a unique natural products relational database that distills the world literature on the chemical constituents, activity, and pharmacology of plant parts and extracts.[8] Its capabilities are vast and replace the type of literature search one used to do "by hand" or with weaker computer instruments. Ready access to those data greatly extends knowledge of the specific plants on which our studies center, helps us to understand more fully the physiologic outcomes of plant use, and suggests direction for refining laboratory investigations.

INTERRELATIONS AMONG INDIGENOUS MEDICINES, DIET, AND DISEASE

In addition to pharmacologic assessment of these plants through laboratory study and literature review, it is important to consider the varied contexts in which they are used. Review of data collected during the first field study made us aware of the overlapping contexts in which individual plants are used. We and others have remarked that very little is known about the pharmacology of food plants and have argued that, given the blurred boundaries between medicines and foods, investigation of the pharmacologic qualities of medicines is not complete without attention to all contexts of

Table 8.6
Activity of Plant Extracts against *Plasmodium falciparum* Cell Cultures

Genus and Species	Hausa Name	Part	I	II	III	III
				NaCl	Chlor	
Acacia nilotica Del. Fabaceae	Gabaruwa	root	+	+	-	+
Agelanthus dodoneifolius P& W Loranthaceae	Kauci	whole	+	-	-	+
Artemisia maciverae Hutch.&Dalz. Asteraceae	Tazargade	whole	+	-	+	-
Cassia occidentalis L. Fabaceae	Majamfari	root	+	-	+	+
		leaves	+	+	-	+
Centaurea perrottetii DC. Asteraceae	Dayi	whole	+	-	+	-
Chrozophora senegalensis A. Juss. Euphorbiaceae	Damagi	whole	+	+	-	+
Cyperus articulatus L. Cyperaceae	Kajiji	root	+	-	+	+
Diospyros mespiliformis Hochst. Ebenaceae	Kanya	leaves	+	-	-	+
Erythrina senegalensis DC Fabaceae	.Minjirya	root	+	-	+	-
Feretia apodanthera Del. Rubiaceae	Kurukuru	leaves	+	-	-	+
Ficus ingens Miq. Moraceae	Kawari	bark	+	-	-	-
F. polita Vahl. Moraceae	Durumi	leaves	+	+	-	+
F. ovata Vahl. Moraceae	Cediya	bark	+	-	+	+
Momordica balsamina L Cucurbitaceae	Garahunu	whole	+	-	-	-

Table 8.6 (Continued)

Genus and Species	Hausa Name	Part	I	II	III	III
				NaCl	Chlor	
Piper guineense Schum. & Thonn. Piperaceae	Masoro	fruit	+	+	-	-
Psidium guajava L. Myrtaceae	Gwaiba	leaves	+	+	-	+
Securinega virosa Baill. Euphorbiaceae	Tsa	leaves	+	+	-	+
Sorghum spp. Poaceae	Dawa	root	+	-	-	-
Syzygium aromaticum Merr.&Perry Myrtaceae	Kanumfari	clove	+	+	+	+
Thonningea sanguinea Vahl. Balanophoraceae	Kulla	root	+	+	+	+
Xylopia aethiopica A. Rich. Annonaceae	Kimba	fruit	+	-	+	-
Zingiber officinale Rosc. Zingiberaceae	Cittar Aho	rhizome	+	-	+	+

Source: Adapted from Etkin 1994c.

exposure to those plants (Etkin and Ross 1991; Johns 1990). Diet is important additionally because plants consumed as food tend to be ingested regularly and in relatively large volume compared, for example, to use of those same plants as cosmetics or in occasional rituals (Etkin 1994c; Etkin and Ross 1991). Further, we have argued elsewhere that Hausa knowledge of some plants as medicines has helped to identify those plants for inclusion in diet (Etkin and Ross 1994).[9]

Table 8.7 illustrates some of the multicontextual aspects of plant utilization, combining the results of both studies. Of 54 commonly used Hausa antimalarials, 82 percent (n = 44) also appeared in diet, and among those there was 89 percent concordance (n = 39) that the same plant structure (root, leaves, etc.) served as both antimalarial and food. Further, among those 39 plants, 67 percent (n = 26) were maximally available during the period of highest risk of malaria infection. The last, summary column of Table 8.7 that refers to categories A, B, and C allows one to quickly review not only overlapping contexts of use as medicine and food, but also whether availability coincides with the period of greatest malaria risk—in other words whether ease of collection/acquisiton maximizes exposure to pharmacologically remarkable plants. We will return to this point after reviewing some general interactions between nutrition and disease, followed by specific comments relevant to malaria infection.

Nutrition and Disease

The bulk of clinical, epidemiological, and biochemical evidence regarding interactions between nutrition and disease point to synergism between malnutrition and infection. This is recorded as increased susceptibility to infection secondary to diminished immune function; compromised skin integrity and reduced gastric acidity; exaggerated symptomatology; depression of nutrient intake due to anorexia; precipitation of frank nutrient deficits with increasing parasitemia; increased metabolic requirements (cellular hypermetabolism); fever-related pathologic changes leading to nutrient excretion via urine; and reactions linked to the mobilization of proinflammatory cytokines (Beisel 1995; Hoffman-Goetz 1986; Pelletier 1994; Stephensen et al. 1994; Ulijaszek 1990). These physiologic parameters are overlaid by such cultural variables as conscious underfeeding of ill children and therapeutically inspired food proscriptions (Burghart 1990; Duggan et al. 1986; McKay 1980).

Less is known of the antagonistic relationships between nutrition and infection, although a number of special cases have been described. Diets consisting almost entirely of milk suppress a variety of infections: rheumatic heart disease of streptococcal origin, likely attributed to the antimicrobial actions of oleic acid; malaria, due to low levels of PABA, riboflavin, and vitamin E; *Giardia lamblia*, due to a human-specific lipase; and malaria, tuberculosis, *Entamoeba histolytica*, and others due to the presence in milk of partially saturated lactoferrin and transferrin in sufficiently high concentrations to compete with parasites for iron. In plants, naturally occurring chelators such as tannins, phytates, citric acid, and other constituents of humic acid may sequester sufficiently large pools of serum iron (Bunnag et al. 1992; Emery 1982; Golenser et al. 1995; Graf and Eaton 1990) to suppress some infectious agents, an effect that might be offset in the case of malaria by the antioxidant actions of phytate, or enhanced by simultaneous consumption of vitamin C. Similarly, low levels of iron and other nutrients have been implicated in suppression of those same infections among people experiencing temporary and long-term food shortages (Bates et al. 1987; Eaton et al. 1976; Gillin et al. 1983; Harvey et al. 1989; Murray et al. 1982).

But what can one say of the pharmacologic effects of routine diets on the occurrence or expression of infection? There exists an atheoretical and disaggregated literature on "food pharmacology" that records physiologic activities for specific foods and projects that information onto populations whose epidemiologic circumstances may not be known but who consume those

Table 8.7
Commonly Used Hausa Antimalarial Plant Medicines

Genus and Species	Hausa Name	Medicinal Application for Malaria	Dietary Use	A	B	C
Abrus precatorius L. Fabaceae	Idon Zakara	Whole plant for periodic fever and jaundice	Whole plant edible; sweet leaves for flavoring	+	+	+
Acacia albida Del. Fabaceae	Gawo	Bark for fever and jaundice	--	-	-	-
Acacia nilotica Del. Fabaceae	Gabaruwa	Fruit pulp and pods for fever	Leaves, fruit, and seed are edible; gum is chewed	+	+	+
Adansonia digitata L. Bombacaceae	Kuka	Leaves, fruit, seeds, bark for fever; bark for jaundice	Fruit, seeds, leaves, young root, and bark are edible	+	+	+
Amaranthus hybridus L Amaranthaceae	Alaiyaho	Leaves for anemia	Seeds and leaves in soup; leaves as greens	+	+	+
Anogeissus leiocarpus G&P, Combretaceae	Marke	Leaves for jaundice; bark for fever	Infusion of bark and stems is a beverage; edible gum	+	+	-
Agelanthus dodoneifolius Polh. & Wiens., Loranthaceae	Kauci	Whole for hematuria	--	-	-	-

Species / Family	Local name	Medicinal use	Food use	A	B	C
Artemisia maciverae Hutch & Dalz, Asteraceae	Tazargade	Leaves and stem for fever and pediatric malaria	Added to foods for fragrance	+	+	-
Azadirachta indica A. Juss., Meliaceae	Darbejiya	Leaves and bark for fever; all parts for periodic fever	Flowers are stomachic	+	-	-
Balanites aegyptica Del. Zygophyllaceae	Aduwa	Root for periodic fever; fruit for fever; leaves for jaundice	Fruit, seeds, leaves, flowers, and resin are edible	+	+	+
Bauhinia reticulata DC. Fabaceae	Kargo	Leaves, root, and bark for fever; root for splenomegaly	Leaves and pods are edible	+	+	+
Cadaba farinosa Forsk. Capparidaceae	Bagayi	Whole plant for anemia	Leaves in sweet snacks; stem chewed for sweet taste	+	+	+
Cassia goratensis Fresn. Fabaceae	Runhu	Leaves and fruit pod for fever	Leaves and fruit are edible; leaf infusion is a beverage	+	+	+

In column A, + denotes that this antimalarial plant is also used for food.
In column B, + denotes that the same structure serves as food and antimalarial medicine.
In column C, + denotes that the plant part from column B is maximally available during the period of high malaria risk.

Table 8.7 (Continued)

Genus and Species	Hausa Name	Medicinal Application for Malaria	Dietary Use	A B C
Cassia occidentalis L. Fabaceae	Majamfari	Leaves for periodic and other fevers, and jaundice; root for fever and liver disorders	Leaves and unripe fruit are edible; root stimulates appetite; seeds in beverage	+ + +
Cassia tora L. Fabaceae	Tafasa	Leaves for fever	Leaves as greens; seeds are edible and used in beverage	+ + +
Celosia trigyna L. *C. isertii* C.C. Towns. Amaranthaceae	Nannaho	Whole plant for periodic and other fevers	Leaves for soup and greens	+ + +
Centaurea perrottetii DC. Asteraceae	Dayi	Whole for splenomegaly	--	- -
Chrozophora senegalensis A. Juss., Euphorbiaceae	Damagi	Leaves for fever	--	- -
Cochlospermum tinctorium Rich., Cochlospermaceae	Rawaya	Bark and root for jaundice	Root imparts yellow color to food	+ + -
Commiphora kerstingii Engl., Burseraceae	Dali	Leaves for jaundice	--	- -

Species / Family	Local name	Medicinal use	Food use	A B C
Corchorus tridens L. Tiliaceae	Turgunnuwa	Leaves and seeds for splenomegaly	Leaves in soup	+ + +
Cyperus articulatus L. Cyperaceae	Kajiji	Rhizome for intermittent fever	--	- - +
Diospyros mespiliformis Hochst., Ebenaceae	Kanya	Bark for anemia; leaves for fever	Fruit raw and in gruel; Young leaves are edible	+ + +
Eragrostis ciliamensis Lutati, Poaceae	Bunsurum Fage	Whole plant for fever	Seeds are edible	+ + +
Erythrina senegalensis DC., Fabaceae	Minjirya	Bark and root for jaundice, anemia; bark for fever	--	- - -
Feretia canthioides Hiern., Rubiaceae	Kurukuru	Leaves for fever	--	- - -
Ficus ingens Miq. Moraceae	Kawari	Bark for anemia, jaundice, fever	Young leaves edible	+ - -

In column A, + denotes that this antimalarial plant is also used for food.
In column B, + denotes that the same structure serves as food and antimalarial medicine.
In column C, + denotes that the plant part from column B is maximally available during the period of high malaria risk.

Table 8.7 (Continued)

Genus and Species	Hausa Name	Medicinal Application for Malaria	Dietary Use	A	B	C
Ficus ovata Vahl. Moraceae	Cediya	Leaves for fever and jaundice; bark for spleno/hepatomegaly	Young leaves in soup; fruit is edible	+	+	+
Ficus polita Vahl. Moraceae	Durumi	Leaves for fever	Young leaves in soup	+	+	+
Guiera senegalensis JF Gmel., Combretaceae	Sabara	Leaves for fever and as vehicle for other medicines	Leaves in soup and gruel	+	+	+
Hibiscus sabdariffa L. Malvaceae	Yakuwa	Seeds, fruit, and leaves fever	Leaves and calyces are vegetables; fruit, seed, and seed oil are edible	+	+	+
Lasarifolia Roem. & Schultes, Convolvulaceae	Duman Rafi	Whole plant for fever	--	-	-	-
Momordica balsamina L. *M. charantia* L., Cucurbitaceae	Garahunu	Whole plant for fever and anemia	Leaves are vegetable	+	+	+
Moringa oleifera Lam. Moringaceae	Zogale	Leaves for fever and jaundice	Leaves in soup and as vegetable; fruit pod, root, and seed are edible	+	+	+

190

				A	B	C
Nauclea diderrichii Merr., Rubiaceae	Tafashiya	Leaves and root for fever, jaundice, and hemoglobin uria; bark for periodic fever and jaundice	Fruit is edible; stem infusion as beverage	+	-	-
Parkia filicoidea Welw. Fabaceae	Dorawa	Leaves and fruit for fever; bark for jaundice	Leaves, fruit, seeds, and flower are edible; bark infusion as beverage	+	+	+
Piper guineense Schum. & Thonn., Piperaceae	Masoro	Fruit for fever, jaundice, anemia	Fruit is common flavoring	+	+	-
Prosopis africana Taub. Fabaceae	Kirya	Leaves and bark for fever	Seeds are edible	+	-	-
Psidium guajava L. Myrtaceae	Goba	Leaves for jaundice and anemia; bark for jaundice; root for pediatric malaria	Fruit is edible	+	-	-
Sclerocarya birrea Hochst., Anacardiaceae	Danya	Fruit for hemoglobinuria	Fruit and seeds are edible	+	+	+

In column A, + denotes that this antimalarial plant is also used for food.

In column B, + denotes that the same structure serves as food and antimalarial medicine.

In column C, + denotes that the plant part from column B is maximally available during the period of high malaria risk.

Table 8.7 (Continued)

Genus and Species	Hausa Name	Medicinal Application for Malaria	Dietary Use	A	B	C
Securidaca longipeduncu-ulata Fres., Polygalaceae	Sanya	Root for periodic fever; seeds and root for fever	Bark infusion is a beverage	+	+	-
Securinega virosa Baill. Euphorbiaceae	Tsa	Root for anemia	--	-	-	-
Sesamum radiatum Schum. & Thonn., Pedaliaceae	Karkashi	Whole plant for jaundice	Leaves and seeds in soup	+	+	+
Sorghum spp. Poaceae	Dawa	Seed for anemia and as vehicle for fever and malaria medicines; root for hematuria and anemia; stalk, leaf, and sheath for pediatric malaria	Seed is staple for flour	+	+	-
Striga hermontheca Benth. Scrophulariaceae	Soki	Whole plant for anemia and jaundice	Whole plant cooked with vegetables and legumes to soften	+	+	+
Strychnos spinosa Lam. Loganiaceae	Kokiya	Fruit and root for fever	Fruit and leaves are edible	+	+	+

192

Species, Family	Local name	Medicinal use	Food use	A	B	C
Syzygium aromaticum Merr. & Perry, Myrtaceae	Kanumfari	Flower bud for fever, jaundice, anemia	Flower bud is common flavoring	+	+	-
Tamarindus indica L. Fabaceae	Tsamiya	Leaves, fruit, bark, and root for fever; leaves and bark for jaundice; flowers for spleno/hepato-megaly	Leaves, fruit and seed oil are edible	+	+	+
Thonningia sanguinea Vahl., Balanophoraceae	Kulla	Root for fever, jaundice, anemia	Root is common flavoring	+	+	-
Xylopia aethiopica A. Rich, Annonaceae	Kimba	Fruit for fever, jaundice, anemia	Fruit is common flavoring	+	+	-
Ximenia americana L. Olacaceae	Tsada	Leaves, young stems, and root for fever	Leaves, fruit, and seed oil are edible	+	+	+
Zingiber officinale Rosc. Zingiberaceae	Cittar Aho	Root for fever, jaundice, anemia	Root is common flavoring	+	+	-

In column A, + denotes that this antimalarial plant is also used for food.
In column B, + denotes that the same structure serves as food and antimalarial medicine.
In column C, + denotes that the plant part from column B is maximally available during the period of high malaria risk.

193

plants as food and/or medicine. For example, extracts of garlic (*Allium sativa* L.) and onion (*A. cepa* L.) are anthelminthic (Peña et al. 1988); West African black pepper (*Piper guineense* Schum. & Thonn.) has antiviral activity (Abila et al. 1993); ginger (*Zingiber officinale* Rosc.), cinnamon (*Cinnamomum verum* J. Presl), and turmeric (*Curcuma longa* L.) are antimicrobial (Mascolo et al. 1989; Rafatullah et al. 1990).[10] The difficulty lies in tying these observations to real populations with known disease history and rigorously testing such hypotheses. The edited volumes *Plants in Indigenous Medicine and Diet* and *Eating on the Wild Side* (Etkin 1986a, 1994a) are organized explicitly around this goal, and the studies reported therein provide direction for this type of inquiry. We use that same framework for reporting results of our investigations of Hausa plant medicines and foods.

Malaria in Northern Nigeria

Malaria is endemic throughout northern Nigeria, and in Hurumi the risk of infection is greatest during August to October, a pattern typical of much of the sub-Saharan savanna, which is dominated by a unimodal pattern of rainfall (Wernsdorfer 1980). In this region the annual cycle includes 3 to 4 months of rains and an 8–9-month dry season. In most years the onset of rains in June is followed by the progressive development of microenvironments that support mosquito breeding, so that by August mosquitoes abound in numbers sufficient for the sustained growth of malaria parasites and their continued transmission to susceptible human hosts. Nonetheless, the reported incidence of fulminant and debilitating plasmodial infection is relatively low for this region.[11] This apparent suppression of malaria infection may be ascribed to a number of factors, one of which—the efficacy of indigenous antimalarials—was discussed earlier in this chapter. The potential contribution of diet to malaria suppression is discussed below.

Malaria Epidemiology and Dietary Patterns: 1975–1976

Reflecting the dependence on local subsistence through the 1970s, dietary patterns in Hurumi were distinguished by marked seasonal fluctuations in the availability of foodstuffs. For example the principal staples, millet (*Pennisetum* spp.) and guineacorn (*Sorghum* spp.), were sown in early June, harvested from mid-September through November, and subsequently stored in granaries. The chief legumes cultivated are groundnut (*Arachis hypogaea* L.) and cowpea (*Vigna unguiculata* Walpers), generally sown in late June to early July and harvested the same time as the later-maturing sorghums. Maximum availability and lowest market costs for all of these products coincided with their harvest, and their supplies gradually diminished through the end of the dry season and beginning of the rainy months, with market prices for their replacement increasing commensurately. The exception to this pattern

Figure 8.2
Calorie Sources Other Than Grains, 1975–1976

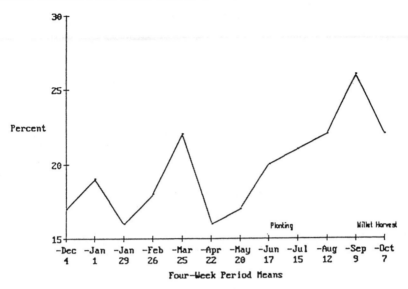

Note: The frequency with which nongrain foods contributed to diet is expressed as a percentage of total caloric intake. The mean caloric value of nongrain foods is 22 percent, ranging between 16 and 28 percent. Means are presented for four-week periods.

of fluctuating availability for the primary foodstuffs was cassava (*Manihot esculenta* Crantz), which was available year-round (protected from livestock, it can endure as a transannual, providing edible rootstock for as long as three years).

The patterning of types and quantities of foods consumed in Hurumi corresponded closely to fluctuations in availability and costs. Variability was greatly diminished immediately following the harvest, when grains were readily available for consumption in the form of thick porridges favored by Hausa as the appropriately energy-dense base around which the primary (evening) and some other meals are contrived. Dietary elaboration was increasingly pronounced through the progression of the dry season and commencement of rains. This took the form of an increased variety of foods eaten and of their sources and preparation styles. Figure 8.2 depicts the frequency with which nongrain foods contributed to total caloric intake and illustrates increasing dietary reliance on nongrain foods as the next harvest approached.

This dietary elaboration is explained by both ecological and cultural features; its implications are multiple. The depletion of staples stored from the previous harvest contributed to greater reliance on market purchases of raw grains and on foods purchased from extrahousehold sources, typically market vendors and village women who sell prepared main dishes and snacks. These

Table 8.8
Food Uses of Local Semi-Wild Medicinal Plants

FOOD TYPE		plants (n=61)	percentage
MEALS	soups	20	32.8
	gruels	7	11.5
	misc. midday secondary	12	19.7
	misc. midday primary	10	16.4
SNACKS	prepared mixture	12	19.7
	raw	5	8.2
	sweet beverages	2	3.3
	milk	4	6.6
EMERGENCY		7	11.5

Source: Adapted from Etkin and Ross 1994.

sources amplified the range of variability in the household's diet beyond what would otherwise have been only those products reaped during the previous harvest. Moreover, the frequency and duration of market attendance increased during the dry season. The population was thus exposed to a greater array of foods from other areas and increased purchases beyond necessities for household meals. Another factor that encouraged dietary variability toward the end of the dry season is a larger number of ceremonies that, in the public celebration of life-cycle events, involve intra- and intervillage food exchanges and redistributions. Although grains predominated in the diet throughout the year, the steady increase in market costs—which reached a maximum during the latter part of the rainy season—dissuaded many people from replacing their diminished grain stores. Instead, they relied on other, less-preferred but readily obtained foods.

Another feature of dietary elaboration that characterized the rainy season is the increased availability of "semi-wild" plants.[12] We refer to these as "vegetables" to underscore their role in Hausa diet, for which they are marked primarily by their foliage (although young stems, calyces, buds, fruits, and flowers are indicated in some cases). These are to a large extent "free goods," since those growing on public grazing land, paths, and other nonprivate property can be collected without permission or obligation. Tables 8.2 and 8.8 document the significance of semiwild plants for Hausa medicine and diet (Etkin and Ross 1994). These plants were most prominent in diet during the last two months of the rainy season (only some are dried for consumption throughout the year). That timing can be explained by three interrelated factors. First, these plants were more readily available then; compared with grains, they matured and were available for collection or market purchase earlier and were less expensive. Second, these vegetables, added to cereal-based mixtures, helped to extend remaining grain stores during the period of shortest supply. Third, they provided a welcome substitute for cassava, which was itself a substitute for the declining grains and had become, by Hausa standards, tedious. Cereal-based dishes were augmented by the addition of vegetables and by the substitution of cassava for at least one meal, usually at midday, in order to reserve grains for the most important, evening meal. The aggregate effect of these seasonal changes was increased consumption of vegetables through the progression of the rainy season.

The leaves of some species were especially favored as centerpiece for several popular dishes, including, from Table 8.7, *Amaranthus hybridus*, *Cadaba farinosa*, *Cassia tora*, *Hibiscus sabdariffa*, *Momoradica balsamina*, *M. charantia*, and *Moringa oleifera*. Other leaves that figure more prominently for soups and as seasonings include, from Table 8.7 *Adansonia digitata*, *Artemisia maciverae*, *Corchorus tridens*, *Celosia trigyna*, *C. isertii*, *Ficus ovata*, *F. polita*, *Guiera senegalensis*, *Parkia filicoidea*, *Sesamum radiatum*, and *Tamarindus indica*. Figure 8.3 demonstrates this increased use of vegetable foods in household diet as the annual cycle approaches the next harvest.

Further, most of the plants listed in Table 8.7 are also used medicinally, other than for malaria. Notable in this regard is *Guiera senegalensis*, one of whose Hausa names, "mother of medicines" (*uwar magunguna*), reflects its use as both principal and vehicle in various medicinal preparations. The likelihood that the use of several of these plants would influence malaria infection is heightened by their indication for the prevention and treatment of other rainy season diseases such as *sanyi* and *raba*, complex symptom clusters whose etiology is ascribed to dampness and the chill of wet clothing and house floors.

As noted earlier, during 1975 and 1976, the period of highest malaria risk coincided with the end of the rainy season, when increases in vegetable consumption and decreases in grain utilization were most marked. Figure 8.4 demonstrates that during the period of maximum malaria risk, the quantity of grains consumed reached its lowest point and the amount of vegetables consumed reached one of its highest points. We suggest that these interrelated aspects of dietary patterning may have antagonistic effects on malaria infection, thereby helping to explain why, despite the high risk, plasmodial infections that occurred tended to be relatively moderate.

MALARIA, MEDICINE, AND MEALS

From a pharmacologic perspective, dietary and other uses of antimalarial plants should be interpreted as additional exposure to constituents of po-

Figure 8.3
Frequency of Vegetable Use in Diet, 1975–1976

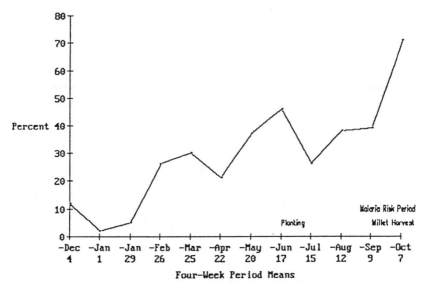

Note: This is expressed as a percentage of days in a four-week period in which vegetables
appeared in household diets. The mean percentage is 28, ranging between 2 and 71. Grain
in some quantity appeared in all household diets for every day examined and would, at
100 percent, appear above the top of the graph as a horizontal line.

tential therapeutic efficacy. That is, the consumption of oxidizing and otherwise antiplasmodial plants in both medicinal and dietary contexts during
a time when risk of malaria infection was highest may have had a compound
effect in limiting this infection.

Additionally, the reduction in grain consumption that coincided with increased use of vegetables may curtail parasitemia. We draw here on the
observations of Murray et al. (1982), who noted recrudescence of plasmodial
infections among populations in famine-relief programs. It is possible that
the apparent protection against malaria occurred because of deficits in vitamin E (an antioxidant) (Eaton et al. 1976), and that this balance was over-
turned on supplying those populations with vitamin E–rich grains. Or iron
may be the critical nutrient. In any case, the observation holds that the
circumstances of grain deprivation coincide with suppressed malaria infection.

We proposed that what appeared to be paradoxically low levels of fulminant malaria in Hurumi could be attributed at least in part to the combined effects of decreased consumption of grains rich in vitamin E and iron
and increased consumption of vegetables and medicines that generate oxidants and/or otherwise impede plasmodial development.

Figure 8.4
Daily Per Capita Consumption of Grains and Vegetables, 1975–1976

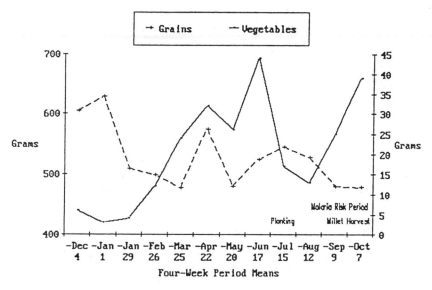

Four-Week Period Means

Dietary Update, 1987–1988

During our follow-up study in Hurumi we noted marked diminution in the seasonal constraints on resources that had characterized dietary patterns 12 years earlier. This is due in part to increased availability of a range of foodstuffs through expanded regional markets, attendant upon the growth of transportation networks and other infrastructural developments. There was substantial evidence of increasing participation of Hurumi residents in the larger economy—more took part in short-term migration to urban areas, bringing back to Hurumi cash and new food preferences; a greater number were selling and buying foodstuffs, both more often and more regularly throughout the year. Further, cassava cultivation and consumption declined dramatically for the most recent period; whereas cassava provided as much as 14 percent of all calories consumed during its peak consumption period in 1975–1976, it represented no more than 2 percent of all calories consumed during the 1987–1988 period (the respective weekly means being 6.1% and 1.6%). This reflects changes in food preference as well as such environmental variables as unfavorable growing conditions and plant diseases. The full impact of these dietary shifts is beyond the scope of this chapter, but we do need to underscore two aspects that are relevant to our earlier model of a seasonally changing diet and its potential impact on malaria.

The first aspect of changing diet pertains to grain consumption. Although there were no marked cyclical reductions for the 1987–1988 research period, the overall yearly consumption of grain was relatively low, in fact comparable

Figure 8.5
Grams of Vegetables Consumed per Capita per Day, 1975–1976 and 1987–
1988

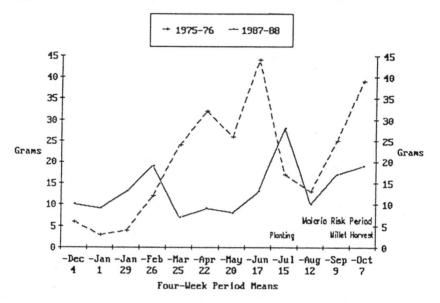

to the diminished rates of grain consumption that characterized the 1975–
1976 high-malaria-risk season. (The 48-week mean was 450 grams per capita
for 1987–1988.) The lower consumption of grain was accounted for in part
by the year-round substitution of legume-based midday meals and the more
frequent inclusion of imported, and costly, polished rice.

The second aspect of dietary change is of greater concern for the continued relevance of our model. Here, we note for 1987–1988 a marked reduction in the quantity of semi-wild vegetables consumed (Figure 8.5). This
decrease, particularly during the period of malaria risk, can be partly attributed to replacement of cassava-based dishes with more favored legume- and
grain-based dishes, and a concomitant reduction in vegetable-based dishes.
It is interesting that while the quantity of vegetables in the diet diminished,
the incidence of population exposure to at least some of these products was
comparable for the two research periods, illustrating the continued importance of vegetables as dietary supplements. Whether this dietary change that
attends economic and infrastructural changes portends a trend that may affect malaria expression is at this stage only conjecture. Indeed, most recent
reports from our Nigerian colleague suggest an ever more complex environment characterized both by the wax and wane of regional markets, creating
conditions in which people actually rely more on foods from local sources,
and the expansion of antimalarial programs that include the widespread but
sporadic use of biomedical prophylaxis. While the exploration of this dy-

namic awaits further fieldwork, the dietary and medicinal pharmacologic model suggested by our earlier work continued to inform our investigations through the most recent field research and helps to shape future inquiry as well.

SUMMARY AND CONCLUSIONS

For the present discussion, a model that integrates features of disease ecology and plant pharmacology was applied to investigate how certain foods and medicines might interact with malaria infection. Elsewhere, we used this framework to investigate how foods and medicines might influence gastrointestinal disorders (Etkin and Ross 1982), as well as to expand the number of overlapping contexts beyond the two considered here (including also plants used as cosmetics and for personal hygiene) (Etkin 1994c). Collectively these studies illustrate how the pharmacologic potential of botanicals is extended through their use in various contexts. By focusing on these plants for investigations of biocultural adaptations to disease, we conceptualize them broadly as ingestible plants rather than exclusively as "medicines," "foods," or something else.

This chapter evaluates the continued utility of our model for dietary shifts as adaptations to both the fluctuating availability of plants and the seasonal occurrence of malaria infection. In sum, we note that a number of Hausa medicinal plants used to treat malaria infection are also important dietary constituents. Laboratory investigations of Hausa antimalarials suggest their efficacy. Moreover, the plasmodiostatic activity demonstrated for some of these plants might be amplified by a diminished consumption of grains. An examination of local diets during 1975 and 1976 revealed that both increased use of medicinal plants as food and diminished consumption of grains coincided with the period of greatest risk of malaria infection. From our more recent study, we document changes in the local diet—most significant, a decrease in the quantities consumed of plants that provided the focus of our earlier investigations. These observations, cast in a broad ecological framework, provide a basis from which we can explore the potential implications of other dimensions of change.

ACKNOWLEDGMENTS

For both field studies and in our present work we are grateful for the contributions of Ibrahim Muazzamu. We acknowledge the collective wisdom and goodwill of the people of Hurumi Village, for their courtesy and cooperation during both field studies, and for their continued participation in our absence. This work was supported in part by grants awarded to Nina L. Etkin by the National Science Foundation (BNS-8703734), the Social Science Research Council, the Fulbright Senior Research Scholars Program, the Bush Foundation, the University of Minnesota, and the Social

Science Research Institute of the University of Hawaii; to Paul J. Ross by the National Science Foundation (SOC 74–24412), Sigma Xi, and Washington University; and to both authors by faculty research appointments in the Department of Pharmacognosy and Drug Development, Ahmadu Bello University, Zaria. We also thank the Kano State Department of Health and Wudil Local Government. Dr. Daniel Klayman (+) of Walter Reed generously provided samples of *Artemisia annua* (used as a control in studies of antimalarial activity against *P. falciparum* cultures).

NOTES

1. During both studies, voucher specimens were collected for all plants discussed. These have been taxonomically identified by botanists at the Missouri Botanical Garden in St. Louis, Kew Royal Botanic Garden in London, and Ahmadu Bello University Herbarium in Zaria, Nigeria. The full catalogue is now part of the permanent African reference collection of the Missouri Botanical Garden Herbarium. Plants designated for phytochemical and pharmacological investigation were collected in bulk, air-dried in the field, and sent to our laboratory in the United States.

2. By 1988 both a paved road and piped water had reached a neighboring village 2 kilometers away, and plans exist to extend these amenities across a wider radius. A few farmers occasionally hired tractor labor and draft oxen, and the manual operation of irrigation for *fadama* (river-edge garden plots) has been virtually replaced by petrol-powered generators.

3. This makes evident the high level of personal and social control that characterizes Hausa interpersonal relations. There is a constant concern that malevolence born of envy or spurned affection will invite the disaffected to engage in sorcery against one's person, property, or family. So, too, one desires protection against witches, who are insidious because one can never be sure of their identity among community members. And the malfeasance wrought by spirits is legion in a world where one must appease one's personal spirits and deflect harm from others. This of course, oversimplifies, but the point is that these imperceptible entities are actively engaged as a matter of course in the daily goings on of Hausa.

4. Residents of Hurumi are predominantly and devoutly Moslem, as testimony to which the sovereign presence of Allah permeates all aspects of life. Traditional Islamic medicines include plants, but more commonly take the form of prayer, recitation and writing of Koranic passages, and the fabrication of amulets and other propitiatory instruments.

5. We are aware that a better research design would have used a larger, randomized survey sample and would have measured quantities of foods actually consumed by each individual. However, our experiences—including a pilot study—during 6 months' residence in the village prior to initiating the dietary survey revealed that the more rigorous methodology was impossible. This reflects the intrusive nature of such measures, the marked emphasis on privacy that Hausa apply to eating, and the great amount of time entailed in conducting such surveys (which would have necessitated the exclusion of other aspects of the study). In light of this, the dietary survey proceeded with acknowledged compromises; any resultant shortcomings are offset by the depth of detail in the data and their high degree of reliability.

6. This initiative gained special momentum after the (re)discovery in the 1970s

of the Chinese Qinghaosu, an extract of *Artemisia annua* L. (Asteraceae), whose powerful antimalarial action ultimately was explained by oxidative activity (Hien and White 1993; Klayman 1993; Meshnick 1994).

7. These investigations of in vitro antiplasmodial activity were conducted in the laboratories of Dr. John Eaton, University of Minnesota Medical School.

8. The NAPRALERT database is maintained and housed by the Program for Collaborative Research in the Pharmaceutical Sciences within the Department of Medicinal Chemistry and Pharmacognosy, College of Pharmacy, University of Illinois at Chicago.

9. Our position is supported by our medicinal plant inventory, which is more comprehensive of local flora than our corollary catalogues for economic plants and foods and which subsumes plants from those other categories. A second point is that all the criteria that Hausa use to judge the suitability of plants for food are influenced by long-term experience with botanicals used in medicinal preparations. But food plants—even those drawn from among medicinals—are appraised for qualities of satiety and taste and only casually understood with reference to health value. For this reason, while knowledge of medicinal plants guides the selection of foods, the opposite is not true: knowledge of a food will not inform its medicinal use because whereas texture, taste, and even toxicity are all integral to food selection, these qualities are subordinated to their medicinal properties (Etkin and Ross 1994:95–96).

10. See Etkin (1997) for discussion of how and why particular foods have again captured the interest of biomedicine.

11. The scope and locus of our study made it impossible to include any clinical examination or to secure blood samples for parasite analysis. In view of that, conclusions regarding the prevalence and severity of malaria infection are drawn from reports of the Nigerian Ministry of Health, the WHO Malaria Research Center in Kano, staff of the district hospital and dispensary, published studies of malaria epidemiology in northern Nigeria (e.g., Abudu 1983; Ayeni et al. 1987; Schram 1971; Stock 1983), and, for 1987–1988, the village and hospital epidemiological surveys.

12. Heavily populated and intensively farmed for generations, the region in which Hurumi is located (the Kano Close-Settled Zone) is actually home to no plants that are, technically, wild. But the deliberate management of noncultivated species on farm borders and public lands and those not removed during the weeding of farms properly evokes the term "semi-wild."

REFERENCES

Abbink, J. 1995. "Medicinal and Ritual Plants of the Ethiopian Southwest: An Account of Recent Research." *Indigenous Knowledge and Development Monitor* 3: 6–8.

Abila, B., A. Richens, and J. A. Davies. 1993. "Anticonvulsant Effects of Extracts of the West African Black Pepper, *Piper guineense.*" *Journal of Ethnopharmacology* 39:113–17.

Abudu, F. 1983. "Planning Priorities and Health Care Delivery in Nigeria." *Social Science and Medicine* 17:1995–2002.

Adam, J. G., N. Echard, and M. Lescot. 1972. "Plantes Médicinales Hausa de l'Ader (République du Niger)." *Journal d'Agriculture Tropicale et de Botanique Appliquée* 19(8–9):259–399.

Agwu, I. E., and P. A. Akah. 1990. "*Tabernaemontana crassa* as a Traditional Local Anesthetic Agent." *Journal of Ethnopharmacology* 30:115–19.

Akerele, O. 1987. "The Best of Both Worlds: Bringing Traditional Medicine up to Date." *Social Science and Medicine* 24:177–81.

Anyinam, C. 1995. "Ecology and Ethnomedicine: Exploring Links between Current Environmental Crisis and Indigenous Medical Practices." *Social Science and Medicine* 40:321–29.

Apisariyakul, A., N. Vanittanakom, and D. Buddhasukh. 1995. "Antifungal Activity of Turmeric Oil Extracted from *Curcuma longa* (Zingiberaceae)." *Journal of Ethnopharmacology* 49:163–69.

Armelagos, G. J., T. Leatherman, M. Ryan, and L. Sibley. 1992. "Biocultural Synthesis in Medical Anthropology." *Medical Anthropology* 14:35–52.

Ayeni, B., G. Rushton, and M. L. McNulty. 1987. "Improving the Geographical Accessibility of Health Care in Rural Areas: A Nigerian Case Study." *Social Science and Medicine* 25:1083–94.

Bastien, J. W. 1995. "Cross Cultural Communication of Tetanus Vaccinations in Bolivia." *Social Science and Medicine* 41:77–86.

Bates, C. J., H. J. Powers, W. H. Lamb, W. Gelman, and E. Webb. 1987. "Effect of Supplementary Vitamins and Iron on Malaria Indices in Rural Gambian Children." *Transactions of the Royal Society of Tropical Medicine and Hygiene* 81:286–91.

Beisel, W. R. 1995. "Infection-Induced Malnutrition: From Cholera to Cytokines." *American Journal of Clinical Nutrition* 62:813–19.

Benie, T., A. El Izzi, C. Tahiri, J. Duval, and M.-L. Thieulant. 1990. "*Combretodendron africanum* Bark Extract as an Antifertility Agent. I: Estrogenic Effects in vivo and LH Release by Cultured Gonadotrope Cells." *Journal of Ethnopharmacology* 29:13–23.

Borris, R. P., and J. M. Schaeffer. 1992. "Antiparasitic Agents from Plants." In *Phytochemical Resources for Medicine and Agriculture*. H. N. Nigg and D. Seigler, eds. New York: Plenum Press, 117–58.

Browner, C. H., B. R. Ortiz de Montellano, and A. Rubel. 1988. "A Methodology for Cross-Cultural Ethnomedical Research." *Current Anthropology* 29:681–89.

Bunnag, D., A. A. Poltera, C. Viravan, S. Looareesuwan, K. T. Harinasuta, and C. Schindléry. 1992. "Plasmodicidal Effect of Desferrioxamine B in Human Vivax or Falciparum Malaria from Thailand." *Acta Tropica* 52:59–67.

Burghart, R. 1990. "The Cultural Context of Diet, Disease, and the Body." In *Diet and Disease in Traditional and Developing Societies*. G. A. Harrison and J. C. Waterlow, eds. Cambridge: Cambridge University Press, 307–25.

Busson, F., P. Jaeger, P. Lunven, and M. Pinta. 1965. *Plantes Alimentaires de l'Ouest Africain*. Paris: Ministère de la Coopération.

Caceres, A., O. Cano, B. Samayoa, and L. Aguilar. 1990. "Plants Used in Guatemala for the Treatment of Gastroinestinal Disorders. 1. Screening of 84 Plants Against Enterobacteria." *Journal of Ethnopharmacology* 30:55–73.

Chadwick, D. J., and J. Marsh, eds. 1994. *Ethnobotany and the Search for New Drugs*. CIBA Foundation Symposium 185. Chichester: Wiley.

Chawla, A. S., and M. Kumar. 1991. "Antimalarial Agents from Plants." *Indian Drugs* 29:57–60.

Chunhuei, C. 1994. "Integrating Traditional Medicine into Modern Health Care Systems." *Social Science and Medicine* 39:307–21.

Clark, I. A., G. Chaudhri, and W. B. Cowden. 1989. "Some Roles of Free Radicals in Malaria." *Free Radical Biology and Medicine* 6:315–21.

Counts, D. R., and D. A. Counts. 1989. "Complementarity in Medical Treatment in a West New Britain Society." In *A Continuing Trial of Treatment: Medical Pluralism in Papua New Guinea.* S. Frankel and G. Lewis, eds. Dordrecht: Kluwer, 277–94.

Dalziel, J. M. 1937. *The Useful Plants of West Tropical Africa.* London: Crown Agents for Overseas Governments and Administrations.

Darrah, A. C. 1980. *A Hermeneutic Approach to Hausa Therapeutics: The Allegory of the Living Fire.* Ph.D. dissertation, Department of Anthropology, Northwestern University. Evanston, Ill.: University Microfilms.

Desta, B. 1994. "Ethiopian Traditional Herbal Drugs. Part III: Antifertility Activity of 70 Medicinal Plants." *Journal of Ethnopharmacology* 44(3)199–209.

Docampo, R., and S. N. J. Moreno. 1984. "Free-Radical Intermediates in the Antiparasitic Action of Drugs and Phagocytic Cells." In *Free Radicals in Biology.* W. A. Pryor, ed. New York: Academic Press, 244–88.

Duggan, M. B., J. Alwar, and R. D. G. Milner. 1986. "The Nutritional Cost of Measles in Africa." *Archives of Disease in Childhood* 61:61–66.

Duke, J. A., and A. A. Atchley. 1986. *CRC Handbook of Proximate Analysis Tables of Higher Plants.* Boca Raton, Fla.: CRC Press.

Eaton, J. W., and G. W. Brewer. 1974. "Pentose Phosphate Metabolism." In *The Red Blood Cell*, Vol. 1. D. M. Surgenor, ed. New York: Academic Press, 435–71.

Eaton, J. W., J. R. Eckman, E. Berger, and H. S. Jacob. 1976. "Suppression of Malaria Infection by Oxidant Sensitive Erythrocytes." *Nature* 264:758–60.

Elvin-Lewis, M. 1986. "Therapeutic Rationale of Plants Used to Treat Dental Infections." In *Plants in Indigenous Medicine and Diet: Biobehavioral Approaches.* N. L. Etkin, ed. New York: Gordon and Breach, 48–69.

Emery, T. 1982. "Iron Metabolism in Humans and Plants." *American Scientist* 70: 626–32.

Etkin, N. L. 1979. "Indigenous Medicine Among the Hausa of Northern Nigeria: Laboratory Evaluation for Potential Therapeutic Efficacy of Antimalarial Plant Medicines." *Medical Anthropology* 3:401–29.

———. 1981. "A Hausa Herbal Pharmacopoeia: Biomedical Evaluation of Commonly Used Plant Medicines." *Journal of Ethnopharmacology* 4:75–98.

———. 1986b. "Multidisciplinary Perspectives in the Interpretation of Plants Used in Indigenous Medicine and Diet." In *Plants in Indigenous Medicine and Diet: Biobehavioral Approaches.* N. L. Etkin, ed. New York: Gordon and Breach, 2–29.

———. 1988. "Ethnopharmacology: Biobehavioral Approaches in the Anthropological Study of Indigenous Medicines." *Annual Review of Anthropology* 17:23–42.

———. 1990. "Ethnopharmacology." In *Medical Anthropology: Contemporary Theory and Method.* T. M. Johnson and C. F. Sargent, eds. New York: Praeger, 149–58.

———. 1992. " 'Side Effects': Cultural Constructions and Reinterpretations of Western Pharmaceuticals." *Medical Anthropology Quarterly* 6:99–113.

———. 1994b. "The Negotiation of 'Side' Effects in Hausa (Northern Nigeria)

Therapeutics." In *Medicines: Meanings and Contexts*. N. L. Etkin and M. L. Tan, eds. Amsterdam and Quezon City, the Philippines: University of Amsterdam and HAIN, 17–32.

———. 1994c. "Consuming a Therapeutic Landscape: A Multicontextual Framework for Assessing the Health Significance of Human-Plant Interactions." *Journal of Home and Consumer Horticulture* 1(2/3):61–81.

———. 1995a. "Antimalarials of Plant Origin." Invited Plenary Address, "Biochemical Co-Evolution Symposium." Presented at the Annual Meeting of the Society for Economic Botany, Ithaca, New York, 21–25 June.

———. 1995b. "Plants as Antimalarial Drugs: Relation to G6PD Deficiency and Evolutionary Implications." Invited Plenary Address Presented at the Symposium "G6PD Deficiency: Evidence for Adaptation and Health Consequences." Cortona, Italy, 3–5 July.

———. 1997. "Medicinal Cuisines: Diet and Ethnopharmacology." *International Journal of Pharmacology* 34:313–26.

———. ed. 1986a. *Plants in Indigenous Medicine and Diet: Biobehavioral Approaches.* New York: Gordon and Breach.

———. ed. 1994a. *Eating on the Wild Side: The Pharmacologic, Ecologic, and Social Implications of Using Noncultigens.* Tucson: University of Arizona Press.

Etkin, N. L., and J. W. Eaton. 1975. "Malaria-Induced Erythrocyte Oxidant Sensitifity." In *Erythrocyte Structure and Function*. G. J. Brewer, ed. New York: Liss, 219–32.

Etkin, N. L., and P. J. Ross. 1982. "Food as Medicine and Medicine as Food: An Adaptive Framework for the Interpretation of Plant Utilization among the Hausa of Northern Nigeria." *Social Science and Medicine* 16:1559–73.

———. 1991. "Should We Set a Place for Diet in Ethnopharmacology?" *Journal of Ethnopharmacology* 32:25–36.

———. 1994. "Pharmacologic Implications of 'Wild' Plants in Hausa Diet." In *Eating on the Wild Side: The Pharmacologic, Ecologic, and Social Implications of Using Noncultigens*. N. L. Etkin, ed. Tucson: University of Arizona Press, 85–101.

Etkin, N. L., P. J. Ross, and I. Muazzamu. 1990. "The Indigenization of Pharmaceuticals: Therapeutic Transitions in Rural Hausaland." *Social Science and Medicine* 30:919–28.

Fitzpatrick, D. F., S. L. Hirschfield, and R. G. Coffey. 1995. "Endothelium-Dependent Vasorelaxation Caused by Various Plant Extracts." *Journal of Cardiovascular Pharmacology* 26(1):90.

Franquemont, C., E. Franquemont, W. Davis, T. Plowman, S. King, C. R. Sperling, and C. C. Niezgoda. 1990. *The Ethnobotany of Chinchero, an Andean Community in Southern Peru*. Chicago, Ill.: Field Museum of Natural History.

Friedman, M. J. 1981. "Hemoglobin and the Red Cell Membrane: Increased Binding of Polymorphic Hemoglobins and Measurement of Free Radicals in the Membrane." In *The Red Cell*. G. J. Brewer, ed. New York: Liss, 519–31.

Gilles, H. M., and D. A. Warrell, eds. 1993. *Bruce-Chwatt's Essential Malariology*. 3rd edition. London: Edward Arnold.

Gillin, F. D., D. S. Reiner, and C.-S. Wang. 1983. "Human Milk Kills Parasitic Intestinal Protozoa." *Science* 221:1290–92.

Golenser, J., E. Marva, M. Kamil, E. Hempelmann, A. Cohen, R. Har-El, and M.

Chevion. 1991. "Free Radicals and Malaria." *South African Journal of Science* 87:584–87.

Golenser, J., A. Tsafack, Y. Amichai, J. Libman, A. Shanzer, and Z. I. Cabantchik. 1995. "Antimalarial Action of Hydroxamate-Based Chelators and Potentiation of Desferrioxamine Action by Reversed Siderophores." *Antimicrobial Agents and Chemotherapy* 39(1):61–65.

Goonasekera, M. M., V. K. Gunawardana, K. Jayasena, S. G. Mohammed, and S. Balasubramaniam. 1995. "Pregnancy Terminating Effect of *Jatropha curcas* in rats." *Journal of Ethnopharmacology* 47:117–23.

Graf, E., and J. W. Eaton. 1990. "Antioxidant Functions of Phytic Acid." *Free Radical Biology and Medicine* 8:61–69.

Green, E. C. 1988. "Can Collaborative Programs between Biomedical and African Indigenous Health Practitioners Succeed?" *Social Science and Medicine* 27: 1125–30.

Hammerschmidt, D. E. 1986. "Chinese Diet and Traditional Materia Medica: Effects on Platelet Function and Atherogenesis." In *Plants in Indigenous Medicine and Diet: Biobehavioral Approaches*. N. L. Etkin, ed. New York: Gordon and Breach, 171–85.

Harvey, P. W. J., P. F. Heywood, M. C. Nesheim, K. Galme, M. Zegans, J.-P. Habicht, L. S. Stephenson, K. L. Radimer, B. Brabin, K. Forsyth, and M. P. Alpers. 1989. "The Effect of Iron Therapy on Malarial Infection in Papua New Guinea Schoolchildren." *American Journal of Tropical Medicine and Hygiene* 40: 12–18.

Hebbel, R. P., J. W. Eaton, M. Balasingam, and M. H. Steinberg. 1982. "Spontaneous Oxygen Radical Generation by Sickle Erythrocytes." *Journal of Clinical Investigation* 70:1253–59.

Hien, T. T., and N. J. White. 1993. "Qinghaosu." *Lancet* 341: 603–8.

Hoffman-Goetz, L. 1986. "Malnutrition and Immunological Function with Special Reference to Cell-Mediated Immunity." *Yearbook of Physical Anthropology* 29: 139–59.

Iauk, L., E. M. Galadi, S. Kirjavainen. 1993. "Analgesic and Antipyretic Effects of *Mucuna pruriens*." *International Journal of Pharmacognosy* 31(3):213.

Johns, T. 1990. *With Bitter Herbs They Shall Eat It: Chemical Ecology and the Origins of Human Diet and Medicine*. Tucson: University of Arizona Press.

Kagawa, K., K. Togura, and K. Uchida. 1993. "Platelet Aggregation Inhibitors in a Bhutanese Medicinal Plant, Shug Cher." *Chemical and Pharmaceutical Bulletin* 41(9):1604.

Kaufmann, J. C., and M. Elvin-Lewis. 1995. "Towards a Logic of Ethnodentistry at Antongobe, Southwestern Madagascar." *Economic Botany* 49:213–22.

Kinghorn, A. D., and M. F. Balandrin, eds. 1993. *Human Medicinal Agents from Plants*. Washington, D.C.: American Chemical Society.

Kitayaporn, D., K. E. Nelson, P. Charoenlarp, and T. Pholphothi. 1992. "Haemoglobin-E in the Presence of Oxidative Substances from Fava Bean May be Protective against *Plasmodium falciparum* malaria." *Transactions of the Royal Society of Tropical Medicine and Hygiene* 86:240–44.

Klayman, D. L. 1993. "*Artemisia annua*: From Weed to Respectable Antimalarial Plant." In *Human Medicinal Agents from Plants*. A. D. Kinghorn and M. F. Balandrin, eds. Washington, D.C.: American Chemical Society, 242–53.

Lanhers, M.-C., J. Fleurentin, and P. Dorfman. 1991. "Analgesic, Antipyretic, and Anti-Inflammatory Properties of *Euphorbia hirta*." *Planta Medica* 57(3):225.

Last, M. 1990. "Professionalisation of Indigenous Healers." In *Medical Anthropology: Contemporary Theory and Method*. T. M. Johnson and C. F. Sargent, eds. New York: Praeger, 349–66.

Longhurst, R. 1984. *The Energy Trap: Work, Nutrition and Child Malnutrition in Northern Nigeria*. Ithaca, N.Y.: Cornell University Program on International Nutrition.

Macfoy, C. A., and E. I. Cline. 1990. "*In vitro* Antibacterial Activity of Three Plants Used in Traditional Medicine in Sierra Leone." *Journal of Ethnopharmacology* 29:323–27.

Mao, A. A., A. Wetten, and P. D. S. Caligari. 1995. "In vitro Propagation of *Clerodendrum colebrookianum* Walp., a Potential Natural Anti-hypertension Medicinal Plant." *Plant Cell Reports* 14(8):493.

Mascolo, N., R. Jain, and F. Capasso. 1989. "Ethnopharmacologic Investigation of Ginger (*Zingiber officinale*)." *Journal of Ethnopharmacology* 27:129–40.

McKay, D. A. 1980. "Food, Illness, and Folk Medicine: Insights from Ulu Trengganu, West Malaysia." In *Food, Ecology and Culture*. J. R. K Robson, ed. New York: Gordon and Breach, pp. 61–66.

Meshnick, S. R. 1994. "The Mode of Action of Antimalarial Endoperoxides." *Transactions of the Royal Society of Tropical Medicine and Hygiene* 88(S1):31–32.

Meshnick, S. R., T. W. Tsang, F. B. Lin, H. Z. Pan, C. N. Chang, F. Kuypers, D. Chiu, and B. Lubin. 1989. "Activated Oxygen Mediates the Antimalarial Activity of Qinghaosu." In *Malaria and the Red Cell*. J. W. Eaton, S. R. Meshnick, and G. J. Brewer, eds. New York: Liss, 95–104.

Murray, M. J., A. M. Murray, N. J. Murray, M. B. Murray, and C. J. Murray. 1982. "Adverse Effects of Normal Nutrients and Foods on Host Resistance to Disease." In *Adverse Effects of Foods*. E. F. P. Jelliffe and D. B. Jelliffe, eds. New York: Plenum Press, 313–21.

Oliver, B. 1986. *Medicinal Plants in Tropical West Africa*. Cambridge: Cambridge University Press.

Palanichamy, S., and S. Nagarajan. 1990. "Antifungal Activity of *Cassia alata* Leaf Extract." *Journal of Ethnopharmacology* 29:337–40.

Paranjpe, P., and P. H. Kulkarni. 1995. "Comparative Efficacy of Four Ayurvedic Formulations in the Treatment of Acne Vulgaris: A Double-blind Randomised Placebo-Controlled Clinical Evaluation." *Journal of Ethnopharmacology* 49: 127–32.

Pelletier, D. L. 1994. "The Potentiating Effects of Malnutrition on Child Mortality: Epidemiologic Evidence and Policy Implications." *Nutrition Reviews* 52(12): 409–15.

Peña, N., A. Auró, and H. Sumano. 1988. "A Comparative Trial of Garlic, Its Extract and Ammonium-Potassium Tartrate as Anthelmintics in Carp." *Journal of Ethnopharmacology* 24:199–203.

Peters, W., and W. H. G. Richards, eds. 1984. *Antimalarial Drugs I: Biological Background, Experimental Methods, and Drug Resistance*. Berlin: Springer-Verlag.

Pollack, V., R. Segal, and J. Golenser. 1990. "The Effect of Ascaridole on the *in vitro* Development of *Plasmodium falciparum*." *Parasitological Research* 76:570–72.

Prietze, R. 1913–1914. "Arzneipflanzen der Haussa." *Zeitschrift fur Kolonialsprachen* 4:81–90.

Rafatullah, S., M. Tariq, M. A. Al-Yahya, J. S. Mossa, and A. M. Ageel. 1990. "Evaluation of Turmeric (*Curcuma longa*) for Gastric and Duodenal Antiulcer activity in rats." *Journal of Ethnopharmacology* 29:25–34.

Ross, P. J., N. L. Etkin, and I. Muazzamu. 1996. "A Changing Hausa Diet." *Medical Anthropology* 17:143–63.

Schram, R. 1971. *A History of the Nigerian Health Services*. Ibadan, Nigeria: Ibadan University Press.

Simmons, E. B. 1976. *Calorie and Protein Intakes in Three Villages of Zaria Province, May 1970–July 1971*. Zaria, Nigeria: Institute for Agricultural Research, Ahmadu Bello University.

Stephensen, C. B., J. O. Alvarez, J. Kohatsu, R. Hardmeier, J. L. Kennedy, and R. B. Gammon. 1994. "Vitamin A is Excreted in the Urine during Acute Infection." *American Journal of Clinical Nutrition* 60:388–92.

Stevenson, D. R. 1986. "High Blood Pressure Medicinal Plant Use and Arterial Pressure Change." In *Plants in Indigenous Medicine and Diet: Biobehavioral Approaches*. N. L. Etkin, ed. New York: Gordon and Breach, 252–65.

Stock, R. 1980. "Health Care Behavior in a Rural Nigerian Setting, with Particular Reference to the Utilization of Western-Type Health Care Facilities." Ph.D. dissertation, Department of Geography, University of Liverpool. University Microfilms.

———. 1983. "Distance and the Utilization of Health Facilities in Rural Nigeria." *Social Science and Medicine* 17:563–70.

Teng, C. M., F. N. Ko, and S. M. Yu. 1994. "Inventory of Exogenous Factors Affecting Platelet Aggregation Isolated from Plant Sources." *Thrombosis and Haematosis* 71(4):517.

Trager, W., and J. B. Jensen. 1976. "Human Malaria Parasites in Continuous Culture." *Science* 193:673–75.

Ulijaszek, S. J. 1990. "Nutritional Status and Susceptibility to Infectious Disease." In *Diet and Disease in Traditional and Developing Societies*. G. A. Harrison and J. C. Waterlow, eds. Cambridge: University of Cambridge Press, 137–54.

Vennerstrom, J. L., and J. W. Eaton. 1988. "Oxidants, Oxidant Drugs, and Malaria." *Journal of Medicinal Chemistry* 31:1269–77.

Wall, L. L. 1988. *Hausa Medicine: Illness and Well-Being in a West African Culture*. Durham, N.C.: Duke University Press.

Wernsdorfer, W. H. 1980. "The Importance of Malaria in the World." In *Malaria* Vol. 1: *Epidemiology, Chemotherapy, Morphology and Metabolism*. J. P. Kreier, ed. New York: Academic Press, 1–93.

World Health Organization. 1978. *The Promotion and Development of Traditional Medicine*. World Health Organization Technical Report no. 622. Geneva: WHO.

Wyatt, G. B. 1977. "Health in Melanesia." In *The Melanesian Environment*. J. H. Winslow, ed. Canberra: Australian National University Press, 459–62.

Wu Leung, Wo-T. 1968. *Food Composition Table for Use in Africa*. Bethesda, Md.: U.S. Department of Health, Education, and Welfare.

Zhang, Q. S., X. Ye, and Z. J. Wei. 1995. "Recent Progress in Research on *Tripterygium*: A Male Antifertility Plant." *Contraception* 51(2):121.

PART III

EMBODIED MIND: METAPHORS OF PAIN, PLACEBO, AND SYMBOLIC HEALING

Lévi-Strauss (1967) describes in some detail how the shaman and the mythology shared by him and the patient alter physiological processes through the control of mental processes, dissolving the boundary between self and other and offering reintegration to the patient. The "shaman provides a language" (p. 198) and, like the psychoanalyst, allows the conscious and the unconscious to merge. He does this through a shared symbolic system and that is why a cured individual improves the mental health of the group. Because of this, the patient performs a very important social function; he provides a definition for normalcy and validates the system by calling into play the group's sentiments and symbolic representations to have them "become embodied in real experience" (pp. 180–82). For these healers, the mind, the body, and the experiential field are one.

The key to this social process is the relationship between the process and the consequences of healing, one of the great foci from which we have much to learn from non-Western medicine. Figure III.1 sketches a few of the paths of consequences in the healing process. The patient experiences something amiss: his stomach hurts, he feels lonely and depressed, he develops a sore on his lip or a pain in his head. These symptoms may well, by themselves, have a series of consequences for the patient (path 1)—in the simplest case, they may frighten him and cause stress. In Figure III.1, this fear is a "conceptual consequence," and the stress is a "physiological consequence" of the fear (path 7). Stress, producing an experience itself (path 8), can compound fear, and therefore the system contains a feedback loop. The universal human response to such a situation is a kind of analysis we call diagnosis. Either alone or in consultation with family or therapist, the patient develops an explanation for his experience (path 2). Diagnosis has two types

Figure III.1
Paths of Consequence in the Healing Process

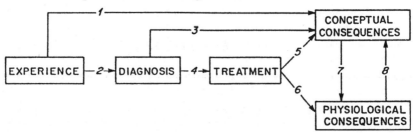

of consequence. The first is directly conceptual (path 3) and may vary greatly in degree. The diagnosis may be soothing ("Oh, it's just a fever sore") or terrifying ("Oh, it's skin cancer"). A soothing diagnosis may "damp down" the feedback loop, whereas a terrifying one may intensify it.

The second consequence or diagnosis (path 4) is treatment, which has two types of consequences, conceptual and physiological. Of course different treatments can have different kinds and degrees of physiological consequences. There is here, however, a particularly interesting interaction between the two types of consequences. The ointment may contain an astringent that will help heal the sore; the evidence of healing can encourage the patient, reducing his anxiety via pathways 6-8-7. This process is often generalized so that people develop a kind of faith—"Ointments heal sores"—which can itself be generalized—"Medications heal illnesses"— which can simultaneously induce healing via pathways 5-7-8.

This entire process is deeply embedded in culture. Sickness, a fundamental assault on person and society, is a matter of the deepest human concern; affecting life and death, it can induce deep emotional arousal. Not surprisingly, the act of healing, often including intensely dramatic ritual, shares qualities of the "numinous" in religious experience—it can be ineffable, absolute, and undeniable (Rappaport 1979:211–16). In simpler terms, the experience of healing can be highly marked.

We begin this section considering the shaman, not only in the sense mentioned above, but as the purveyor of archetypes of thought which, in Western culture, we have relegated to the realms of literature and art. Our anxiety-suppressing methods of studying shamans and their healing art might not be the best way to learn about shamanic healing or about ourselves (Romanucci-Ross, Chapter 9). Roberts develops a persuasive argument for the symbolic character of medicines, showing how a specific agent (the charred bones of immolated arsonists) represents a vast cosmological system in Tabwa therapeutics and witchcraft. In Lévi-Straussian terms mentioned above, we find an actual representation of metaphors for illness and cure acted upon to restore harmony to the community—disharmony or disorder had resulted from deviant behavior. Moerman examines "placebo surgery" and some bimodal aspects of coronary bypass surgery, that is, "real" changes in function strongly aided by a placebo effect. He argues that even in demonstrated physiological change there is room for explanation provided by a metaphoric structure surrounding the medical event.

Significant pain, Kugelman notes, gets woven into complex narratives that reflect and influence how people explain, treat, and "make sense" of their suffering in the trajectory of their lives. The varied discourses of pain emphasize the need for its medical recognition, not only of its spiritual and emotional aspects, but the physical reality as experienced by the sufferer. Ng, Dimsdale, and colleagues present us with the results of their study, demonstrating that while there were no differences in the amount of narcotics *self-administered* (by patient), there were significant differences in the amount of narcotic *prescribed* by physicians among Asians, blacks, Hispanics, and whites. Their study would appear to indicate that pain *is* medically recognized and relegated to concepts about racial and ethnic attributes, at least in some medical contexts—not, of course, what patients had in mind.

None of this is to suggest that the physiological consequences of medical treatment are not important; path 6 of Figure III.1, the central domain of biomedicine, is a fundamental one (see Part II of this book for detailed treatments of this path in non-Western medical traditions). It *is* to say that paths 1, 3, 5, and 7—that is, the conceptual consequences of sickness, diagnosis, and treatment—and their interactions are extremely important in understanding and controlling sickness. An integrated biohuman medical paradigm requires that all of these relationships be understood simultaneously. And biohuman medicine requires that they all be controlled to optimize the healing process.

REFERENCES

Lévi-Strauss, C. 1967. *Structural Anthropology*. Garden City, N.Y: Doubleday.
Rappaport, R. 1979. *Ecology, Meaning, and Religion*. Richmond, Calif.: North Atlantic Books.

9

THE IMPASSIONED KNOWLEDGE OF THE SHAMAN

LOLA ROMANUCCI-ROSS

The shaman can best be understood as a healer of the mind/body as well as the "body politic," or community. This is achieved through his or her status as the interpreter of symbols, those cultural instruments for perceiving and arranging reality. As interpreters in understanding the manifold meanings of sign and signifying function, they also play a role in the integration and use of symbols as generators and stylizers of patterns of systems, principally religious and medical, but also social, economic, and political. They are, therefore, significant vectors of a force that compels mind, matter, and experience (Romanucci-Ross 1980b). Enigma in a symbol, as Ricoeur (1970) suggested, does not block understanding but rather promotes it. One might also note that enigma is often a stimulus to innovation.

The shaman then, in shamanic cultures, emerges as "larger than life." This adds to therapeutic power as s/he (which will be abbreviated to "he" in this text) experiences mind and body metamorphoses in the patient-shaman encounter; the audience (family and others) is very much involved emotionally in this "medical event." As this psychosomatic drama unfolds, we learn what the society considers important in communication of assertions about the connectivity of all relationships from intrapersonal, to interpersonal, to communal, to the relations between humans and the rest of the universe. Where knowing and feeling are not viewed as distinctive processes, the shaman, whether he is being discursive or "iconic," is the community intellectual. Oral traditions, through the shaman, are passed along in rich contextual and personal pathways of meaning.

Possessing the ultimate power to heal or prevent illness and disaster, the

This chapter includes a number of concepts previously presented in Romanucci-Ross 1989. Permission granted by Istor Books.

shaman is a specialist in the combinatorial arts, that is, in the conjunction and disjunction of all objects and events in the universe, and he is keeper of the lore, which includes the collective psychology. As such, he is part of the group but apart. He must live morally, yet his art has important elements of the Dionysian, wild and orgiastic. He must be known for sexual absti- nence, yet he relates to the world in a mode we consider erotic.

Knowledge comes to him during events of tremendous feeling—pain, ec- stasy, and seizures, illness and trauma, at times self-inflicted. Other conduits for knowing are plants and animals and deceased predecessors. In trances or in other altered states brought about by self-inflicted suffering, the sha- man experiences "torture," "being cut to pieces," which lead to death and resurrection. In a hallucinating or "other-conscious" state, he goes on to the celestial sphere or may pursue his dreams in other places.[1] (Though Mela- nesia in the South Pacific is not considered a culture area known for classic shamanism, I nevertheless collected accounts from *tamberan* men whose ac- quisition of healing power and knowledge derived from elements mentioned above.)[2] For excellent recent accounts of what remains of "classic" shaman- ism and the changing images of the shaman in Eurasia, see Hoppál.

IMPASSIONED COGNITION

What does it mean to say that cognition can be "impassioned"? Does it mean knowing "objectively" with an overlay or a veneer of feeling? Or is it the grasping of an idea in a highly emotive state with an overlay of concen- sually validated knowledge? Or is it that moment of understanding we call "insight" which, as Lonergan (1965) asserts, comes suddenly and unex- pectedly as a release from the tension of inquiry which, pivoting as it does between the concrete and the abstract, must be described as a function not of outer circumstances but of inner conditions?

Cognition and affect are both socially constructed, but their being consid- ered separate or unified is *also* a social and cultural construct. Linguistically coded systems of classification order the Western universe; our linguistic codes include highly concentrated symbols in a closed universe of discourse, for example mathematical systems. Images are also a repository of informa- tion, although we tend not to think of them in that way. And, if we would emphasize "perceptual codes" as much as linguistic codes, we might then be forced to develop an "interlingual code" as suggested by Kosslyn (1980) because the structural differences between visual and verbal representations would be problematic for direct translation. Yet images can act as surrogate percepts, evoking as many responses as the actual object (Locke 1687).

Because we have favored the disjunction of cognition and affect, we still "seek" the lost map to the territory of shamanism. Our notion of "person" has also been an impediment. A "person" in Western culture is an abstrac- tion, a point in social space for the premises and corollaries of rights and duties; completely a cultural construct, the notion of "person" *(persona)* has been constructed as a mask for ritual (Kant 1797; Mauss 1925). That our ego-psychology has been dominated by these concepts and that it contrasts with other possibilities for concepts of "the person" can be readily appreciated in the reading of any complete ethnographic description of a "primitive" society. In these accounts person as indistinguishable from lineage or clan is seen almost immediately in the ease with which one slips into a kinship slot or other status slots with nonnegotiable privileges and duties from the moment of birth (see Romanucci-Ross 1985:81–95). Even those individuals who are labeled as having recognizable powers to heal or harm by touch or glance—the bringers of rain and hail or those who can change themselves to animals and then back to humans—are characterized by age, sex, personality, and social circumstances (Romanucci-Ross 1969; Nutini and Roberts 1989). (See note 1.)

Universal Themes

To know of the bloodsucking witches *(tlahuelpuchi)* in Tlaxcala, Mexico, is to find striking parallels with tales of vampirism in Europe and to think in terms of "universals." It brings one to the more fundamental question of the nature of "magic" knowledge. Since the road to such power is most often one of asceticism (self-denial) and self-torture, one might interpret the cutting up of the body and removal of limbs and organs "experienced" by the Siberian shaman as a dispersion of the self. Whether or not one accepts Roheim's analysis that magic may be "oral, anal, urethral, narcissistic or phallic," or a "revolt against the gods," one certainly feels comfortable with his notion that magic is "a great reservoir of strength against frustration and defeat" and a pitting of the self against the social and natural world (Roheim 1953).

Sources of shamanic symbols are found in the cyclicity of death and renewal in the universe, that structure which is permanent throughout changing manifestations of a phenomenon. The shaman has the map-series of abstractions shared within his own culture and, after mystical experiences, can translate these into concrete events. The shaman knows how ideas are to be conjoined and how to define the range onto which selected domains are mapped. Voyager returned from mystical experiences or trances, he brings back wondrous reports of the strange and thereby can redefine the range or alter the map.

Throughout the endeavor he indulges in an open and notorious fashion in poetry (simile, metaphor, allegory) as he describes "reality." For himself and his patients (individual and audience) he analogically overcomes great difficulties and obstacles in his "travels," assisted by dreaming and trance. His trials match those of the Greek classic heroes: traversing high gorges and narrow bridges, escaping quickly between huge rocks that will close

together, and so forth. These are universal themes in the making of a shaman, and paradigms within visionary experiences "validate"[3] the knowledge
brought back to those who await revelations. Long sea voyages, disasters,
one-eyed monsters, devastating winds and evil adversaries to be overcome
have always been part of voyages of self-discovery, metaphors of finding
oneself entrenched in the tradition of many cultures.

Seeking solitude, the shaman is provided a context for creativity by his
culture. In magical flight from creatures of his own kind, he goes to other
worlds and returns with his own version of them. In and out of vastly different worlds with ease (the art is to be inside but also outside everything),
the shaman can have his own subcultural ontology, epistemology, and ethics,
unifying real world and dreams and distorting data so that it flows into some
channels but not others.

The shaman relates to the world in a mode that is erotic, using a sensual
language; he is between Logos and Eros, between Apollo and Dionysius;
both the former and the latter are inseparable, each a set. Have we not *created*
a "problem" by breaking up each set into separate polarities? Do we not
therefore assess his sensual language in terms of a framed performance rather
than the range of his total competence?

We bring our words to our world of symbolic relations. Spoken and written
words (mainly, if not solely) touch off our images and systems of iconics.
Some would discuss symbols only in terms of language, and indeed, I think,
in Western culture, we do parallel symbols with the poetic imagination in
which we freely admit to grasping reality through emotions.

If we want to hypothesize that both shaman and poet know and use the
unconscious, we might refer to Coleridge, who admitted to looking at nature
and "asking for a symbolical language for something within me that already
and forever exists" of *Anima Poetae* (p. 34). In the *The Ancient Mariner*, he
employs the archetype of rebirth which has a long trajectory in classical
literature. Aeneas had long before offered Proserpine a golden bough, and,
guided by Sybil, he visits his father in the underworld, a landscape of darkness, void but with sunless lakes. From his father he received a prophecy
and a vision of his descendants before being dismissed through the ivory
gate of dreams. Dante's Hell is equally a dismal hole. Shivering with cold,
the voyager is not living, but also not dead. From Hell to Paradise is an
ascent through light of increasing intensity (Canto X). Here again we find a
plunging into the depth and the center (which are in you) for knowledge of
self and destiny. The whole of paradise is an emotion of "knowing" vast
order and harmony with the ranging vision of the flight of the eagle. Universal shamanic themes also include one chosen for his or her capacity for
ecstatic experience—a *maestro*, who leads and shows the way, who descends
into mystical death and ascends to celestial journeys, and returns to another
time *(illo tempore)*. (Dante chose Virgil as the *maestro*.)

Knowledge as illumination can be found from Dante to Rimbaud, and worlds of heroic deeds are in the many recurrent transformations of the Prometheus Unbound theme. Orpheus with his charmed music demonstrates the power of persuasion by incantation. Returned from the underworld, Orpheus is torn to pieces (once more, in our idiom, dispersion of self). In the literature of Christianity we find descents and ascents, temptations and tortures, and dismemberments caused by demons.

Even in everyday life, for example in New Guinea (Romanucci-Ross 1985) and from other societies of similar complexity, we find existential states and sets of behavior that have permeable boundaries: fish are transformed women; animals may speak, shed their skins, and become human; the sea and stones may cause pregnancy. One experiences feelings, and the sea and the wind act them out in a poetic imagination where knowing and feeling are not separate. So that as Bogoraz (1925) notes of the Chuckchees, "one may discuss the mathematics, physics, art and philosophy of shamanism."

"Intellectualized" Passions

Heirs to the metapsychology of Freud, we are believers in the layered trinity of mind, the marketplace model of "the-more-you-take-the-less-there-is" also known as "the limited good," unaware perhaps that Ricardo and the rent economists provided this lump-sum, fixed pool of economic resources assessment as a model. Perhaps if psychoanalysis were being assembled now *de novo*, we might choose the Keynesian economic model, and the "more-the-more" or "pump priming" model, based on Keynes, to expand the economy. (Economic models seem to have been considered quite appropriate as models for dynamics of the human spirit, cast an analytic eye on G. H. Mead, for example.) Furthermore, the eclectic epistemes of Sigmund Freud included his very personal interpretations of some aspects of the classic literature of the Western world and ethnology of his time—now much ignored except by the curiosity-shopping intellectual. Mixing all this with the scientism of the medicine of his time, Freud also equated illness and creativity. Fortified by psychoanalytic principles, many investigators return now to "interpret" original material in the field—this is *our* impassioned cognition. The shaman, then, who also had undergone his suffering willingly, awaits to be pronounced psychotic by many anthropologists and psychoanalysts. We found creativity and pronounced it illness. But the ability to dissolve ego boundaries is not the same as lack of ego boundaries (Roheim 1953).

The early methodologists of psychoanalysis, in their emphasis on the emergence of their "method" from medical science, were (and still are) reticent to acknowledge its many precursors. Following Biasin, it is suggested that it has been amply demonstrated that Freud did not come out of a void but was rather the culmination of a whole trend in the culture of the

nineteenth century (see Gadda and Whyte). From Platner, who coined the
term unconscious *(Unbewusstsein)* in 1776, through Schelling, Schopenhauer,
Nietzsche, von Hartman, and Carl Gustav Carus (we add Groddeck, who
had earlier coined Freud's "Id" as "It"), Freud received more than sufficient
material on "the unconscious," on mental illness, on family relationships, on
dreams, and so on to schematize and reduce to his "medical" terms. This
in itself would not deprive psychoanalysis of its possible therapeutic value
(which has not yet been demonstrated). The point here is that psychoanalysis is a macrocultural "judgment" that does not make sense outside its
universe of discourse (i.e., European cultural systems and their derivates).
One might therefore be justly puzzled by Norman O. Brown's "shattering
experience" when he "took a steadfast unflinching look at the Western
tradition of morality and rationality" and "what Freud had to say" (Brown
1959:3). "Shattering" only if one does not recognize that a phenomenon is
brilliantly explained because its very soul and substance was used to structure the theory that would then explain the phenomenon.

Devereux (1967) has asserted that the scientific study of man is impeded
by the anxiety-arousing overlap between subject and observer, and that
countertransference is the most crucial data of social science. The data of
the behavorial sciences are the behavior of the observed along with the
disturbances produced by the observational activities of the observer. Anxieties and defense maneuvers of the investigator give rise to research strategies and "decisions" that culminate in observer attribution of meaning.
Countertransference is the sum total of all those distortions in the psychoanalyst's perception of and reaction to his patient that cause him to react to
his patient as though he were an early *imago* and then act in the analytic
situation in terms of his usually infantile unconscious needs, wishes, and
fantasies (Devereux 1967).

What is the "stimulus value" of the shaman when he is taken out of his
total universe of discourse for interpretation? Devereux emphasizes that we
tend to discourage inquiry into the more anxiety-probing facts. We have
examples from the literature of anthropologists who tried to become "insid-
ers" of shamanic esoterica but eventually had to break away (Peters 1981).
Scientists are expected to justify the prevailing ideology and how one is to
think about things. We tend to note what is most different from our daily
lives and such anthropological data can elicit intense anxiety (Devereux
1967).

In the most enduring of his "combinatorial arts," the shaman (like the
poet) has an interest in relating and/or conjoining "person" and the mystical
body of society to achieve resurrections for mankind. Art in the form of
drama rich with visual and auditory symbols and/or language is the means
of sharing this moral commitment. In these dramatic "plots" passion determines behavior, reinforcing the old and perhaps introducing, on occasion,
the new. What is sometimes called catharsis transforms the aesthetic expe-

rience into moral (and political?) insight, shaping the body politic in community interaction.[4]

We can hope to go beyond partial understanding of shamanism by accepting its terms and permises for meaning and to be at least conscious of our own. Note the words with which we describe our modalities of knowing: "cognition" derives from the Latin *cogito*, which means "I shake together"; *intellego* means "I select among," *scio* (from which we get our word "science") means "I separate." As we shake, select, and separate, we seek aggregates that please our aesthetics, that is, our cultivated and "cultured" sense of form, beauty, and elegance. Shamanic societies have a cultural aesthetic, perhaps more relational than discriminatory, and perhaps more inclusive than boundary-seeking, that has shaped another modality of knowing and living in this world—their own structuring for science and morality as well as art forms.

NOTES

1. Recent research suggests a physiological basis for shamanic ecstasy. We refer to "endogenous morphine-like substances" (a description which collapses verbally into "endorphins") in the body, enkephalin and functional aspects of the neuroendocrine opioid system as these relate to perception and to kinesis. Such assumptions need not detain us here as our concern is with the external pathways (rhythmicity, dance, song, communality), and presumably these would affect all human beings in a similar fashion (Jilek 1982).

2. Kampo, of the Admiralty Islands of New Guinea, told me of how he received the gift of healing from a bush spirit *(marsalai)*. First he had traveled in dreams (under a large tree). In these dreams he again met this same *marsalai* named Pewaseu, who gave him five pieces of ginger root, with which, and by pronouncing the name Pewaseu, he could cure anything. But for five days he could eat only fire ("It's just like eating yams!"); after this, he was told, he would have power (Romanucci-Ross 1963–1967).

3. Richard de Mille's interpretation of "validity" and "authenticity" are pertinent here. "A report is judged valid when it agrees with what we think we know" ... "authenticity refers to the provenance of the report. Did it arise from the persons, places, and procedures it describes?" (De Mille 1980:44).

4. See Else (1938), the major proponent of the transformation (in Western literature) from aesthetics to morality. To add a few sources from divergent ideologies: St. Thomas Aquinas, Augustine, Corinthians XV:22, Marx, Freud, and Durkheim, for example.

REFERENCES

Augustinus, St. 1962. *The City of God (De Civitate Deo)*, trans. John Healey. New York: E. P. Dutton.

Biasin, G. 1975. *Literary Diseases: Theme and Metaphor in the Italian Novel*. Austin: University of Texas Press.

Bogoraz, W. 1925. "Ideas and Concept of Space and Time." *American Anthropologist* 27(2):205–66.

Brown, N. O. 1959. *Life against Death: The Psychoanalytic Meaning of History.* New York: Random House.

Carus, K. G. 1962. *Symbolik der menschlichen Gestalt.* Stuttgart: n.p.

Coleridge, S. T. 1895. *Anima Poetae,* ed. E. H. Coleridge. London:W. Heinemann.

De Mille, R. 1980. *The Don Juan Papers: Further Castaneda Controversies.* Santa Barbara, Calif.: Ross-Erickson.

Devereux, G. 1967. *From Anxiety to Method in the Behavioral Sciences.* The Hague: Mouton.

Durkheim, E. 1912 (1961). *The Elementary Forms of Religious Life.* New York: Collier Books.

Eliade, M. 1964. *Shamanism: Archaic Techniques of Ecstasy.* New York: Pantheon Books.

Ellenberger, H. 1970. *The Discovery of the Unconscious.* London: Allen Lane.

Else, G. F. 1938. "Aristotle on the Beauty of Tragedy." *Harvard Studies in Classical Philology* 44:179–204.

Freud, S. 1953–1974. "Interpretation of Dreams." In *Standard Edition of Freud's Works.* vols. 4–5. J. Strachey, ed. London: Hogarth Press.

———. 1953–1984. *Moses and Monotheism.* vol. 9. J. Strachey, ed. London: Hogarth Press.

Fromm, E., and M. Maccoby. 1971. *Social Character in a Mexican Village.* Englewood Cliffs, N.J.: Prentice-Hall.

Gadda, C. 1958. *I Viaggi la Morte.* Milton: Garzanti.

Groddeck, G. 1961. *The Book of the It.* New York: Vintage Books.

Hoppál, M., ed. 1984. *Shamanism in Eurasia, Parts I and II.* Gottingen: Herodot.

Jilek, W. G. 1982. "Altered States of Consciousness in North American Indian Ceremonials." *Ethos* 10(4):317–43.

Kant, I. 1790 (1970). *Critique of Judgment.* New York: Free Press.

———. 1797 (1996). *Metaphysics of Morals.* trans. Mary Gregor. Cambridge: Cambridge University Press.

Kaufman, W., ed. 1959. *Nietzsche.* New York: Viking Press.

Keynes, J. M. 1936. *The General Theory of Employment, Interest and Money.* New York: Harcourt.

Kosslyn, S. M. 1980. *Image and Mind.* Cambridge, Mass: Harvard University Press.

Locke, J. 1687 (1993). *Essay on Human Understanding.* Vol. 2. Boston: C. E. Tuttle.

Lonergan, B. B. 1965. *Insight: A Study of Human Understanding.* New York: Philosophical Library.

Marx, K. 1859 (1904). *The Critique of Political Economy.* Trans I. N. Stone. Chicago: International Library Publication Co.

Mauss, M. 1925. *Essai sur le don: forme et raison de l'echance dans les sociétiés archaiques. Anné Sociologique* 1:30–186.

Nutini, H., and J. Roberts. 1989. *The Social and Psychological Context of Bloodsucking Witchcraft in Rural Tlaxcala.* Princeton, N.J.: Princeton University Press.

Peters, L. 1981. *Ecstasy and Healing in Nepal: An Ethnopsychiatric Study of Tamang Shamanism.* Malibu, Calif.: Undena Publications.

Ricardo, D. 1815. *Essay on the Influence of a Low-Price of Corn on the Profits of Stock.* London: n.p.

Ricoeur, P. 1970. *Freud and Philosophy: An Essay on Interpretation*. Trans. Denis Savage. New Haven, Conn.: Yale University Press.

Roheim, G. 1953. *Magic and Schizophrenia*. Bloomington: Indiana University Press.

Romanucci-Ross, L. 1963–1967. *Field Notes and Research Notations on the New Guinea-Admiralty Islands Expedition for the American Museum of Natural History*. Washington, D.C.: Smithsonian Institution, Margaret Mead Collection.

———. 1969. "The Hierarchy of Resort in Curative Practices: The Admiralty Islands, Melanesia." *Journal of Health and Social Behavior* 10:201–9.

———. 1973. *Conflict, Violence and Morality in a Mexican Village*. Palo Alto, Calif.: Mayfield. 2d ed., Chicago: University of Chicago Press, 1985.

———. 1979. "Melanesian Medicine." In *Culture and Curing: Anthropological Perspectives on Traditional Medical Beliefs and Practices*. Pittsburgh. University of Pittsburgh Press, 115–38.

———. 1980a. "Anthropological Field Research: Margaret Mead, Muse of the Clinical Experience." *American Anthropologist* 82(2):304–17.

———. 1980b. "On the Researching of Lost Images." *Anthropology and Humanism Quarterly* 5(1):14–20.

———. 1985. *Mead's Other Manus: Phenomenology of the Encounter*. South Hadley, Mass.: Bergin & Garvey.

———. 1989. "The Impassioned Cogito: Shaman and Anthropologist." In *Shamanism: Past and Present*. M. Hoppal and O. J. Sadovszky, eds. Los Angeles/Fullerton: Istor Books, 35–47.

Ross, W. D. *Kant's Ethical Theory*. Oxford: Oxford University Press.

Strauss, A., ed. 1964. *George Herbert Mead on Social Psychology*. Chicago, Ill.: University of Chicago Press.

Thomas Aquinas. 1990. *The Treatise on Law (Summa Theologiae)*. Trans. R. J. Heale. Notre Dame, Ind.: University of Notre Dame Press.

Whyte, L. L. n.d. *The Unconscious before Freud*. New York: Doubleday Anchor Books.

10

ANARCHY, ABJECTION, AND ABSURDITY: A CASE OF METAPHORIC MEDICINE AMONG THE TABWA OF ZAIRE

ALLEN F. ROBERTS

In memory of Minnie G. Curtis

THE EVENT

On 10 October 1960, two young men named Kiyumba and Mulobola[1] rode their bicycles from Kirungu to Chief Kaputo's village, ostensibly to purchase reed mats to resell at Kirungu market. In fact, their intention was to steal tax moneys held by the chief's clerk; Kiyumba would set fire to the chief's residence, and while everyone's attention was fixed on the blaze, Mulobola would break into the clerk's and steal the funds. Kiyumba did his part, not realizing that the chief himself was napping inside. Women saw him and sounded the alert. Mulobola, frightened by the ensuing commotion, took flight, while Kiyumba was captured by the chief's men. Kiyumba was thrashed till he admitted his plan and told where his partner would probably be waiting for him, on the road back to Kirungu. Mulobola, too, was apprehended, and both were beaten senseless. Chief Kaputo sent his car to fetch his judge, then visiting a nearby village; the judge later told me that by the time he arrived at the chief's, the thieves were in a pitiful state. He could do nothing, at that point, to alter the course of the event.

Accounts vary as to what occurred next. The official inquest[2] found that "in a paroxysm of anger," Chief Kaputo Lambo ordered that the two men be burned alive. As though summing up the event, the report concludes that "a very important detail should not be overlooked...: Kiyumba was found bearing an MNC Lumumba card." My informants skipped over this detail. The judge said that he saw Kanengo, the chief's counselor and a noted practitioner of traditional medicine (*mfumu*, pl. *wafumu*), take a long, sharp knife and lead young men from the village in carrying the two thieves to the bridge across a nearby stream. The judge later learned that the two had been burned alive. As Nzwiba, another practitioner and close informant, said, "This [the culprits' ashes] is what is called *kapondo*. *Wafumu* practitioners from all over went and got *vizimba* medicines then. Many, many went there, and those who have *kapondo* will show it to you if you ask, and will say it came from that time at Chief Kaputo's. If you say you want to buy some, ah, you buy it."[3]

THE HISTORICAL CONTEXT

With Independence on 30 June 1960, the Congo began a series of convulsions, relatively mild at first, that would lead to unparalleled tragedy. A week after Independence, the Force Publique mutinied; several days later, before a rumored intervention by the Soviet Union could occur, United Nations troops arrived in the Congo; and almost concurrently, Katanga seceded. Through July and August, Katangans lived in fear of an expected invasion by the Congolese National Army (ANC); in August, Kasai also seceded and sought federation with Katanga. In September, the ANC occupied several key centers in Kasai, and many civilians were killed. President Kasavubu divested Prime Minister Lumumba of his powers, and vice versa; Colonel Mobutu declared both parties "neutralized" till the end of the year. On 10 October, Lumumba was confined to his official residence, with UN troops assuring his security by occupying the gardens around the house, while ANC forces menaced all within the periphery of the property they surrounded.

Tabwa living along the southwestern shores of Lake Tanganyika were within the old province and new state of Katanga and were among the earliest and most ardent supporters of Tshombe's breakaway government, providing several of its first ministers and other high officials. The tumultuous nature of these first months of double independence was the backdrop for the questioning of much more local authority; unrest would grow among Tabwa around Kirungu, as factions long denied power within the colonial hierarchy of chiefs attempted to wrest control from their adversaries. With international, national, regional, and local tensions so high, an attempted robbery was not especially remarkable; the judiciary could not focus attention upon such an event in such times. Instead, the Belgian Magistrat Instructeur noted that one of the perpetrators had allegedly possessed the party identity card of those against whom Katangans were fighting for independence, and the matter was dropped without Chief Kaputo, his counselor Kanengo, or anyone (but the two thieves) receiving the least punishment.

THE ACTORS

It is difficult to say much about the two thieves. Present-day residents of Chief Kaputo's village remember the event, but nothing of the young men; I did not contact their families. Although others in the area who engaged in overtly political, insurrectionist actions during these same years are well known and still celebrated locally, these two are not. It seems most likely that the general state of alarm prevailing throughout Katanga and the attraction of a strongbox containing 8,000 francs in tax receipts proved too great a temptation for the two, who sought only private gain. They were not (or were not allowed to become) "social bandits"—men acting with public (or at least factional) approbation in social protest against forces commonly perceived as "the oppressor" (see Hobsbawn 1965, 1981). The magistrate, trying to justify (or at least to pass over) both their assassinations and the lack of pursuit by an overtaxed Katangan judiciary, seems to imply that they *were* social bandits, acting in the name of a political party subversive to the Katangan state. Rather, they were deemed criminals by Chief Kaputo's people, men without regard for order as personified by the chief whose life they had wantonly threatened in the course of their attempted robbery.

Chief Kaputo Lambo (dead in the mid-1960s) was known as an irascible fellow whose ambitions for power within his local political arena knew few bounds. He tried to replace an inferior chief in the colonial hierarchy whose insistence of superiority by tradition and precolonial history had long chafed him; when this effort was foiled, with great loss of face, Kaputo saw to it that he was physically abused by soldiers. It is still believed that Kaputo had great medicines at his disposal, including an ability to send "lion" to maim or kill his enemies. Such powers are associated with Kanengo, his closest henchman.

Until his death in the late 1970s, Kanengo was widely renowned for two capacities: his knowledge of Chief Kaputo's history, for which he was consulted in all affairs in which the legitimacy of the chief's rule was questioned; and his knowledge of medicines. When my wife and I knew him, he was living in exile from Kaputo's chiefdom after protracted quarrels with the man who succeeded to the chair at the death of Kaputo Lambo. As a gauge of his marginality, Kanengo's house—far from any village and located deep in a swamp—was the only round (hence, "traditional") one we saw in four years among the Tabwa. He was known as the greatest practitioner of *mfumu* in the area, and the most difficult cases were taken to him. A kinsman of his who had violent psychotic episodes was kept in stocks in the same yard in which others—there for treatment, or living with Kanengo—were seated or seeing to everyday chores. Kanengo told us that he had tried all his means to heal the young man, but was resisted at every turn; we were left with the distinct impression that the old man would "solve" the problematic case whether or not the disturbed nephew survived his cure. He suggested that my wife (an anthropologist studying traditional medicine, who as a paramedic ran a small clinic of Western medicine) give injections of his traditional medicines to his kinsman and other difficult cases. This and his attempt to involve us in his conflict with the seated Chief Kaputo (by telling others *we* wanted to divest him of power, and as expatriates would see that it happened) left us very uneasy in our dealings with Kanengo.

Kanengo was also one of only two Tabwa we ever knew who was reputed to have been (or perhaps to still be) in the Kazanzi society (BaKazanzi). This society was introduced to the central Luba around the turn of the nineteenth century by Luba traders visiting the Songye (Reefe 1981:118) and spread to the lands along the Luvua and Lukuga rivers (Lebaigne 1933).[4] It was popular among northern Tabwa (or "Holoholo") at the turn of the twentieth century (Schmitz 1912:278) and was encountered among ("Luba-ized") western Tabwa (or "Hemba") slightly thereafter (Colle 1913:528). An elderly informant once came upon a seance of the society at Chief Rutuku's near the Lubilaye (and counts himself lucky to have escaped unscathed!), but said that the society never spread farther south than that. The BaKazanzi may have survived the first decades of the 1900s, but in an attenuated form, being replaced by new religious organizations more apt in the context of established colonialism (e.g., BuGabo, Ukanga). It did not disappear altogether. As one old man remarked with acerbity, "It lasted long after the Belgians came; even when they finally left [in 1960], they didn't know how to 'see' sorcerers, so how could they 'see' Kazanzi adepts?"

Among Luba, the Kazanzi eliminated avenging ghosts by disinterring corpses, burning fagots in the opened graves to prevent the spirits' return, and incinerating the remains for later use as medicines (Lebaigne 1933; Joset 1934). All Tabwa I questioned contended that Kazanzi adepts among them killed and ate sorcerers identified by diviners and/or the poison oracle (and denied that war enemies, the elderly, slaves, or others of "lowly condition" would also be consumed, as stated in Colle 1913:540). With macabre detail, Tabwa recount how adepts would be summoned by a chief to eliminate one designated a sorcerer. Using the strength of their medicine called *niembo* or *buyembe* (as in Colle 1913:541; Burton 1961:171), they would secrete medicines in the headpad the victim used to carry loads, and this would cause the soul (*roho* in Swahili, *mutima* in KiTabwa) to leave the body. The sorcerer would be powerless against this, and his/her body would then go to the Kazanzi camp. The adepts, their faces crimson with *nkula* powder ground from Pterocarpus bark (this a "symbol of blood" [*mfano ya damu*], as I was told), would dance about and start to dissect the victim, beginning with the legs, as the victim looked on vacuously. When the sorcerer finally fell, his/her flesh would be eaten, openly, it was said, in contrast to the secret manner in which sorcerers consume the flesh of their victims. Colle reports that as they did this, they would imitate the hyena's cry (1913:539). The bones would be burned and used as medicines. BaKazanzi also danced, publicly performing incredible feats such as piercing their cheeks. In the past, they held regular ceremonies during the dark of the moon (Schmitz 1912: 281).

THE ACTION

The execution of the two thieves at Chief Kaputo's is most easily explained as the result of "a paroxysm of anger"; that the chief's house was set afire, and that he himself was asleep inside at the time, would seem due cause for retribution. The severity and form of the method, the choice of executioner, and the ultimate meaning of the act as reflected in what became of the relics are not so simply explained.

A common Tabwa adage is that "theft and sorcery are of one path." The perpetrators of either manifest a disregard for others' sanctity, act in contradiction to community, and therefore taunt and threaten social life. Sorcery for Tabwa is a "solar" activity; God and the sun are both said to be sorcerers in their lack of limit (hence, figuratively, of pity [*uruma*]) and through their association with death. God is said to feast upon humans "like goats," and the sun kills crops (and hence humans) when it shines unabated. Yet the sun is recognized as necessary to life, the order of which is synonymous with a god called *Leza Malango* ("Almighty Intelligence").

Opposed to these phenomena is the marked discontinuity of the life cycle. Kinship is considered a phenomenon expanding outward from a central point where there emerged, either from a deep body of water or a subterranean passage, the first human beings. As generations passed, humankind spread out to populate the lands surrounding this point. Such a concept is given representation (or found) in spirals such as that of *mpande* conus shell disks, once an important symbol of chiefship and still revered as an ancestral shrine item.[5] The *mpande* is of a paradigm with the moon, as is most clearly indicated in a Tabwa myth in which they can be interchanged (A. F. Roberts 1980:426–27). Each turn of its spiral is analogous to the "belt" of a chief; succession is called "to wear the belt" *(kuvaa mukaba)*, and the succession of generations can be imagined as concentric circles, each succeeding generation encompassing previous ones. A paradox of existence is that while life is eternal in that the "belt" is always inherited (except in the case of executed sorcerers), it is finite in that each individual is born and dies (ibid.: 98–101). Sorcery is an action opposing such expansion, as those who superficially appear supportive kinsmen or neighbors nefariously rob their victims of vitality and finally "eat their flesh." Sorcerers, when caught and executed, are not succeeded, and every attempt is made to obliterate them physically and from memory (*kufuta*). Thieves with so little regard for life and property would be meted out condign punishment, and Tabwa are hard pressed or loath to draw a distinction between sorcerers and thieves in cases of the sort.

Kanengo was the executioner of the two young men, a role for which his cultic background had prepared him technically and for which his personality

was attuned. Several of the traits characteristic of Kazanzi adepts are especially apt in this case, and may be elaborated.

Colle reported that as the BaKazanzi partook of their ghastly repast, they
uttered the cry of the hyena. A reference to this animal, in turn, allows a
clearer understanding of the place of Kazanzi adepts in their contemporary
society. Specifically, *baendo* joking partners, who see to the burial of members of their opposite clans, are called "hyena"; and the classificatory grandchildren who orchestrate the burial of a chief are assigned the term even
more explicitly. Those who act as *baendo* and bury someone one day will
receive the same service from their opposites another. The cutting insults
they offer must be tolerated, as they, too, will be returned on a later occasion.
This sort of exchange is called *vizambano*, and the image Tabwa evoke in
explaining the term is of boys wrestling, first one on top of and pinning the
other, then the one on the bottom reversing his partner. Such alternation
finds its obvious analogy in that of the seasons, and the fierce but jocular
behavior of the "hyena" is that of dry-season heroes seeing to the bloody
business of change.

The burial of a chief is performed in a lunar idiom, the period of his reign
analogous to the light of the moon, his death to the tenebrous two or three
days prior to the new moon. It is no coincidence that the Kazanzi adepts,
too, chose this time for their celebrations. For Tabwa, moonlight is thought
auspicious, as it allows one to discern predators lurking on the periphery of
the community or along one's path; on the other hand, the dark of the moon,
called *kamwonang'anga*, is a liminal time, fraught with danger. The name
means "the one seen by the *ng'anga* or practitioner": the moon is "still
there," but can only be seen by those with supernatural vision. The moon
is a *mulozi* or sorcerer then, as it effects its apparent journey from the east,
where its final sliver was seen, to the west, where it will newly appear; during
kamwonang'anga, Lake Tanganyika, whipped by high winds, unleashes its
most treacherous furies, and the most pernicious beasts are in evidence. In
contrast, game and fish may be seen in especially large numbers, but they
will elude their pursuers; they have been "closed" by the moon, as people
say (A. F. Roberts 1980:111–18). The moon, then, usually lights a person's
way, or "leads" the person, just as a chief is ordinarily the "father of his
people" and looks to their succor. Yet, on a regular basis, the hidden side
of the moon—like that of a chief—will predominate. As Father Theuws has
written of beliefs held by people closely related to the Tabwa, "the moon
is ambiguous as is life itself: ... to be and become, to live and to die are
but two faces of the same reality" (1968:11). Tabwa chiefs are leaders of
their people but they are also deemed the greatest sorcerers of the land.
Theirs is the marginality of privilege. They do not kill and eat victims like
other sorcerers, but they do condone the practice in their community. It is
said that sorcerers will bring a portion of the meat of their victim to the
chief, who will sell it to other sorcerers, thus drawing a direct profit. For

Tabwa, lunar and solar tropes are used to order and understand life, but neither is univocal; each has two sides, and when the positive of one predominates, often it does so in contradistinction to the other, and vice versa.

THE HYENA AND ITS METAPHORIC SIGNIFICANCE

The spotted hyena, *Crocuta crocuta*, is a *solar* animal, and so opposed to the moon and those of its idiom. A Tabwa myth tells of a hyena fetching the sun and bringing it to the universe. The sun is said to be unchanging, hence unmarked (whereas the moon has phases and period); unlike the moon, it is sexless and not personified. The trait of the spotted hyena making it most sunlike through metaphor is its apparent lack of sexual dimorphism. Observers as early as Aristotle commented upon this, and as noted in the twelfth-century *Bestiary*, the spotted hyena's "nature is that at one moment it is masculine and at another moment feminine, and hence it is a dirty brute" (White 1960:3).[6] Beidelman has reviewed the spotted hyena's other odd characteristics noticed by many African observers and given moral sense via metaphor: they have an odd posture and gait, with front legs longer than back; their "grotesque and somewhat humanoid calls [have been] described by some writers as demonic"; they "paste" an odoriferous substance from anal glands to mark territory; and they chew up and digest bones left as refuse by other predators, so that their droppings may be white—and "hot," as Tabwa say—as a consequence (Beidelman 1975:190; see also Sapir 1981). Important for Tabwa in conjunction with this last is the hyena's *malosi*, the singular vision that they believe allows the beast to see carrion at great distances; metaphorically, this would assist "hyena" in perceiving sorcerers. Like hyenas, Kazanzi adepts are reputed to have exhumed corpses, especially of those "proven" sorcerers by the poison oracle, and to have obliterated them (just as hyenas consume bones, the final vestige of vital form). Finally, hyena anal hairs *may* have been a transform for the *kizimba* of the rainbow-producing serpent, Nfwimina. If for Kaguru such "liminal qualities make hyena the witches of the animal world" (Beidelman 1975: 190), for Tabwa these same allow "hyena" to turn *against* the sorcerers with whom they are somewhat consonant. Sorcerers in the social realm, like hyenas in the natural, are betwixt or altogether outside of the categories by which life is ordered (cf. Turner 1967:97 and passim). Being quintessentially "between," they bespeak transition, both negative (sorcerers robbing the vitality of crops or kin) and positive ("hyena" restoring order by destroying sorcerers).

After a Tabwa chief is buried,[7] classificatory grandchildren—whose "souls are red" like the camwood powder and Lady Ross's turaco plumes they sport—are said to lust for blood, and a moment called *kisama* is begun. All goods on their way back from the watercourse beside or under which they have buried the chief are broken or confiscated; chickens, goats, and even small children are slaughtered; and adult kinsmen of the chief are captured, mistreated, and held for ransom. The chief's surviving kinsmen hasten to placate them, and, their rampage stopped, the same "grandchildren" choose a successor. It is they who sing "he returns, he awakens, he awakens" as they circle the hut where the successor is hidden, bidding him to "reappear" like the new moon.

In this act they echo the role of the cosmic serpent Nfwimina, which stops the rains with the rainbow, yet assures their return with the smoke of the dry season's last and most important bushfires. Tabwa place a medicine bundle at a point in the woods which they intend to make the center of a fire lit from several sides; it is hoped that all four cardinal winds will join to bring the fire to a flaming circle, trapping game at the center where the medicines have been hidden. An element of this *nsipa* bundle[8] is the belt of an executed sorcerer *(mukaba wa mulozi)*, and the pyric circle of the bush-fire repeats its message of destruction and contraction, so opposed to the expansion of the generations. Another *kizimba* used in the bundle is that of Nfwimina, the solar serpent; and when the circle closes, annihilating all brought within its constricting perimeter, the column of smoke that rises above the point is said to be Nfwimina itself, standing on the tip of its tail, its head toward the heavens. This moment is one of several vital transformations: wild animals become meat (even "cooked" meat!), and the column of smoke causes clouds to "build" *(kujenga)*, carrying the first rains, which will in turn extinguish the bushfires.

The "hyena" have staged the death of the chief (which is hidden from the populace till the decomposition of the corpse is such that the skull falls from the body), the *kisama* interregnum, and the reapparition, just as the dry-season heroes bring back the wet. "Hyena" had other roles in Tabwa society, in which their dread propensities had an ultimately moral denouement. One didactic tale recorded by Schmitz among northern Tabwa recounts how Kimbwi, the hyena, changed into a person and accepted a baby from a negligent mother intent on going off dancing, only to smash the baby's head on a rock (1912:268). Although there were theriomorphic lions (and Tabwa terrorists who assumed this disguise), aside from random stories in which an odd circumstance might be explained (unconvincingly for many listeners) by sorcerers assuming some other animal's form, Tabwa do not speak of hyena-men. That is, when they speak of "hyena," this is a figurative term, one with social connotations for Tabwa, but not evidence of a belief in metempsychotic transformation to this beast.

As "hyena," then, the Kazanzi adepts—like classificatory grandchildren burying a chief—oversaw a transformation important to the continuity of social life. As a "stabilizing institution," they were " 'saviors to the whole community' " (Reefe 1981:205 citing W. F. P. Burton, p. 118). Unlike the "grandchildren," they were summoned by will rather than circumstance, by a desire to eliminate a sorcerer rather than by the death of a chief. They reduced the sorcerer to nothing. It is not clear whether they engaged in the anthropophagous orgies early missionaries did, and Tabwa still do, attribute to them; this may have been feigned as a part of their showmanship, of which the piercing of their cheeks while they danced was another example. A few colonial authorities denied the existence of the practice (Lebaigne 1933), but most repeated or rephrased the ghoulish details of Father Colle and other missionaries as though absolute truth (e.g., Administrateur Territorial 1919). Such a clear-cut "failure to comprehend that they were dealing with inverted moral orders, rather than descriptions of concrete happenings" (Arens 1979:153), had political motivations and consequences best elaborated elsewhere.[9] More significant was the adepts' obliteration of the sorcerer, their dismembering of the cadaver (or, perhaps, of the yet-living), incineration of its bones, and their transmutation of the circumstance and substance into an elemental meaning for use in medicines. The disruptive were then brought back into order and put to the service of the community, I would suggest, in the same way that the smoke from the last and most intense bushfires, catalyzed by the *nsipa* bundle with its *vizimba* of a sorcerer's belt and Nfwimina, brings the clouds of the season's first rains.

THE MEANING

The elements of Tabwa traditional medicine are of two clear-cut categories, *miti* ("trees" in KiTabwa) plant substances, and *vizimba* (s. *kizimba*), or what Richards has called "activating agents" (1969). These latter are mostly parts of animals, references to place (e.g., a pebble from the mountaintop wherein resides an Earth spirit) or to circumstance (e.g., a piece of root traversing a path upon which one has tripped). A few may be termed relics in that they are parts of human beings whose essence or history may be typified. To possess knowledge of these is suspicious; to *use* them, much more so, and always subject to situational interpretation, either condemned as sorcery or deemed pardonable when resorted to in "self-defense."

As C. D. Roberts has written, "the transformative capacity of any kizimba is referred to by people not as its 'strength' (*nguvu*), but as its 'meaning' (*maana* in Swahili)" (1981). When the two thieves were burned alive, their bones were taken and used as the *kapondo kizimba*. Different informants explain *kapondo* in various ways, according to their level of esoteric knowledge and their descriptive flair; an overarching or underlying meaning can be discerned in them all. Kiuma, a chief's son in his 60s who is *not* a practitioner, said that *kapondo* is when someone dies alone in the bush of hunger or lack of care; this, he stated, is what Nfwimina is, and furthermore both are the same as a woman who has never menstruated or had children, a "woman-man." Others, among them practitioners, articulate this knowledge, distinguishing among these parts; all *are* related, and a relic of a *musala* or amenorrheal woman *is* a transform of the *kizimba* of Nfwimina, the rainbow-breathing solar serpent (whose story Kiuma did not know; see A. F. Roberts 1980: 244–49). These are related to but not the same as *kapondo*. Another nonpractitioner said that this was someone who lives alone in the woods without fields or a house, and who steals from others; such a person's "head is not right" *(kichwa si sawa, hata)*. He went on to describe a case of this when he was a boy, of a woman who lived in the hills like an animal, with hair and fingernails exaggerated to the point of bestiality. As an aside, it may be added that Kanengo (the executioner of the two thieves) once said that crazy people are like Mbote "pygmies": they run about in the woods and will sleep anywhere.

Other Examples of Alienation

Practitioners offered more elaborated explanations. Kabemba (the only person whom we ever met with *muyembe* medicines like Kanengo's said *kapondo* is a person walking alone, fallen upon and killed for no reason. Kalwele (a renowned practitioner living at Chief Kaputo's) said this is someone who has been "taken" by a possessing spirit *(pepo)*, a usage repeated by others (see C. D. Roberts 1981); when I said that the same term had been used in reference to the two thieves, he noted that to burn a chief's house, one must have been possessed by a bad spirit or *shetani* (from "Satan"). All of these explanations bespeak mental and/or social alienation, hence absurdity, discordance. Yet by being contrary to reason, by being antistructural, they are part of a greater whole demanding dialectic to define reason.

The word *kapondo* is from a verb meaning to pound, grind, or crush, as one does with manioc or corn in a mortar.[10] Derivatives bridging metaphorically from this root range in sense: "to dispirit," "to be shunned," "a night thief," "a woman who eats well without the knowledge of her husband" (who presumably does not), "din or tumult." All touch upon reduction and disindividualization.

Most informants' exegeses, like these dictionary definitions, deal with solitude, isolation, or seclusion. Dying alone is absurd, since a "proper" death is in the arms of kinswomen whose warmth and ministrations reflect the afflicted person's lifelong participation in kinship and other close relations. Dying of hunger while alone underscores the abjection, for Tabwa are diligent farmers and responsible providers who would not be so careless with self or others—even complete strangers—except in the most dire of circumstances. Such a person is *lost*, from human contact and the succor it implies. Being killed while a solitary traveler, for no reason due to past history, is equally absonant with a social universe in which all acts are willed and have a history that is determinable through divination, if not already common knowledge. Kiuma's assertion that *kapondo*, Nfwimina the solar serpent, and the amenorrheal woman are all the same plays upon the unmarked nature of them all.

The alienation in the examples given is more evident when individuals are deranged (their "heads are not right") or possessed by spirits to the exclusion of an ordinary self. Eating alone is a rejection of the commensal norm important to Tabwa for everyday survival and proclaimed as an attribute of Tabwa chiefs (Kaoze 1950) as opposed to Luba or Luba-ized ones, who eat in seclusion. Tabwa see this as the height of greed, which, as a threat to life, is a definitive characteristic of sorcery; to choose to eat alone, then, is evil, while to be forced to eat alone is pitiable. Din and tumult are opposed to harmony in the aural realm, just as solitude is a "pounding down" (also from *kapondo*) of the obligations and prerogatives that make an individual *distinctive* within a community interrelated by kinship, marriage, and neighborliness.[11]

The two thieves at Chief Kaputo's displayed a singular disregard for person and property. The firing of *anyone's* house is a heinous act, and when the residence is the chief's, brings an added sense of anarchy. Solitude, eating alone, and din are all of a paradigm with anarchy, each having its own context against which it is the disorderly foil. The thieves' anarchy was checked, however, by the old "hyena," Kanengo the aged Kazanzi adept, and his young followers. *Kapondo*, too, represents this completion, this ultimate restoration of order after absurdity.

The substances which are made *vizimba* are employed as I understand tropes in rhetoric to be used.[12] Roots by the thousand cross one's path, yet a particular one on a particular occasion "causes" one to stumble; a piece of this root is taken for use in medicines, as the reduction of that set of circumstances which includes the trip and the tripping, but also such other elements as a sense of destiny, the interference of vengeful ghosts or sorcerers, pain (in the toe), and the knowledge that such a seemingly inconsequential injury can lead (through secondary infection) to eventual loss of limb or life. Through a synecdochal process, the particular root is chosen that represents the whole of these circumstances, and it will "foreground those aspects of the whole that are not only distinctive but are also taken as essential or directly relevant to the topic" (Sapir 1977:16). It is still a piece of root (without regard to botanical identity) and as such metaphorically joins the separate domains "root" and "fate" or whatever ultimate meaning the *kizimba* possesses.

The charred bones of the two thieves are still just that as well: charred bones like all other; but their transmutation has led to a sense beyond that of ordinary skeletal remains. This is a sense which may be derived from other circumstances than the anarchic threat as in the event described here. Each of these others will be synecdochically reduced, then each stands metaphorically in relation to the others, through the common mediator of the *kizimba* (see Figure 10.1: A:K, B:K, C:K = synecdoche, AK:BK:CK = meta-

Figure 10.1
Origins of the Kapondo Kizimba

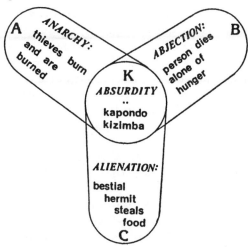

phor; K + L + M + other *vizimba*: amulet X = metonomy). The *kizimba*
has a single meaning (in this case, *kapondo*'s absurdity, I would assert), although each *kizimba* is a paradigm for its various sources; *kapondo* can then
be mixed metonymically with other *vizimba*/paradigms in the preparation of
complex medicines (where "metonym" implies the juxtaposition within a
single domain—the medicine bundle or amulet—of distinct items).

THE EVENTUAL USE

Substances used as *vizimba* are often difficult to obtain and may be purchased from distant practitioners at significant expenditure of money, time,
and energy. Only a tiny quantity is required (perhaps a cubic centimeter of
charred bone, for instance) and this will serve many, many times, since each
medicine bundle or amulet contains the merest shaving of the bone, a dust-
ing from something else, a smudge of yet another. In other words, these
elements or their combination are not iconic, and one cannot know their
identity and meaning unless told.

The *kapondo kizimba* is an ingredient in important concoctions, the con-
stitutions of which were revealed to us only after several years of working
with the same practitioners. It is an element of the *kiito* medicine horn of
Tabwa snare hunters, and used to be employed in the *kinkungwa* horn of
members of the now-defunct Mowela big-game hunting guild. It is added
to medicines prepared "to throw someone in the bush" (*kumutupa mutu mu
pori*), that is to rid the patient of an avenging ghost. It can be employed in
the *mwanzambale* protective amulet, as *muyembe* practitioner Kabemba ex-

plained, and this *kizimba* in conjunction with the many others of the device will make a solitary person seem as though many. "If you are alone and someone comes to test (*kupima*) the strength of his medicines against the strength of yours [as sorcerers do in trying to conquer even the hardiest of practioners], they will see that in your medicines many things are mixed, each and every quality or meaning." In other words, the solitude of the *kapondo*'s source is put to use, to make hunted animals bereft of direction or wiles, or to thwart aggressive sorcerers by having "solitude" under control and "closed" within one's amulet.

There are other, less salubrious uses. As Nzwiba explained,

Now these *vizimba* that they go and take from your fellow man, ah we see this tends to be sorcery. For they take the kizimba from that one who has died, and they invoke it: "Now, you kizimba, I want so-and-so to be killed." So it is certain that afterwards he will die, the kizimba will agree that the person will die.... For instance, if he had taken a kapondo kizimba, a bone or something of someone who has died, he puts this with other medicines and begins to invoke there, saying, "This man has not done right by me, I want him to die the same way you died," then won't he die? Because he has prayed to the person who has already died to do this, he [the victim] will die or have another kind of accident.... because the one who died agrees to the business for which it has been called.[13]

Any of these uses may be deemed sorcery, depending upon the situation. Hunters are said to ensorcell (*kuloga*) their game, and amulets like *mwan-zambale* are considered to be protective by their possessors, but offensive by critics. The absurdity of *kapondo*—its meaning *(maana)* as a constituent of medicines—is brought to bear on animal or human targets, plucking them from their apparent destinies and assuring them another fate they desire less, yet one which allows the greater community to continue in restored harmony. Individuals who possess and deploy *kapondo* are intervening in the course of events, and such hubris must always have its detractors as well as its supporters among those denied and gaining advantage, respectively. The hubristic, in turn, are *of* society but not altogether *in* society. Like the hyena, they are masters of transformation and transition, necessary yet dread.

ACKNOWLEDGMENTS

Four years' anthropological fieldwork was undertaken from late 1973 to late 1977 with financial support from the National Institute of Mental Health (no. F01–55251–01-CUAN), the Committee on African Studies and the Edson-Keith Fund of the University of Chicago, and the Society of the Sigma Xi. A first draft of this paper, entitled "*Kapondo*: The Use of Potitical Synecdoche in Tabwa Traditional Medicine," was prepared for the "Sovereignty, Sickness and Health in Africa" panel of the 1981 African Studies Association meetings, chaired by Randall Packard. As this work has evolved, helpful comments have been received from J. Knight, O. Kokole,

D. Merten, D. Moerman, R. Packard, T. Reefe, and C. Roberts, some of which have been incorporated here. Despite such generosity, all responsibility for this paper's content remains my own.

NOTES

1. All names have been changed except that of Kirungu, the central town of Tabwa lands along the southwestern shores of Lake Tanganyika in the Zaire Republic. Common Tabwa names have been chosen and are employed in the writing of C. D. Roberts (1980, 1981) and of the present author to refer to the same individuals.

2. A single document concerning this incident was discovered quite by chance in the archives of the Bureau des Affaires Culturelles, Division Régionale des Affaires Politiques in Lumbumbashi: W. DeBruyn, Magistrat Instructeur, "Avi d'ouverture d'instruction," Parquet du Tanganika, Etat du Katanga, 7 November 1960.

3. Nzwiba, interview of 14 May 1976 at Nanga; other relevant interviews with the chief's judge, Kanengo, and other interested parties were conducted on a visit to Chief Kaputo's in March 1977.

4. I disagree with Reefe's assertion that "the presence of the bambudye and bakasandji secret societies and subsequent transformation of oral traditions in frontier areas to the Luba, like those of northern Tabwa, suggest that the loyalty of distant client-lineages and villages was changing into a more substantial sense of belonging to a common polity" (1981: 153). Although there *is* a linguistic and cultural *aire* of which Luba, Tabwa, and other groups are members, among whom ideas and practices have long been traded easily, evidence that these chiefdoms (e.g., Tumbwe's) were "client-lineages and villages" of a centralized Luba empire is scant and unconvincing. Rather then belonging to "a common polity," that there were Tabwa Kazanzi adepts may reflect the borrowing of beliefs and behavior patterns deemed powerful because of their alien origin. The most effective medical practitioners, practices, and substances known to Tabwa that my wife and I consulted still come from Luba, beyond the hills and rivers to the west (or, less frequently, from across Lake Tanganyika).

5. Other spirals important to Tabwa cosmology are discussed in A. F. Roberts (1980:353–74).

6. Female spotted hyenas have an elongated clitoris visually identical to the male's penis, and a sham scrotum; the clitoris becomes erect during greeting, as does a male's penis, and field biologist Kruuk admits that he can distinguish between male and female adolescents only through close anatomical inspection (1974:210–11). The vagina is at the end of the clitoris, and coitus occurs when, in estrus, the entrance swells and the clitoris does not become erect; these points are reviewed in A. F. Roberts 1980:265–74.

7. Although many Tabwa ceremonies and rituals are no longer practiced as they were precolonially, most informants believe that chiefs are still buried in the manner mentioned here, and a *kisama* interregnum follows; no direct observation was possible.

8. *Nsipa* is a term used for the bundle of medicines buried in a central place in

a new village to attract residents and to keep them content in staying. Cunnison (1956) has described these among southern Tabwa along the Luapula.

9. In a paper entitled " 'Sinister Caricatures': 'Cannibalism' Among Belgians and Africans in the Congo," the Kazanzi society among colonized and the Mitumbula among colonizers was contrasted as to political history and essence (see Roberts 1993).

10. Van Acker 1907:54; Van Avermaet and Mbuya 1954:533–34; White Fathers 1954:619; Kajiga 1975:611; Johnson 1971:384. In KiTabwa-*ponda* can also mean "to insult, to dance fast"; *muponda* is the wild dog, *Lycaon pictus*, and *kiponda* a "night thief," according to Van Acker. In both KiLuba and CiBemba (which in turn are closely related to KiTabwa), derivatives refer to rebellion, insurrection, and the "underground" *(maquis)*.

11. Not coincidentally, Tabwa and others in the area used to create a din when the moon was "eaten" during eclipse. See Heusch 1972:72–82, for an elegant discussion of how this is an action to "separate the sky and the earth," to maintain the discrete nature of cosmic principles.

12. I rely here upon J. David Sapir's "Anatomy of Metaphor" (1977), in which he holds that "metaphor states an equivalence between terms taken from separate domains"; "metonymy replaces or juxtaposes contiguous terms that occupy a distinct and separate place within what is considered a single semantic or perceptual domain"; and "synecdoche, like metonymy, draws its terms from a single domain; however, one term always includes or is included by the other" (p. 4). Figure 10.1 is also derived from his (p. 20).

13. The place and meaning of invocation in the Tabwa medical process, as well as the usefulness of the rhetorical analogy in the explication of the process, will be expounded upon in the writings of C. D. Roberts.

REFERENCES

Administrateur Territorial. 1919. Untitled administrative report from Albertville, 22 January 1919. Archives of Sous-Région du Tanganika, Kalemi, Zaire.

Arens, W. 1979. *The Man-Eating Myth*. New York: Oxford University Press.

Beidelman, T. 1975. "Ambiguous Animals: Two Theriomorphic Metaphors in Kaguru Folklore." *Africa* 45(2):183–96.

Burton, W. F. P. 1961. *Luba Religion and Magic in Custom and Belief*. Tevuven: Annales du Musée Royal de L'Afrique Centrale, Sciences Humaines, no. 35.

Colle, P. 1913. *Les Baluba*. 2 vols. Anvers: Albert Dewit.

Cunnison, I. 1956. "Headmanship and the Ritual of Luapula Villages." *Africa* 26(1): 2–19.

DeBruyn, W. 1960. "Avis d'ouverture d'instruction." Judicial report, Parquet du Tanganika, Etat du Katanga, 7 November 1960. Archives du Bureau des Affaires Culturelles, Division Régionale des Affaires Politiques, Lubumbashi.

Heush, L. de. 1972. *Le roi ivre, ou l'origine de l'etat*. Paris: Gallimard.

Hobsbawm, E. 1965. *Primitive Rebels*. New York: Norton.

———.1981. *Bandist*. New York: Pantheon.

Johnson, F. 1971. *A Standard Swahili-English Dictionary*. London: Oxford University Press. (1st ed., 1939.)

Joset, G. A. 1934. "Etude sur les secrets secretes de la circonscription de Kinda, district du Lomami—territoire des Baluba." *Bulletin de la Société Royale Belge de Géographie* 58(1):28–44.

Kajiga, B. 1975. *Dictionnaire de la langue swahili*. Goma: Librarie des Volcans.

Kaoze, S. 1950. "Histoire des Bena-Kilunga." In *Une société de l'est du Zaire, les Tusanga depeints par eux-mêmes*. G. Nagant, ed. Paris: Ecole Pratique des Hautes Etudes.

Kruuk, H. 1974. *The Spotted Hyena: A Study of Predation and Social Behavior*. Chicago: University of Chicago Press.

Lebaigne, L. 1933. "Sectes Secretes." Administration report from Albertville, 13 July 1933. Archives of Sous-Région du Tanganika, Kalemie.

Reefe, T. 1981. *The Rainbow and the Kings: A History of the Luba Empire to 1891*. Berkeley: University of California Press.

Richards, A. 1969. *Land, Labour and Diet in Northern Rhodesia*. London: Oxford University Press.

Roberts, A. F. 1980. "Heroic Beasts, Beastly Heroes: Principles of Cosmology and Chiefship Among the Lakeside BaTabwa of Zaire." Ph.D. diss., University of Chicago.

———. 1982. " 'Comets Importing Change of Times and States': Ephemera and Process Among the Tabwa of Zaire." *American Ethnologist* 9(4):712–29.

———. 1993. "Sinister Caricatures: 'Cannibalism' Among Belgians and Africans in the Congo." Wenner-Gren Conference, "Rethinking Cannibalism," Uppsala University, Sweden. New York Wenner-Gren Foundation. Unpublished paper.

Roberts, C. D. 1980. "*Mungu na Mitishamba*: Illness and Medicine among the BaTabwa of Zaire." Ph.D. diss., University of Chicago.

———. 1981. "*Kutambuwa Ugonjuwa*: Concepts of Illness and Transformation among the Tabwa of Zaire." *Social Science and Medicine* 15B:309–16.

———. In press. "Emblems and Imagery: Analysis of a Tabwa Diviness Headdress." In *Verbal and Visual Arts in Africa*. D. Ben-Amos, ed. Bloomington: Indiana University Press.

Sapir, J. D. 1977. "The Anatomy of Metaphor." In *The Social Use of Metaphor: Essays on the Anthropology of Rhetoric*. In J. David Sapir and J. Christopher Crocker, eds. Philadelphia: University of Pennsylvania Press, 3–32.

———. 1981. "Leper, Hyena, and Blacksmith in Kujamaat Diola Thought." *American Ethnologist* 8(3):526–41.

Schmitz, R. 1912. *Les Baholoholo*. Anvers: Albert Dewit.

Theuws, T. 1968. "Le Styx ambigu." *Bulletin du Centre d'Etudes des Problémes Sociaux Indigénes* 81:5–33.

Turner, V. 1967. *The Forest of Symbols*. Ithaca, N.Y.: Cornell University Press.

Van Acker, A. 1907. *Dictionnaire kitabwa-francais, francais-kitabwa*. Musée Royal du Congo Belge, *Annales*, series 5, Ethnographie-Linguistique.

Van Avermaet, E., and B. Mbuya. 1954. *Dictionnaire kiluba-francais*. Musée Royal du Congo Belge, *Annales*, Sciences de l'Homme, Linguistique.

White, T. 1960. *The Bestiary*. New York: Putnam.

White Fathers. 1954. *Bemba-English Dictionary*. Capetown: Longmans, Green.

11

PHYSIOLOGY AND SYMBOLS: THE ANTHROPOLOGICAL IMPLICATIONS OF THE PLACEBO EFFECT

DANIEL E. MOERMAN

How can we account for the effectiveness of non-Western medical treatment? What can we learn about the effectiveness of Western healing through comparative study? One of the foremost dilemmas in ethnomedicine is understanding how it is that the manipulations of the shaman or healer actually influence the physiological state of the patient. Many studies, including several of my own, have devoted much energy to the study of the effectiveness of native pharmacology. The standard exercise is to show that pharmaceuticals in use have "appropriate" physiological impact. And many tribal peoples cooperate with this exercise by having enormous pharmacopoeias at their disposal. Wyman and Harris (1941) reported 515 species of medicinal plants for the Navaho alone. My compilation of native American medicinal plants includes 2,865 different plant species from 941 genera used by 219 different cultures in 25,025 different ways (Moerman in press). In a less-standard exercise, comparing those medicinally *used* plants with *available* plants, I have been able to demonstrate substantial selectivity among families by Native Americans. The three most heavily utilized families (Asteraceae, Rosaceae, Lamiaceae) account for 26 percent of medicinal items in my compilation, but only 18 percent of the 21,641 species of plants in North America (Kartesz 1994). The three least heavily used families, in terms of their availability (Poaceae, Cyperaceae and Fabaceae) account for 4 percent of items in my list, but 18 percent of the species in FNA (for details of this argument, see Chapter 4 of this volume, "Poisoned Apples and Honeysuckle"). But we can also be certain that neither native therapists nor their patients saw pharmaceuticals as any more important in therapy than the song, dance, and din that accompanied treatment. While several investigators (most notably Victor Turner) have provided brilliant symbolic analyses of these more dramatic aspects of treatment, few have attempted to understand the healing quality of such symbolic dimensions to treatment.

This bimodal quality of native treatment often baffles Western observers. One notes approvingly the intelligent study, the deliberate consideration, and the long empirical tradition employed as the Navaho healer gathers 30 or 40 herbal medicines—many of them "rational," "effective" drugs. But despair follows when the subsequent infusion is fed to and washed over the patient—*and* a dozen singers and friends who are participating in the ritual. What kind of effectiveness is this? The Navaho healing ritual, focused on a sweat-emetic rite and coupled with chants and beautiful sand paintings, is said by Reichard to be like "a spiritual osmosis in which the evil in man and the good of deity penetrate the ceremonial membrane in both directions, the former being neutralized by the latter" (1970:112). Such a rich metaphorical structure, part of the whole Navaho cosmological system, is simultaneously healing and barely intelligible to the Western "biomedical" understanding.

BIMODAL QUALITY OF WESTERN BIOMEDICINE

Yet there is an impressive array of evidence of similar processes, with similar effects, in our medical practice. This bimodality in treatment is probably universal. My argument is

- that the *form* of medical treatment as well as its content can be effective medical treatment,
- that medical treatment must be understood bimodally, in terms of both its specific and general dimensions,
- and that we have only a rudimentary capacity for simultaneously understanding both modes.

In Western medical and surgical contexts, what I refer to as general medical therapy is usually referred to as the "placebo effect." Various investigators (Beecher 1961; Frank 1975:195) attribute between 35 and 60 percent of the effectiveness of contemporary biomedicine to this placebo effect. In the shaman's context, some investigators attribute *all* effectiveness to general medical therapy, although this clearly devalues empirical pharmacological traditions dating back to Middle Paleolithic times (Solecki 1965).

Even though the general effectiveness of treatment is recognized occasionally as a substantial component of the healing process, biomedicine founders in its attempts to account for the phenomenon. This follows, I suggest, from the naive dualism of contemporary medical science, which characteristically assumes a fundamental mind-body dichotomy in its conceptualization of the human organism. And since disease is an affliction of the "body," whereas perception (of treatment) is an aspect of the "mind," and since the only available mediators of this dichotomy are as ineffable and "unscientific" as the "soul," biomedicine tends simply to ignore, or even deny, the significance of general medical therapy (see Engel 1977; Goodwin, Goodwin, and Vogel 1979).

Even in neuroendocrinology, where recent ingenious work has shown that the hypothalamus, a central portion of the brain, is simultaneously a central portion of the endocrine system (the "body"), authors have insisted on maintaining this naive dualism; the hypothalamic neurons that produce hormones (which regulate pituitary function) are routinely called "transducer cells" (Wurtman 1971). There is a wide range of phenomena that compels us to reject this dualism. In addition to the findings of neuroendocrinology, we might mention phenomena as diverse as "psychosomatic" illness, biofeedback (Stoyva et al. 1972), host-pathogen interaction (Solomon 1969), Eastern meditative techniques (Datey et al. 1969) and, just for fun, fire handling (Brown 1984; Kane 1976). Fortunately, some recent writers in psychoneuroendocrinology are challenging these dualisims with more elegant and complex formulations (Watkins 1995). General medical treatment as I have defined it falls within this class wherein conceptual, meaningful, cultural, categorical events influence physiological processes.

Anthropologist James Fernandez has eloquently demonstrated the power of the metaphor, a "strategic predication" that can move us, that is, change our behavior (1971:43). I argue that metaphor can heal, that meaning mends. I will consider in some detail one case in which we can see some consequences of meaningful human performance in Western biomedicine.

Placebo Surgery

One of the most common causes of death in the United States is myocardial infarction, or heart attack. The traditional biomedical understanding of this disease is that it is caused by ischemia, a lack of adequate blood flow to some region of the heart, which is in turn caused by atherosclerosis, which is a buildup of lipids or fatty tissues in the coronary arteries which carry blood to the heart. The lipid buildup or atherosclerotic plaque causes lesions on the blood vessels. The heart attack is typically understood to be caused by thrombosis, that is, blockage of the narrowed artery by a blood clot (a thrombus). The clots are said to form near sites of such fixed lesions; they are often not actually seen since, it is said, "spontaneous thrombolysis" (break down of the clots) occurs in two-thirds of cases. In any event, these clots block the artery; the heart muscle, deprived of oxygenated blood, dies. The heart goes into fibrillation, and the patient dies.

In milder forms, coronary arteriosclerosis may lead to angina pectoris, a pressing pain beneath the sternum, which often radiates out to the left arm. Small doses of nitroglycerin dissolved under the tongue provide dramatic and rapid relief from the severe pain of angina. This has been the medical treatment of choice for over 100 years. The drug has a potent relaxing effect on smooth muscle tissue, notably of the blood vessels, and it rapidly reduces blood pressure. In addition, recent research shows that the drugs seems to mimic the action of an endogenous "relaxing factor," comprised largely of nitric oxide and produced by the endothelial cells, a component of the vascular tissue (Abrams 1988; Ignarro 1989). The relaxation of the blood vessels presumably allows blood to flow more freely to the heart, alleviating the pain.

But angina pectoris, a grave and dangerous symptom of serious underlying pathology, is highly responsive not only to nitrates but to inert treatment as well. This is quite surprising, as the theory of sclerotic arteries and blood clots would seem to leave little place for such unlikely findings. Benson and McCallie reviewed the literature on placebo effectiveness in angina (1979); examining the histories of a series of treatments subsequently demonstrated to be inactive and then abandoned, they note a consistent pattern: "The initial 70 to 90 percent effectiveness in the enthusiasts' reports decreases to 30 to 40 percent 'base-line' placebo effectiveness in the skeptics' reports" (Benson and McCallie 1979:1424). Thus, for this grave condition, skeptics can heal 30 to 40 percent of their patients with inert medication, enthusiasts 70 to 90 percent. Either case, given the standard explanation of lesions, clots, and epithelium, seems remarkable.

The logic of this theory has yielded several other interesting approaches to angina. The surgical metaphor, by analogy with the manipulation characterized by splinting limbs, removing broken teeth, or cleaning wounds, is a powerful one for a people confident of the physical basis of illness. The placebo consequences of surgery were noted a generation ago by Beecher (1955, 1961) and have more recently been elaborated by Frank (1975). And, in recent years, a number of surgical procedures have been developed to deal with angina. Since the problem (pain and ultimately infarction) is presumed to be due to a constricted blood supply, why not reroute some blood supplies, "bypassing" the constricted areas and "revascularizing" the muscles at risk? Several indirect revascularization techniques involving rerouting various arteries were developed in the 1930s by Beck and in the 1940s by Vineburg (Meade 1961:480–515). Although Beck's procedure attained modest popularity, the first widely used surgical approach to angina was the bilateral internal mammary artery ligation (BIMAL). The internal mammary (or thoracic) arteries arise from the aorta and descend just inside the front wall of the chest, ultimately supplying blood to the viscera. Following anatomical research by Fieschi, an Italian surgeon, which indicated connections between various ramifications of these arteries and the coronary circulation, several other Italian surgeons developed a procedure in which the arteries were ligated below the point where these branches presumably diverged to the myocardium, in order to enhance this flow and supplement the blood supply. The operation was first performed in the United States by Robert

Table 11.1

Improvement of Patients Undergoing Actual and Sham Bilaterial Internal Mammary Artery Surgery

	Actual surgery				Sham surgery			
	Study number				Study number			
Improvement	1	2	Row Total	Percent	1	2	Row Total	Percent
Substantial	5	9	14	67%	5	5	10	83%
Slight	3	4	7	33%	2	0	2	17%
Total	8	13	21	100%	7	5	12	100%

Sources: Study 1: Cobb et al. 1959. "Substantial improvement" = subjective improvement greater than 40 percent. Study 2: Dimond et al. 1960. "Substantial improvement" = subjective improvement greater than 50 percent.

Glover and J. Roderick Kitchell in the late 1950s (Glover 1957; Kitchell, Glover, and Kyle 1958). It was quite simple, and since the arteries were not deep in the body, could be performed under local anesthesia. The physicians reported symptomatic improvement (ranging from slight to total) in 68 percent of their first sample of 50 patients in a two-to six-month follow-up. The operation quickly gained some popularity.

This situation, a simple technique requiring only local anesthesia to treat a grave disease, laid the basis for a remarkable and nearly unique scientific study. Two research teams independently carried out double-blind studies comparing the BIMAL with a sham procedure in which the entire operation was carried out except that the arteries were not ligated (Cobb et al. 1959; Dimond et al. 1960). In both studies, patient follow-up was carried out by cardiologists unaware of which patients had undergone arterial ligation and which had not. In both studies the sham-procedure patients reported the same substantial subjective relief from angina as BIMAL patients (see Table 11.1). Most patients, with ligation or without, reported substantially reduced need for nitroglycerin. Both studies concluded that the results of the operation could be accounted for by placebo effects, and therefore should be discontinued. It was; Dr. Dimond reported subsequently that this paper was "generally credited with the successful burial of internal mammary artery ligation" (Dimond 1978 [personal communication]).

In sum, the surgery did not work for the reasons that it was performed and it quickly disappeared from the surgeon's repertoire. The question for us is, how *did* it work, how did it relieve this severe systemic pain?

A major breakthrough in the surgical approach to angina came in the 1960s with the development of "direct" revascularization, in which veins from elsewhere in the body (now routinely the saphenous vein from the leg) are grafted directly into the aorta and then into the appropriate coronary arteries beyond their obstructions.

Contemporary Use of Coronary Bypass Surgery

While it is hard to know exactly how many of these operations are done, authoritative estimates suggest that some 228,000 were performed in 1986, up from 114,000 in 1979 (Feinleib et al. 1989). Given the increasing rate at which the operation is being repeated a second or even third time for the same person—currently 10 to 20 percent of the caseload at many large centers (Grondin et al. 1989)—and given the increasing proportion of the population that is in the greatest risk years, and given that these operations cost in the vicinity of $20,000 each, this is at least a $5 billion-a-year business, and growing. Although the operation has become very popular, it remains highly controversial. Many surgeons are, clearly, deeply committed to the tremendous value of the procedure. Its logic is obvious, its effects dramatic.

Numerous studies indicate that the operation is highly successful, reducing symptoms (i.e., pain) in 80 to 90 percent of patients with severe stable angina pectoris. However, there are other measures of the effectiveness of such a procedure. In several very large controlled trials, only small subsets of surgically treated patients have been shown to survive longer than medically treated patients. In a trial carried out by the Veteran's Administration, survival after seven years of surgically treated patients was 77 percent and of medically treated patients 70 percent; that difference was not statistically significant. After 11 years, even that difference had narrowed; surgical patient survival was 58 percent and medical patient survival was 57 percent. Similar results were achieved in the more recent European Coronary Surgery Study. After 7 years, the surgical group survival rate was 87 percent while the medical group survival rate was 79 percent; after 12 years, surgical patient survival was 71 percent while medical group survival was 67 percent (Gersh et al. 1989). There are a few subgroups of patients, for instance those with restrictions of the left main coronary artery or those with three-vessel disease and left ventricular dysfunction, for whom surgery improves chances of survival. Unfortunately, the degree of left ventricular disfunction is the best predictor of death during surgery (Bonow and Epstein 1985). One large study has shown that although the operation clearly alleviates symptoms, it has little rehabilitative effect on patients. Among 350 patients studies, "There was no improvement in return to work or hours worked after surgery" (Barnes et al. 1977; see also Smith, Frye, and Peihler 1983 for a review of several such studies, all with similar results). Another recent study has shown that of a group of 88 patients recommended for bypass graft surgery, 74 were referred for continued medical treatment in a second-opinion program. "Sixty of these 74 patients chose this option and continued to receive medical therapy without any fatalities during a follow-up period of 27.8

months" (Graboys, Headley, Lown et al. 1987:1611; see also McIntosh 1987).

But the most interesting aspect of coronary artery bypass surgery is that several authors have noted that "some patients undergoing coronary artery bypass have improvement of angina despite the fact that all grafts are occluded" (Gott et al. 1973:30). A study examined 446 bypass patients who underwent coronary arteriography subsequent to their surgery. Of these, 54 had no functioning, patent grafts. Both groups displayed similarly impressive functional improvement. The authors conclude that coronary bypass surgery patients "experience impressive symptomatic improvement regardless of completeness of revascularization . . . [and] the late survival of unsuccessful revascularization patients is more favorable than predicted from previous natural history data. [This] suggests that factors other than coronary bypass surgery may play a role in the long-term survival of coronary artery disease patients undergoing surgery" (Valdes et al. 1979).

One authority concluded, gently enough, that "the situation is complex and . . . increased blood flow to the ischemic [occluded] region is not the only possible explanation for symptomatic improvement" (Ross 1975:503). Other explanations have been proposed, including the notions that surgery actually causes minor myocardial infarctions ("heart attacks"), or that surgery denervates the angina-producing region.

How Does Heart Surgery Work?

This means that although the surgery works, *it does not necessarily work for the reasons for which it is done.* The rationality of the procedure for the preponderance of patients is apparently unconnected with its effectiveness. In the 1880s, when James Mooney analyzed the use of a series of Cherokee drugs, he concluded, "We must admit that much of their practice is correct, however false the reasoning by which they have arrived at this result" (Mooney 1891: 328). A similar situation apparently applies to these cases of heart surgery.

How can cutting two little incisions over the second intercostal space alleviate the pain of angina pectoris? How can coronary bypass patients with occluded grafts experience this profound relief? The logic of these procedures is persuasive, if erroneous. And it is this logic that is propounded to the patient by the surgeon. And, thereby, an obvious remaining explanation for the effectiveness of bypass surgery, or BIMAL, is general or placebo effectiveness. Bypass surgery, especially, is, from a patient's point of view, a cosmic drama following a most potent metaphorical path. The patient is rendered unconscious. His heart, source of life, font of love, racked with pain, is *stopped.* He is, by many reasonable definitions, dead. The surgeon restructures his heart, and the patient is reborn, reincarnated. His sacrifice (roughly $20,000) may hurt as much as his incisions. Remembering that angina can be a remarkably stable nonfatal condition (Gott et al. 1973) and considering the substantial subjective components in pain itself, it seems reasonable to conclude that the general metaphorical effects of this surgery are as decisive in its anomalous effectiveness as are graft-patency rates (Frank 1975).

Recent research on the etiology of coronary artery disease has shown that angina and infarction may be caused by coronary artery spasm (Maseri et al. 1978; see also Goldberg 1983 for a comprehensive review), which may in turn be caused by neurological impulses or emotional stresses. Angina and heart attacks are not random mechanical events but rather the results of neurological or mental processes—the process is a complex one open to cortical influence, increasing our confidence that it is subject to symbolic and meaningful influences.

In modern Western biomedicine as well as in tribal healing, whether by design or default, the *form* of medical treatment, internal or surgical, can itself be effective medical treatment. Recall the characteristic American medical treatments of the period immediately preceding the biomedical revolution of the 1880s: most conditions were treated with calomel (mercurous chloride), a powerful purgative, or with venesection, minimally a symbolic operation, the laying on of steel (Shryock 1966:245). These two treatments probably had some specific physiological impact as might modern medical treatments for cancer that also employ powerful purgatives. Such stress might trigger a general immunological response. But in all likelihood, the decisive elements in any effectiveness the physician had was a consequence of the dramatic, general and metaphorical elements these treatments contained. Such effectiveness adheres to modern treatment.

HEALING AND PHILOSOPHY

We have no generally accepted theoretical paradigm within which we can evaluate and interpret such human experience. Even the growing literature on holistic medicine seems essentially empirical, cataloging experience on biofeedback, host-pathogen interactions, "stress" and illness, and so on (Pelletier 1977). And consonant with that empiricism is a kind of religiosity: those who venture beyond the empirical seem almost inevitably to begin speaking of archetypes, gods, or souls (Hillman 1964). Even the more scholarly of them, we feel, are straining against the temptation to break into song.

Dualism

This follows, I think, from a naive dualism, the ethnometaphysic of our time. With a thinking and unextended mind, and an unthinking and extended body, in Descartes's formulation, there is no ground for interaction of these human quanta, or onta, save some ephemeral mystical spiritual soul

(Stent 1975). A variant and, I suggest, increasingly popular form of this dualism involves a more complex conceptualization of the organism, one where
the person has a "mind and a body" but the body also has a "mind of its
own." Thus a student once explained the placebo effect to me this way:
"The mind tells the body what to do," she said. The body, presumably
listening with its own mind, did what it was told. Much current speculation
about "visualization," "body imagery," and the like employs similar language; for a critique of such thinking, see Robert Kugelmann's chapter elsewhere in this volume.

Philosophical attempts to resolve the dilemma of dualism come in many
forms, one as likely as the next, each reasonable in its own terms, each
fundamentally flawed in terms of the others. Idealism and behaviorism are
two most powerful monisms, each denying one or the other of these quanta.
Although idealism resolves the mind-body dilemma by denying body, it also
denies the reality of the external world; solipsism seems too high a price to
pay for this solution. Much more popular is behaviorism, which resolves the
dilemma by denying mind, by denying mental life. Among the strongest of
such positions is that taken by the philosopher J. J. C. Smart: "When I 'report' a pain, I am not really reporting anything . . . , but am doing a sophisticated sort of wince" (Smart 1959:11). Such a position denies the existence
of an autonomous inner life, not to mention the possibility of culture.

Among several more sophisticated varieties of dualism are parallelism and
interactionism, and several combinations of them. They all seem similarly
open to critical challenge. For a classic philosophical dogfight on the matter,
see *Consciousness and the Brain* (Globus et al. 1976).

Person Theory

A most interesting recent philosophical consideration of this problem is
Brody's (1977) defense of Strawson's (1958), Kenny et al. (1973), and
Grene's (1976) "person theory." This theory simultaneously meets many of
the challenges of the standard philosophical positions and can be extended
to meet many of the concerns of the anthropologist. It is one philosophical
position in this debate that has a central role for culture. At the risk of
oversimplifying, I will briefly summarize Brody's argument and indicate how
it meets the anthropological requirements of a cultural epistemology and
how it provides a framework for understanding what I have called general
medical therapy.

Denying the primitive qualities of the quanta "mind" and "body," this
theory asserts that there are two kinds of entities, "material bodies" and
"persons," to which two kinds of predicates, "mental" and "physical," can
be attached. "Material bodies can correctly have ascribed to them only physical predicates, while persons can have applied to them both physical and
mental predicates" (Brody 1977:93). Kenny says, "To have a mind is to have

the capacity to acquire the ability to operate with symbols in such a way that it is one's own activity that makes them symbols and confers meaning upon them" (quoted in Grene 1976:178). The critical logical feature of this position is that "the concept of person is more basic than the physical and mental predicates ascribed to it" (Brody 1977:93). This is a unitary conceptualization of the human organism which does not have to account for either of those quanta in terms of the other, yet lets us talk about human beings in an intuitively familiar manner. In this formulation, "persons" are understood as animals possessing the capacity to use symbols in special ways, specifically in structuring experience, and generally in participating in culture, an anthropological commonplace. In this context, there is no longer in principle an anomaly in understanding how performance can influence physiological state:

If being a dweller within culture is a special way of being an animal, it should not be anomalous if this characteristic were found to influence other animal capacities—including the capacities to undergo changes in bodily status and function. Experiencing symptom change due to the placebo effect is therefore the bodily expression of the person's participation in the healing context as a culturally determined, symbolic phenomenon. (Brody 1977:102–3)

To be a person is to have a mind. To have a mind is to be able to use symbols. Symbols are most evident in language. Private symbols are impossible in the same sense that private language is impossible—were it private, it would not be language. Therefore being a person is essentially a *social* phenomenon and requires the prior existence of other persons. (I note parenthetically that the quantum "person" need not necessarily be confined to one individual body [Crocker 1976].) "One can ascribe states of consciousness to oneself only if one can ascribe them to others" (Strawson 1958:339); "The ability to use [mental] predicates self-referentially follows from the ability to use them at all" (Brody 1977:111), that is, to use them regarding others. Hence self-consciousness is a differentiating process, a process of noting meaningful contrasts, of noting, in Bateson's phrase, differences that make a difference, not merely an indexing or naming process. Using Kleinman's contrast (1973), we equate "disease" with "difference," and "illness" with "a difference that makes a difference," that is, a meaningful difference. It is at this point that diagnosis, either by the patient (based on widely shared symbolic norms) or by the healer (based on more private, technical, professional, or sacred norms), becomes critical. For it is at this point that the inchoate disease becomes a meaningful quantum illness, hence understandable, and, within the limits of animal mortality, finally controllable. And likewise for the treatment of illness through performance, remembering Fernandez (1971), medical metaphors are those strategic mental predications that can "move" us, that is, manipulate physical predications, in a process we call "healing."

Objections

Consider a curious and poetic objection in an essay by Erde, a philosopher of medicine. He contrasts some contemporary dualisms with a variation of this person theory in a sort of double *reductio ad absurdum* proof. He argues that dualism commits us to much that is incredible, a position with which I would agree. But he further argues that a unitary position does likewise:

[It] implies that the body is animate. . . . [I]f the body is also a character within the drama, if we personify the body and it becomes an agent unto itself, we might understand that it could produce physical illness from within. . . . [T]he implication is that what we call "bodily illness" may be meaningful in the sense made current by Freud regarding neuroses, dreams, and slips of the tongue. . . . [I]f a man is a unity, somatic illness is as meaningful as any illness . . . and should be understood by the sick individual and by the physician even before it is determined whether it should be treated by . . . secondary material means. (Erde 1977:187, 189.)

This, Erde concludes, is "incredible."

It seems to me to be eminently credible, and even, from an anthropological and semiotic point of view, properly intuitive.

MEDICAL THERAPY, SPECIFIC AND GENERAL

From this perspective, I propose these somewhat more formal definitions of specific and general medical therapy. Specific therapy is that healing activity influencing the physical predicates of persons; general therapy is that influencing (wittingly or otherwise) the mental predicates of persons. Such a view places these alternative experiences on an equal ontological footing, compatible and comparable in effect. It also affords a guide to clear talk *about* such experiences. Thus the sentence "I feel better; I have less heart pain" breaks down into "I feel better because I have more blood in my myocardium and because I have a restructured heart." The relative impact of these two predicates on the subject is, in any individual case, open to analysis and, before the fact, each is open to manipulation, control, and skill.

Of course this does not solve the problem of general effectiveness in detail any more than it does for specific effectiveness; how a given drug precisely influences a given organ is a complex research question and the same may be expected in understanding the particular influence of any general therapy. But it *does* mean that there is no obstacle *in principle* to understanding such effectiveness through properly designed studies. Work by Levine and others implicating endorphins in placebo analgesia is a brilliant example of the beginnings of such work (Levine et al. 1978).

Meaning mends. Study meaning, and learn about mending. But study mending and we might learn about meaning. These are some of the implications of the study of physiology and symbols.

ACKNOWLEDGMENTS

I am indebted to John Ross, M.D., who advised me on the details of coronary artery disease and its treatments. Diane Lintner read the manuscript and made very helpful suggestions. Of course all responsibility for the interpretations put forth here is mine.

REFERENCES

Abrams, J. 1988. "Nitrates." *Medical Clinics of North America* 72:1–35.

Barnes, Glenda K. et al. 1977. "Changes in Working Status of Patients Following Coronary Bypass Surgery." *Journal of the American Medical Association* 238: 1249–52.

Beecher, H. K. 1955. "The Powerful Placebo." *Journal of the American Medical Association* 159:1602–6.

———. 1961. "Surgery as Placebo." *Journal of the American Medical Association* 176: 1102–7.

Benson, Herbert, and David P. McCallie. 1979. "Angina Pectoris and the Placebo Effect." *New England Journal of Medicine* 300(25):1424–29.

Bonow, Robert O., and Stephen E. Epstein. 1985. "Indications for Coronary Artery Bypass Surgery in Patients with Chronic Angina Pectoris: Implications of the Multicenter Randomized Trials." *Circulation* 72(suppl. V):V23–30.

Brody, Howard A. 1977. "Persons and Placebos: Philosophical Dimensions of the Placebo Effect." Ph.D. dissertation, Michigan State University, East Lansing. Ann Arbor: University Microfilms.

Brown, Carolyn Henning. 1984. "Tourism and Ethnic Competition in a Ritual Form: The Firewalkers of Fiji." *Oceania* 54:223–244.

Cobb, L. A., G. I. Thomas, D. H. Dillard, K. A. Marendino, and R. A. Bruce. 1959. "An Evaluation of Internal Mammary Artery Ligation by a Double Blind Technic." *New England Journal of Medicine* 260:1115–18.

Crocker, J. Christopher. 1976. "The Mirrored Self: Identity and Ritual Inversion among the Eastern Bororo." *Ethnology* 15:129–45.

Datey, K. K., S. N. Deshmukh, and C. P. Dalvi. 1969. "Shavasan': A Yogic Exercise in Management of Hypertension." *Angiology* 20:325.

Dimond, E. G. 1978. Personal communication.

Dimond, E. G., C. F. Kittle, and J. E. Crockett. 1960. "Comparison of Internal Mammary Artery Ligation and Sham Operation for Angina Pectoris." *American Journal of Cardiology* 5:483–86.

Engel, George. 1977. "The Need for a New Medical Model: A Challenge for Biomedicine." *Science* 196:129–36.

Erde, Edmund L. 1977. "Mind-Body and Malady." *Journal of Medicine and Philosophy* 2:177–90.

Feinleib, Manning, R. J. Havlik, R. F. Gillum, R. Pokras, E. McCarthy, and M. Moien. 1989. "Coronary Heart Disease and Related Procedures: National Hospital Discharge Survey Data." *Circulation* 79(6, pt. 2):I13–18.

Fernandez, James. 1971. "Persuasions and Performances: Of the Beast in Every Body . . . and the Metaphors of Everyman." *Daedelus* 110:39–60.

Frank, Jerome. 1975. "Psychotherapy of Bodily Illness: An Overview." *Psychotherapy and Psychosomatics* 26:192–202.

Gersh, Bernard J., Robert M. Califf, Floyd D. Loop, Cary W. Atkins, David B. Pryor, and Timothy C. Takaro. 1989. "Coronary Bypass Surgery in Chronic Stable Angina." *Circulation* 79 (suppl. I):I46–59.

Globus, Gordon G., Grover Maxwell, and Irwin Savodnik. 1976. *Consciousness and the Brain: A Scientific and Philosophical Inquiry*. New York: Plenum.

Glover, Robert P. 1957. "A New Surgical Approach to the Problem of Myocardial Revascularixation in Coronary Artery Disease." *Journal of the Arkansas Medical Society* 54:223–34.

Goldberg, Sheldon, ed. 1983 "Coronary Artery Spasm and Thrombosis." *Cardiovascular Clinics* 14(1):1–223.

Goodwin, James S., Jean M. Goodwin, and Albert V. Vogel. 1979. "Knowledge and Use of Placebos by House Officers and Nurses." *Annals of Internal Medicine* 91:106–110.

Gott, Vincent L., J. S. Donahoo, R. R. Brawley, and L. S. Griffith. 1973. "Current Surgical Approaches to Ischemic Heart Disease." *Current Problems in Surgery* 10:4–53.

Graboys, Thomas B., Adrienne Headley, Bernard Lown, Steven Lampert, and Charles M. Blatt. 1987. "Results of a Second-Opinion Program for coronary Artery Bypass Graft Surgery." *Journal of the American Medical Association* 258: 1611–14.

Grene, Marjorie. 1976. " 'To Have a Mind . . . '." *Journal of Medicine and Philosophy* 1:177–99.

Grondin, C. M., Lucien Campeau, and J. C. Thornton et al. 1989 "Coronary Artery Grafting with Saphenous Vein." *Circulation* 79(6, pt. 2):I24–29.

Hillman, James. 1964. *Suicide and the Soul*. New York: Harper and Row.

Ignarro, L. J. 1989 "Endothelium-Derived Nitric Oxide: Pharmacology and Relationship to the Actions of Organic Nitrate Ester." *Pharmaceutical Research* 6: 651–59.

Kane, Stephen. 1976. "Holiness Fire Handling: A Psychophysiological Analysis." Paper presented at the annual meeting of the American Anthropological Association, Washington, D.C.

Kartesz, John. 1994. *A Synonymized Checklist of the Vascular Flora of the United States, Canada and Greenland*. 2 vols. Portland, Ore.: Timber Press.

Kenny, A. J. P., H. C. Longuet-Higgins, J. R. Lucas, and C. H. Waddington. 1973. *The Development of Mind*. Edinburgh: Edinburgh University Press.

Kitchell, J. F., R. P. Glover, and R. H. Kyle, 1958. "Bilateral Internal Mammary Artery Ligation for Angina Pectoris." *American Journal of Cardiology* 1:46–50.

Kleinman, Arthur. 1973. "Medicine's Symbolic Reality." *Inquiry* 16:206–13.

Levine, J. D., N. C. Gordon, and H. L. Fields. 1978. "The Mechanisms of Placebo Analgesia." *Lancet* (2):654–57.

Maseri, Attilio, et al. 1978 "Coronary Vasospasm as a Possible Cause of Myocardial Infarction." *New England Journal of Medicine* 229:1271–77.

McIntosh, Henry D. 1987. "Editorial: Second Opinions for Aortocoronary Bypass Grafting Are Beneficial." *Journal of the American Medical Association* 258:1644–45.

Meade, Richard H. 1961. *A History of Thoracic Surgery*. Springfield, Ill.: Charles C. Thomas.

Moerman, Daniel E. In press. *Native American Ethnobotany*. Portland, Ore.: Timber Press.

———. 1989. "Poisoned Apples and Honeysuckles: The Medicinal Plants of Native America." *Medical Anthropology Quarterly* 3:52–61.

Mooney, James. 1891. "The Sacred Formulas of the Cherokees." Seventh Annual Report of the Bureau of American Ethnology, pp. 301–97. Washington, D.C.: Smithsonian Institution.

Pelletier, Kenneth R. 1977. *Mind as Healer, Mind as Slayer: A Holistic Approach to Preventing Stress Disorders*. New York: Delta.

Reichard, Gladys. 1970. *Navajo Religion*. New York: Bollingen Foundation.

Ross, Richard S. 1975. "Ischemic Heart Disease: An Overview." *American Journal of Cardiology* 36:496–505.

Shryock, Richard H. 1966. *Medicine in America: Historical Essays*. Baltimore, Md.: Johns Hopkins University Press.

Smart, J. J. C. 1959. "Sensations and Brain Processes." *Philosophical Review* 68:141–56.

Smith, Hugh C., Robert L. Frye, and Jeffrey Peihler. 1983. "Does Coronary Bypass Surgery Have a Favorable Influence on the Quality of Life?" *Cardiovascular Clinics* 13:253–64.

Solecki, Ralph S. 1965. "Shanidar IV, A Neanderthal Flower Burial in Northern Iraq." *Science* 190:880–81.

Solomon, George F. 1969. "Emotions, Stress and the Central Nervous System." *Annals of the New York Academy of Science* 164:335–42.

Stent, Gunther S. 1975. "Limits to the Scientific Understanding of Man." *Science* 187:1052–57.

Stoyva, Johan, T. X. Barber, L. V. DiCara, et al. 1972. *Biofeedback and Self Control, 1971*. Chicago: Aldine.

Strawson, P. F. 1958. *Persons*. Minnesota Studies in the Philosophy of Science, vol. 2. Minneapolis: University of Minnesota Press.

Valdes, M., B. D. McCallister, D. R. McConahay, W. A. Reed, D. A. Killen, and M. Arnold. 1979. " 'Sham Operation' Revisited: A Comparison of Complete vs. Unsuccessful Coronary Artery Bypass." *American Journal of Cardiology* 43:382.

Watkins, A. D. 1995. "Perceptions, Emotions and Immunity: An Integrated Homeostatic Network." *Quarterterly Journal of Medicine* 88:283–94.

Wurtman, R. 1971. "Brain Monoamines and Endocrine Function." *Neuroendocrine Research Program Bulletin* 9:172.

Wyman, Leland C., and Stuart K. Harris. 1941. "Navaho Indian Medical Ethno-Botany." University of New Mexico Bulletin no. 336. Albuquerque: University of New Mexico Press.

12

NARRATIVES OF CHRONIC PAIN

ROBERT KUGELMANN

In recent years a narrative approach has taken root in the social sciences. This trend recognizes that the important human phenomena are not, strictly speaking, natural events like the movements of planets or clouds, but that they are personal, social, cultural, and historical events. Grief and depression, heart disease and drug abuse, growing up, old, and in love constitute incidents in the ongoing life histories of unique individuals. Moreover, these individuals can and do talk about the important events in their lives, reflect upon them, act upon their understandings, and so forth. Self-awareness, long simply a vexing confounding variable in research, has returned to center stage as one of the things we need to understand.

Pain occurs only to conscious beings, making it an inevitable theme of stories. Watch any child: the slightest cut or bruise becomes the major topic of the day, as the fascinated child endlessly repeats stories of the "owie." Significant pain, whenever it occurs in life, gets woven into narratives that reflect and influence how people explain, treat, and make sense of the suffering, their lives, and their worlds. Chronic pain, to use a contemporary term for pain that typically lasts for more than six months, has its own types of narrative. To them I turn.

CHRONIC PAIN

There are many varieties of chronic pain. I shall address only that pain subsequent to an injury, pain that does not diminish after what is considered a reasonable length of time. This type of chronic pain is quite common, and it results in many workers' compensation cases and disability claims. Chronic pain proves difficult to understand theoretically and difficult to treat medically. There is, by definition, no quick fix for it, and treatment can entail everything: surgery, medication, biofeedback, physical therapy, acupuncture, stress management, and occupational therapy.

All pain, not only chronic pain, defies simple explanation. Whereas earlier in this century the dominant theory was that pain is a sensation like touch or vision, this explanation has fallen away because it does not adequately account for many pain phenomena. Beginning with Melzack and Wall's (1965) gate control theory, theories of pain have come to include psychological and social variables as constituent of pain, not simply as add-ons to a process of sensation (Novy, Nelson, Francis, and Turk 1995). The fact is that there is no one-to-one relationship between tissue damage and pain. Clinical definitions of pain today define pain as a perceptual experience:

An unpleasant sensory and emotional experience associated with actual or potential tissue damage, or described in terms of such damage.

Note: Pain is always subjective. Each individual learns the application of the word through experiences related to injury in early life. . . . If they regard their experience as pain and if they report it in the same ways as pain caused by tissue damage, it should be accepted as pain. (International Association for the Study of Pain 1979: S217)

On the basis of this definition alone, we conclude that in order to understand pain, we need to consider seriously that "subjective report." That report is the narrative.

Medical sociologists and medical anthropologists have made significant contributions to the narrative approach to chronic pain. In particular, Kotarba (1983) investigated the making of chronic pain patients. Jackson, in a study of how the "changes in thinking about pain were correlated with self-reports about improvement" (1992:139), has explored the ways in which a pain clinic challenges the assumptions that many patients bring to such treatment centers. Vrancken (1989) and Csordas and Clark (1992) discuss the diverse explanatory models of pain in a variety of pain centers. Given that the medical and psychological understandings of chronic pain are in flux, that the very existence of a "chronic pain syndrome" is under debate, there are multiple narratives, theoretical as well as personal, that coexist at the present time.

I interviewed 15 patients who were in a pain management program at a rehabilitation hospital. All but one of the patients had been injured on the job. The length of time that they had suffered pain varied, from 9 months to 13 years. With the patients' consent, I audiotaped the interviews. The transcribed interviews constitute the narrative data. I used an open-ended approach to the interviews, simply asking patients to tell me the story of their pain and how it has affected their lives. The basic questions I have brought to the data include:

1. What are the basic plots in these stories of chronic pain? By plot, I

mean, "the arrangement of the incidents" (Aristotle, trans. 1964). I do not assume that there is one plot that accounts for all narratives, nor do I assume that there is one plot to account for any one narrative. With Jackson (1994), I assume that each narrative is potentially "polyphonic" in structure. That is, each narrative can contain many points of view, numerous "I" positions. The narratives, I further assume, reflect the situation of the telling, namely, the pain clinic. Certainly the narratives do reflect the fact that the patients were in the midst of a three-week program designed to teach them how to manage pain more effectively. However the patients evaluated that program, it could and did enter into their conversations.

2. What are the cultural, historical, and social contexts that provided the vocabularies, plot-lines, typical experiences, expectations, social institutions, and systems of knowledge for the patients to make sense of their pain? In particular, how did their participation in the pain management program challenge their preconceived notions of pain and its treatment? This investigation, of course, requires research beyond the interviews themselves, and beyond the psychological understandings of it.

NARRATIVES OF PAIN IN THE CONTEXT OF CULTURE AND HISTORY

These narratives have no ending. The pain was ongoing and likely to remain that way. What I will present are significant events in the narrative plots and the results of a cultural-historical interpretation of the incidents, with an eye toward showing their embeddedness in wider presuppositions about the nature of pain, the body, the self, and society.

In the Beginning: The Accident

Patients said that the pain originated in an accident, either at work or in a motor vehicle. This is hardly surprising, since I was interviewing patients with complaints of back or neck pain. In fact, what could be more matter-of-fact than that pain originates in an accident?

Before the middle of the nineteenth century:

back pain ... was generally believed to be a build-up of rheumatic phlegm in the muscles and both local and systemic treatments were used to remove the phlegm. ... Throughout the 19th century treatment of back pain consisted of general measures against rheumatism such as relief of constipation, counter irritants, blistering and cupping. (Allan and Waddell 1989:2).

In the nineteenth century, with the industrialization of production and transportation, two unprecedented notions took root: "These ideas were that back pain came from the spine and that it was due to trauma" (Allan and

Waddell 1989:2). The key term here for Allan and Waddell is *chronic* back pain. Certainly pain as a result of injury was not an innovation of the nineteenth century, as a glance at the *Iliad* will show. But this change in narrative—from humor to trauma—warrants further discussion, for it implies a change in assumptions about etiology, from one of unbalance to one of mechanical failure. One patient described the beginnings of his difficulties in these words: "I was in a rear-end collision [driving a school bus]. So, I had stopped to let a student off and I was rear-ended by a truck and, of course, you know how physics works, energy isn't lost if . . . and since the bus was still, everything transferred to the front of the bus and myself and students in the first couple of three rows were the only ones who really got hurt." For all these patients the beginning of their difficulties was a discrete mechanical accident. The older etiology was relational in insisting upon correspondences between climate and bodily humors. The newer one emphasizes the body as an isolated physical entity, and it emphasizes chance in calling the initiating incident an "accident." On both counts, the meaningfulness of pain has decreased, for it is not related coherently to a surrounding world (the body is a discrete object) and it is unrelated to the flow of personal life (it was an accident).

This beginning in terms of the body as a physical object does not reflect an eternal structure of the narratives of pain, it reflects a particularly modern understanding.[1] Moreover, the event was explained by means of the conceptual framework of biomedicine. The spine and the nerves were the most prominent physical locations of the cause of pain. This account, learned directly from a physician or chiropractor or assumed on the basis of earlier learning about the anatomy of the body, is also characteristic of the modern epoch. Earlier accounts would have primarily focused on humoral excess as an affective response to environmental conditions.

What we take for granted reveals the ways in which the experience is socially and historically constructed. In this instance the location of the cause of pain in a site in the body, as a piece of information derived from a particular kind of question, grounded in what Foucault (1963/1973) called the "clinical gaze," directs action and self-conception along certain lines. The practical consequences of this explanation of the cause of pain were many of the subsequent events in the narratives. These sequelae include: the seeking of medical intervention in the expectation of surgery and medication; rest and inactivity to prevent further injury and pain; a passivity of the self vis-à-vis the pain; a belief that pain is a technical problem to be fixed.

Becoming a Patient

An incident in the plot occurring in all of these narratives (a necessary incident, insofar as I interviewed only people in a pain management program) was entry into the social role of a patient. A sick or injured person becomes a patient when he or she consults a physician or other health care provider. This step is the person's entry into that amorphous social institution called the health care industry. If the accident occurred on the job, there was an intermediary step involved, namely, filing a report with the company. At times this was an unproblematic but an important step, for it defined the situation as medical. The filing of a report with the employer enabled the person to receive medical treatment for the injury. But first of all it established the accident, the injury, and the pain as real, that is, as legitimate. Prior to this event the accident and injury had been private matters. The report legitimated them socially, and the person entered the sick role. Thus the person acquired a new social status, with certain rights and responsibilities. For most of the patients it meant that they continued to be paid despite the fact that they were not working. But the sick role demanded of them that they seek medical care in an effort to get well and return to work.

Medicine as the legitimating institution for health and sickness has a history. Reiser (1978) notes that in the seventeenth century, the patient's narrative was authoritative in determining the existence of sickness, and Duden (1991) shows how in the eighteenth century, sick people did not assume that physicians had a greater ability than they did to know if they were sick. While some may argue that today physicians know more than did their predecessors, what seems less debatable is that today only a physician's word (or that of a physician equivalent) carries social authority. People today do not have the liberty to declare themselves healthy or sick in any socially meaningful way.

In addition to this issue of the status of the word of the patient and of the physician, the sick role status places pain in close proximity to work and productivity. Pain is inevitably associated with the self as useful. Pain challenges the very definition of the modern self as autonomous (Cushman 1990). Many of the patients implicitly held the opinion that their worth as a human being was tied to their ability to work, a common assumption in a society in which personal identity is tied closely to occupational status.

Pain Becomes Chronic

At some point, despite all efforts, the pain would not go away. Then, anxious, depressed, angry, etc., patients began to feel locked inside an invisible trap. They sensed that they had been permanently altered by the accident. At this point they came to realize that their pain did not fit the category in which they had initially located it. Now the pain was chronic. They had believed that pain came and went, but their experience did not conform to that pattern.

At this point, usually after at least six months of treatment without substantial improvement, pain becomes medically defined as "chronic." As Kallinke (1995) indicates, there is nothing definitive about this length of time:

> If the six-month time limit has any meaning at all, it could suggest the approximate time frame in which many people begin to panic and, in the longer run, are often "thrown off track," because Western medicine cannot keep its promise of salvation—to banish illness, suffering, and death. (p. 60)

Moreover, the medical status of "chronic pain" as a disorder remains debated. Two separate federal committees in the late 1980s came to opposing conclusions, one recommending chronic pain as a distinct entity, the other recommending against it as too vague a classification (Osterweis, Kleinman, and Mechanic 1987; Csordas and Clark 1992). Finally, the degree to which chronic pain is primarily a medical problem is unclear, especially in light of the fluctuations in such pain with the economy (Nachemson 1994). Csordas and Clark question the degree to which chronic pain "is a problem of distributive economics as much as one of medicine" (1992:392).

Loss and Grief. For the patients, however, the persistence of pain beyond their earlier expectations produced a situation of loss and grief:

> I was really always an outdoor person, hunting and fishing, and you can't do it anymore, you know. I hadn't tried to go hunting because, you know, I know it would be strenuous on me because of the terrain and stuff I'd have to walk through, and it just, it's heartbreaking, . . . you have your heart set on doing something and you've always done it and you can't do it, it's kind of like a love.

Within the limits set by pain, this patient, a man in his twenties who had worked outdoors since adolescence, grieved the loss of his ability to live as he had. Another patient emphasized the chronicity of her pain, the fact of its ever-presence, its inescapability: "I've had testing and everything is like normal, normal, normal. The pain is like there, there, there. And I don't understand it so." The repetition of "normal, normal, normal" and "there, there, there," said in a monotone voice, sounded like a dirge. Pain refused to recede into the past, so that time, the time of the patient's life, came to a standstill. This grief contained a conflict between the desire to let their former lives sink into the past and a desire to hold on to what has been lost. This formulation is not quite correct, for it might sound as if a person deliberately holds on to pain. But while such a willful act would be rare, it is nevertheless true that there is no pain without consciousness, and that pain entails an attitude of consciousness, namely a repulsion. That pain requires an attitude of consciousness is so despite the fact that pain is not chosen but rather inflicted upon the person. The passivity of the person precedes the reaction of consciousness confronted with pain. Coupled with the temptation to cling to pain was the temptation of suicide, expressed clearly by one patient, who said that suicide always remained "an option" if all else failed.

If one lives in a timeless world, a world in which nothing can happen yet is not eternity, one does nothing. And many of these patients have severely restricted their activities, as one woman recounted:

From May until now, I have not worked. I've laid around the house and taken a lot of pain killers, a lot of, lot of muscle relaxers. . . . No memory. No concentration. I couldn't read. I like to read. I couldn't read. I couldn't concentrate. I couldn't remember. [I didn't do anything] other than television. But I could even drift away through that if I wanted to, but that's the only thing I could focus on and you know, knowing I had to shower. I was doing good if I could shower once a day. That's when I was doing real good and sit just a little bit around the house. [My boyfriend] did everything else.

In the context of the treatment program of the pain clinic, many patients described how terribly out of shape that they had become. They did not feel that they should move, in part out of fear of aggravating their pain or worsening their injury. They retreated from their former life activities in a move of self-protection.

This retreat was at once physical and social. To the extent that they were not physically active, they were socially isolated. To some extent this isolation was reinforced by the physical construction of their social environment in this typically sunbelt-type urban area: To get anywhere, they had to drive or be driven in a car. For many, being in a car was a painful experience they sought to avoid.

The approach of the pain clinic wherein I interviewed patients saw rest and retreat as pathological, if for no other reason than that the lack of activity induced muscular atrophy and thus aggravated pain. However, the treatment of pain with rest has its origins in the nineteenth century with the emergence of orthopedics as a specialty (Allan and Waddell 1989:5). In the shift in explanatory models from humoral excess to spinal damage, irritation was seen as the cause of the pain. The recommendation for rest was part of the medicalization of back pain. Rest has never been an unproblematic recommendation, however. Today, the meaning of rest as a treatment for chronic pain is much in debate. The outcome of the debate will define the narrative of chronic pain in years to come.

The Personal Is Political: Economic and Social Costs of Pain. The changes in life as a result of being in continual pain were manifold. Some of them entailed self-definition. For example, among the men I interviewed, some expressed fears about not being men any more because of the pain. As one man expressed it: "A man needs to play a certain role in his family and anything that decreases that role or limits that role gets him sort of depressed. I mean, you know, you lose a lot." He had applied for Social Security disability benefits. His claim had been denied and was on appeal. He felt torn between a desire to work, his feeling of inability to do so, and a desire to support his family any way he could. Economic worries, and what he described as a lack of understanding from his wife, irritated him and aggravated, from his point of view, his pain. The site of pain, in his lower back, was where the economic, marital, and social dimensions of his life were inscribed. Not all patients responded to the economic costs of pain as did he, but all faced them. What was inescapable was facing the loss of income and loss of social position in the family.

The Search for a Cure

Patients who refuse to give up hope for a cure, despite medical failure and physician conclusion that nothing more can be done, act on a deeply held conviction in modern medicine, however irrationally such patients seem to apply that assumption. Before the advent of scientific medicine, physicians typically understood that there are limits to medical power. Van den Berg summarizes this awareness of limits by paraphrasing a Hippocratic text: "Not to try to cure patients whose ailments are incurable" (1969/1978:9). As contemporary debates over abortion and euthanasia illustrate, no longer are the boundaries of life and death understandable, no longer are there obvious limits to medical intervention.

Becoming Disabled

Inability to work and the receipt of some form of disability assistance plays a major role in these narratives. Essential to the stories was the fact that the patient actually had obtained compensation or was officially declared disabled; that is, the "realness" of the disability was the issue. As one woman stated:

After the first fusion I was okay. I stayed off of work a year, and I went back and I worked just about over a year before the second. I was able to work but . . . no heavy lifting. [The doctor] said something about alternated standing and sitting but there I couldn't do it, so I would like walk around, walk in my work area and then get breaks like every two and a half hours then I would sit down then.

For this woman the disability issue was clear; she had no conflict with her employer, she felt she had been treated fairly, and she anticipated just treatment in the future. For others this event was most problematic, and some described how the conflict over disability exacerbated pain. For example: "I had a rough time when I first got hurt, the lady wouldn't turn in my claim or anything for about three months. So, that stressed me out. I was calling up there and begging her to . . . she'd constantly tell me, I've already done it, I've already done it." It is as if the financial, legal, medical, and social contexts were woven directly into the flesh. They are not separable components but rather one structure.

Becoming an Attorney's Client

Some patients had sought legal counsel because they felt that they were not being treated fairly by their employer, insurance company, or physician. Pain thus has a legal dimension too. This facet was always present, insofar as these patients were in the pain management program because of legal obligations of employer and employee. For some, however, this facet became problematic. Then, the patients felt that they must prove that their pain was real and that they were legitimately disabled. The evidence was in part clinical (i.e., they could testify that their movements were restricted because of pain and a physician could observe this), and it was in part biomedical (X-rays, etc.). As the literature on this point indicates, being in such a position is a temptation to desire, however ambivalently, to maintain oneself as a patient with pain (Chapman and Brena 1989; McAlary and Aronoff 1988). At times in some interviews, this temptation had been taken, even when, at other points in the interview, it was denied.

The historical dimension of this facet of the narratives is that of social welfare (Nachemson 1994). The implication of this history is that chronic pain has woven into its fabric a complex array of legal significations. Chronic pain, despite the fact that it cannot be shared, despite its invisibility to others, is not a private event.

Entering the Pain Clinic

That medical treatment—including surgeries, medication, nerve blocks, and physical therapy—failed, was a conclusion drawn by the patients because they continued to suffer pain. For some, their physicians concurred, according to their account. For others, this was a matter of dispute.

I went back to him and he told me I just needed to learn to live with the pain. And at that point I was so disgusted because it was like, he didn't really care anymore. Or he had just reached whatever level he was capable of handling or whatever. So I decided to myself I was going to go see my chiropractor and see if I could get him to recommend me to another doctor so I could get a second opinion.

As this description shows, this patient questioned her medical status. So long as pain persisted, the status of her condition was to be negotiated. Kotarba found a similar result: "In general, the pain-afflicted person will attempt virtually any treatment that appears likely to offer effective elimination of the pain, if at all economically feasible" (1983:193). He found not only demands by patients for more treatment, but also for certain types of treatment, including acupuncture, behavior therapy, stress management, biofeedback, and hypnosis. While individual methods have had uneven fates over the past two decades, the trend toward multidisciplinary treatment of pain has continued.

Thus constitutive of the experience of chronic pain in the present day is the very existence of pain clinics, last resorts or not. They legitimate and teach a variety of holistic and biopsychosocial models of pain, models that some patients may resist because, in their opinion, it intimates that their pain is "only" psychological (Jackson 1992). The negotiations between the clinic staff and the patients over the meaning of pain was prominent in several of my interviews. For example:

I don't think you actually make it [pain] get worse and better [with biofeedback]. I think you actually put your mind into another area all together to where you're not thinking about it so you don't actually deal with that, 'cause your mind is like totally concentrating on this music. . . . Just for a minute you forget about the numbness and pain or what have you. . . . When you stand up it all comes back. Reality sets in.

This same patient, in the following interview, dismissed the biopsychosocial model entirely, insisting that his pain and numbness stemmed from what he considered a botched back surgery. Other patients found the educational aspect of the pain management program more amenable.

The implication of the multidisciplinary treatment in pain clinics is that patients are encouraged to reckon medically with pain as a biological, psychosocial, and spiritual phenomenon. What is radical in this conception is not that pain has all these dimensions, but that health care professionals claim competence to address them. Thus therapists not only manipulate muscles and coping styles, they invoke, during guided imagery sessions, generic imaginal healing figures into the clinic, invite patients to "fill in the blanks," and envision this figure as Christ or some other higher power. The professional management of such experiences is essential to the pain clinic in the medical world, in a world that had secularized pain over the past few centuries (Caton 1985).

Explaining Pain: Discourse of Physical and Emotional Pain

One aspect of the narratives was not, strictly speaking, an event. It was the explanation of the mechanisms of pain. Explanations of pain are integral to these narratives, for people not only tell stories, they explain what occurs in their stories. For these narratives, then, we must identify the explanatory models (Kleinman 1980) used by the storytellers to generate typical events in the stories. A significant part of the explanatory model followed from the physical origin of pain and from the fact that the patients did not experience pain "only" as physical: They experienced physical and emotional pain.

That pain was first of all "physical" had significant consequences for the narratives. First, there was *the* accident. Then, when medical measures did not relieve the pain, and the pain persisted, emotional pain grew like barnacles on the physical pain. There was an intimate relation between the two pains. For one man, "physical [pain] will cause emotional problems." He said that at one point he was in pain after an injury to a knee and knee surgery. He was taking pain medication but it was not helping him.

I got to where I was just real irritable and if anybody said anything to me and I didn't have the medicine in me I was just ready to knock them on the floor or something. And me and my wife was having excruciating marital problems because the medicine is changing my personality around. And this is where it was getting into emotional pain now because things were really hitting me hard.

His irritability stemmed from his inability to escape pain. Pain was surrounding his life, hemming him in, so he lashed back. Things were "hitting him hard," and his preferred solution, relief through medication, was not working. Thus, in this account, physical pain caused emotional pain. This account mirrors the typical bifurcation of soma and psyche in Western medicine (Gordon 1988). Despite the assertions of biopsychosocial and holistic paradigms, emotional and functional disorders play second-fiddle to "real" disorders (i.e., those in which the body-as-machine can be shown to have broken down).

The temporal sequence in the narratives, in which physical pain preceded emotional pain, was of vital importance to the justification patients often made of the reality of their pain: Emotional pain appears after real pain originating in a real event. Many of these patients had had the reality of their pain questioned, and they reacted strongly to the suggestion that their pain was psychological, because that suggested a lack of sanity or character. However, emotional distress subsequent to an accident and emotional pain (including depression) heaped on physical pain has legitimacy because patients were dealing with real and intractable physical torment.

Ambivalence Toward Drugs and Alcohol. When many of the patients described their physical "and" emotional pains, they addressed simultaneously and spontaneously their use of drugs and alcohol to relieve pain. Nearly all of them saw the use of these agents as a sign of moral weakness (in part because of attitudes at this pain clinic). The setting of the telling of the story—the context was an intense three-week program—influenced the character of the narrative, giving it a confessional connotation.[2] Some confessed to substance abuse, as did one man, a part-time preacher:

My body could not cope with it, and I started getting excruciating headaches. And I was old enough then to drink, so I said, "Well, I'll just drink some and get rid of some of these problems." You got to understand now that my Mom and Dad had not teached me to do that. They taught me that you don't need to drink. . . . And drinking heavy, very heavy, because I had these headaches and I wanted to get rid of them, some way or another. So instead of getting high on life, I'd get high on a bottle of alcohol.

Another man, active in a 12-step program and employed as a substance abuse counselor, stated that his primary disorder was not pain subsequent to an automobile accident, but chemical dependency:

I was working twelve hours a day and going home and taking medication. I'd go off the pain medication in the morning and go back on it around between two and five the next day, but that's the insanity that goes along with the disease [called chemical dependency]. I felt like that if I only took them between those hours, I wasn't abusing. The problem is that that line got crossed, too. For some mornings I got up and felt like warmed over shit and that's when I'd take the pain medication right off. And of course if I could get started, I'd do it during the day.

He said that he had learned this pattern for dealing with pain in a childhood filled with physical and emotional abuse: "If it hurts, don't feel it, do something about it to change it. It's a common pattern of our society, and I've learned it well." As he described it, his clinging to "hatred and resentment" toward his mother set the stage for how he dealt with back pain. Because of his history and his heretofore unwillingness to forgive his abusers, he had been coping with physical and emotional pain with alcohol and drugs. He now viewed this pattern as counterproductive, but indicated that physicians often supported drug abuse (and at other times they could be manipulated into supplying pain medication).

This man expressed well one side of a cultural ambivalence toward pain and pain killers. On the one hand, because anesthetics exist, there is an expectation that all pain can be alleviated. As one woman, an electrical technician, stated: "With all the technology and all the medications you can possibly think of, I'm upset that nobody can give me anything right now. If I abused the drug, it was because I was in pain. But, nobody will say: 'Well, let's have this under control.' " Such an expectation would have been utopian prior to the mid-nineteenth century, when chemical analgesics began to be mass produced. On the other hand, the use of chemicals (including alcohol) to relieve pain is considered dangerous because it leads to addiction, a disorder greatly feared. Addiction as a disease was, along with analgesics, another nineteenth-century innovation (Conrad and Schneider 1992:115). This same woman expressed the ambivalence clearly: "It's like I'm being slowly tortured and it's like everything I need is somewhere, somewhere behind some door. I don't know what's worse, being in pain or being on medication and being addicted." She felt doubly betrayed. She said that her family dealt in illegal drugs, and that through education, she had sought to escape that social milieu. But after the accident at the plant, she felt abandoned by the company, and in order to escape constant pain, she had turned to prescription drugs, illegally obtained. To be an addict is bad, yet the pain—which she described as a constant "toothache" in her arm—was intense.

Addiction was also problematic in these narratives because the clinic sought to reduce or eliminate patient use of pain medication in an effort to have the patients live a productive life despite ongoing pain. As do many such clinics, it has a "work hardening" program, and the overall emphasis is on improving physical conditioning. In these narratives, the addict, a figure of lassitude and self-indulgence, was, in this culture that praises creature comforts, a figure of profound ambivalence. Like chronic pain, with which addiction is intertwined, "substance abuse" is a disorder of uncertain reality. The person with chronic pain faces the suspicion of malingering or milking the system, and the addict the suspicion of not having a disease but being a criminal.

Stress and Pain. "Stress" was often spoken of as a bridge between emotional and physical pain. One patient, the part-time preacher quoted above, stated he had discovered a link between pain in his knee and his emotional life:

What causes the pain to increase is stress, anything that bothers you. . . . I've seen it happen, me and my wife was coming to a little bit of a, uh, not a fight or anything, but just a little argument, and a little stress would come on, and my knee would start throbbing. . . . And the only way to relieve yourself of pain is first of all, think positive, okay. Don't ever think negative. Think positive. Okay, second of all, keep yourself out of stressful situations.

The clinic staff, he asserted, had told him that stress exacerbates pain. Stress is "anything that bothers you," and one is bothered only when thinking negative thoughts. The process in his explanatory model (shared by many of the patients) was: (1) an event occurs that is potentially bothersome; (2) a negative appraisal of the event; (3) "stress," largely in the form of felt muscle tension, builds up; (4) this tension produces increased pain.

This explanatory model was employed by this patient and some others to account for how their own activities or attitudes exacerbated or alleviated pain. This account enabled them to imagine responses to pain other than medication, alcohol, or surgery. They said that either biofeedback or relaxing muscle tension without using biofeedback equipment would ease their pain. For the part-time preacher, the power of relaxation was a major insight gained in the pain clinic: "Next thing I know, I'm relaxed and the pain and the soreness had went away." He was encouraged that he could do things to relieve pain. He stated:

Now I'm on the outside and I'm telling the pain, "Hey, I can control you. In other words, I've got you under control. And if you try to take advantage of me then I'll go into my relaxation period. And I'll let my little healing process take place in my body and you won't be there."

"Stress" as an explanation for disease etiology originated during the same time period that chronic back pain from trauma originated, when the "clinical gaze" (Foucault [1963] 1973) began to locate disease in the interior of the body made visible through anatomy and its accompanying technologies, such as the stethoscope. (Elsewhere in this volume I address stress management as a means of controlling the body, and its application to the treatment of pain is a case in point.) Historically speaking, there is nothing new to the understanding that personal attitude and deportment can affect pain (Illich 1976). What is new is the restriction of the significance of pain to an engineering problem or inadequate "body mechanics" (to use the term the clinic employed to teach correct posture). Feeling the pain of interpersonal conflict becomes described in metaphors of tension or "negative" thinking. When Galenic medicine or traditional Chinese medicine spoke of loss of balance, a relationship with the cosmos was being addressed. The prevalence of metaphors such as stress suggest that we no longer relate to a cosmos. For us, balance means equilibrium of forces,[3] the application of external forces on a body. The use of the metaphors of positive and negative to characterize thought, an electrical or magnetic figure of speech, is to conceive thought as a "force" that increases or decreases "stress." In this effort to banish depression, the alternative suggested by the metaphor is an empty happy face.

The regimen of this pain clinic included physical therapy, occupational therapy, biofeedback training, education in proper body mechanics, and group therapy sessions focusing on stress reduction and related topics. Enhanced physical fitness, relaxation skills, and improved coping skills were the desired outcome of this aspect of treatment. When viewed as a culturally specific way of understanding pain, this emphasis on muscle strength and relaxation is a disciplinary technique to strengthen the self as an autonomous individual. The ultimate goal is for the patients to be more self-sufficient, more in control of their lives, especially of their bodies. Physical therapy, body mechanics, and relaxation training, the heart of the approach to pain at this particular clinic, are techniques of the muscles, the muscles of the autonomous individual. Buytendijk observed: "relaxation of our muscles allows us to forget we have a body" ([1943] 1961:57). These means augment "the mind's dominance and control over the body" (Kirmayer 1988:58). The preacher expressed the aim of the program, using religious terms: "your pain is just part of your body, and if your spirit can take over the physical part of it, the physical part can't win." The techniques of the clinic reinforce a narrative of dualism by developing a separation of self and body that fosters the self's control over the irrational body. The aim is accomplished by teaching skills for the indirect modulation of physical pain by direct control of emotional pain.

Search for Legitimation of Suffering

The desire on the part of patients for relief of pain, which for the most part they expected to find, despite indications to the contrary from the staff of the pain clinic, was at the same time a desire for legitimation of their suffering. They wanted someone, especially someone with authority, namely a physician, to recognize their pain. They felt dismissed, they felt that there ought to be a visible sign that they are suffering.

> Well I know I'm not imagining it, it's what I would say to myself. Well, why doesn't [the physician] do something about it? I try to figure out logically in my mind why this man would sit there and tell me. "You shouldn't have any pain." But yet I'm having a lot of pain. . . . And that's when I decided to myself I'd go to the other doctor that was on my deal and have him just check me over, see what he thought.

What appeared important in the narratives was a search for recognition of the pain's reality, if no cure was forthcoming. Medical recognition, in the context of these clinic-based stories, was especially important.

For some patients, medical recognition was important in legitimating or authorizing disability. The way in which such patients told their story made it the functional equivalent of a legal brief. Through their telling of their story to me, they were arguing with the medical community in order to elicit its support for compensation. Like a plaintiff, patients asserted the truth of their testimony. Like eighteenth-century patients, they knew the reality of their pain; however, the context for the weight of their words had changed. For the health care community, it is not a question of the "reality" of the pain, since it is now the received view that pain can occur whether or not medical investigation turns up any cause for it. But for these patients, as for the culture at large, an emphasis on the psychological or psychiatric means "imaginary" pain.

The Meaning of Pain: Spiritual, Emotional, Physical. A variation on the legitimation theme is the search for meaning. One patient, the part-time preacher who became convinced that pain could be controlled with biofeedback, came to the following conclusion during his stay in the pain management program: "So there's a whole lot that has changed in my life in this last four weeks. The last time we talked I was in the center, remember? Now I'm on the outside."

Another patient, a woman who confessed to using drugs and alcohol to deaden herself to all the pain in her life, decided that the way of Alcoholics Anonymous (AA) was going to offer her greater relief than potential surgeries:

I'm trying not to worry about the future and when I get out of [the pain management program]. That's part of the spiritual program with AA, is letting go and trusting. And that's not been a strong suit of mine. . . . After talking to my friend, we found out my basic problem is a lack of security. I was terrified of being homeless, hungry. It's not the first time it's happened. At least I didn't lose my home this time. But I was drinking then. I was wild, but I'd work two jobs if I had to. And I was [in] a lot better health. . . . [My friend] told me about the God channel. That this is God. This is me and this is another thing that gets in the way of me and God. So, God is a jealous God. Whenever something stays too long, he takes it away. And I feel like all my life I had something taken away.

The injuries and subsequent pain had taken away her livelihood. She was reinterpreting this loss as God's removing obstacles between herself and Him.

In part, this conclusion was a theological justification of suffering. Nevertheless, it was also a step in what Illich calls the art of suffering, which is a cultural task *par excellence*, but which has become problematic. It is difficult today to recognize "in the capacity for suffering a possible symptom of health" (Illich 1976:152).

Work Con Amore as Relief of Pain. One event in the narratives, although not in all of them, was the difference that work *con amore*, with love and devotion, made. One man, who was disabled, severely obese, in part from inactivity, nevertheless was able to work hard on a boat he bought:

Getting the boat was something I enjoyed and wanted to do. . . . Doing something physically that you enjoy doing, that helps out. Seems like you kind of work through the pain, so sometimes it did get pretty heavy for me, so I'd have to quit for a while, and go relax, and . . . I'd lay down and mentally go through the relaxation part of it, and sometimes I'd doze off for a few minutes, or a half an hour, and when I woke up I'd feel perky and I'd feel better. And then go back to doing whatever we needed to be doing out there.

It has been a common observation for at least a century that if a person loves and enjoys whatever work he or she does, then it promotes well-being (Clinical Society 1873) and eases pain. Perhaps this is because in part pain is a phenomenon of isolation. To the extent that a person is isolated, he or she feels more pain. As J. H. van den Berg expressed it: "Pain may be caused by seclusion, by interpersonal dislocation" (1974:225–26). Moreover, not only isolation from other people, but detachment from things aggravates pain. The boat, in this example, connected this man with his father, with his past, and with a future. Perhaps this accounts in part for the observations (Brena 1978; Nachemson 1994) that chronic pain is an epidemic in contemporary industrial countries. That the importance of beloved activities and their loss was expressed like the loss of a loved one in these narratives suggests that the phenomenon of chronic pain is in part a suffering of the loss of social connection, a loss that precedes the onset of pain and that provides the breeding ground for it.

CONCLUSION: THE SOCIAL CONSTRUCTION OF SUFFERING

What these analyses show is not a rigid pattern of experiencing pain and of recounting the story of being in pain, but the complex interplay between the events of life and the social and historical context in which they occur. Pain, at first glance merely a physical symptom, has a cultural history. What I have shown is the extent to which what I find to be most mine, namely, my story, is simultaneously, most ours.

The narrative structures of the chronic pain experience also suggest the difficulties faced by professional care givers who respond to the pain of such patients. If the narrative structures indicate anything, it is the extent to which current social arrangements throw people into an eternity of suffering. Our time is out of joint, not so much with the body as a biological organism, but with the body as a means of our being-in-the-world.

NOTES

1. The older explanatory model still occurs in these narratives, but its occurrence does not have the explanatory power it would have had two hundred years ago. Here are two examples: "Mornings are the worse. Mornings and evenings, rainy days or cold weather days. . . . The day before it rains, you can kind of like tell, it kind of pains in your back, it comes up, like, the spine." "When the weather changes, you're in a lot of pain. Because it's just horrifying, it's just like somebody's in there with an electric shock thing, going, 'Okay, the weather's changed, and now it's time for you to be in pain'. . . . And it was a bad time of year, it was really damp, and that made it even worse."

2. Some patients addressed me as an interested outsider and a psychologist (which is how I presented myself). Several of the patients confided in me about their use of "substances" with the explicit proviso that I not "spill the beans." At other times I was addressed as a representative of psychology or of medicine. In this capacity I was told what "you doctors ought to know." It is important but now always possible to know "who" is being addressed, but as with the context of the telling, the "I"

and the "you" of the story matter. In psychoanalytic terms, the "I" and the "you" are dealt with in terms of transference and countertransference.

3. Illich writes: "Neither the Galenic-Hippocratic representations of balance, nor the Enlightenment utopia of a right to 'health and happiness,' nor any Vedic or Chinese concepts of well-being, have anything to do with survival in a technical system" (1994:9). The metaphor of stress, from this perspective, more honestly reflects our situation than holistic attempts to employ traditional metaphors. And if we attend to the stress metaphor, I contend, it addresses the grief of living without a "cosmos" or, to use Walker Percy's title, of being *Lost in the Cosmos* (1983).

REFERENCES

Allan, D. B., and G. Waddell. 1989. "Understanding and Management of Low Back Pain." *Acta Orthopaedica Scandinavia* 60(suppl. 234):1–23.

Aristotle. 1964. *De Arte Poetica*. Trans. George Olmes. New York: Lubrecht and Kramer.

Brena, S. F. 1978. *Chronic Pain: America's Hidden Epidemic.* New York: Atheneum/SMI.

Buytendijk, F. J. J. 1961. *Pain: Its Modes and Functions.* Trans. E. O'Shiel. Chicago: University of Chicago Press. (Original work published 1943.)

Caton, D. 1985. "The Secularization of Pain." *Anesthesiology* 62:493–501.

Chapman, S. L., and S. F. Brena. 1989. "Pain and Litigation." In *Textbook of Pain,* 2nd ed. P. Wall and R. Melzack, eds. Edinburgh: Churchill Livingstone, 1032–41.

Clinical Society of London. 1873. *Medical Times and Gazette* 1(291). (Summarizes paper by Clifford Allbutt, Overstrain of the heart.)

Conrad, P., and J. W. Schneider. 1992. *Deviance and Medicalization: From Badness to Sickness.* Exp. ed. Philadelphia: Temple University Press.

Csordas, T. J., and J. A. Clark. 1992. "Ends of the Line: Diversity among Chronic Pain Centers." *Social Science and Medicine* 34:383–93.

Cushman, P. 1990. "Why the Self Is Empty." *American Psychologist* 45:599–610.

Duden, B. 1991. *The Woman beneath the Skin.* Trans. T. Dunlap. Cambridge: Harvard University Press.

Foucault, M. 1973. *The Birth of the Clinic: An Archeology of Medical Perception.* Trans. A. M. S. Smith. New York: Random House. (Original work published 1963.)

Gordon, D. R. 1988. "Tenacious Assumptions in Western Medicine." In *Biomedicine Examined.* M. Lock and D. R. Gordon, eds. Dordrecht: Kluwer Academic, 19–56.

Illich, I. 1994. "Brave New Biocracy: Health Care from Womb to Tomb." *New Perspectives Quarterly* 11:4–12.

Illich, I. 1976. *Medical Nemesis: The Expropriation of Health.* New York: Vintage Books.

International Association for the Study of Pain, Subcommittee on Taxonomy. 1979. "Pain Terms: A List with Definitions and Notes for Usage." *Pain* 6:249–52.

Jackson, J. E. 1994. "The Rashomon Approach to Dealing with Chronic Pain." *Social Science and Medicine* 38:823–33.

Jackson, J. E. 1992. " 'After a while no one believes you': Real and unreal pain." In *Pain as a Human Experience.* M.-J. D. V. Good, P. E. Brodwin, B. J. Good, and

A. Kleinman, eds. Berkeley: University of California Press, 138–67.

Kallinke, D. 1995. "Suffering from Pain: Observations by a German Practitioner." *Advances: The Journal of Mind-Body Health* 11:56–65.

Kirmayer, L. J. 1988. "Mind and Body as Metaphors: Hidden Values in Biomedicine." In *Biomedicine examined*. M. Lock and D. R. Gordon, eds. Dordrecht: Kluwer Academic, 57–93.

Kleinman, A. 1980. *Patients and Healers in the Context of Culture*. Berkeley: University of California Press.

Kotarba, J. A. 1983. *Chronic Pain: Its Social Dimensions*. Beverly Hills, Calif.: Sage.

McAlary, P. W., and G. Aronoff. 1988. "A Review of the Chronic Pain and Disability Syndrome: Prevalence, Contributing Factors, Detection, Prevention, and Treatment." In *Pain Centers: A Revolution in Health Care*. G. M. Aronoff, ed. New York: Raven Press, 201–222.

Melzack, R. and P. Wall. 1965. "Pain Mechanisms: A New Theory." *Science* 150:971–79.

Nachemson, A. 1994. "Chronic Pain—the End of the Welfare State?" *Quality of Life Research* 3:S11–S17.

Novy, D. M., D. V. Nelson, D. J. Francis, and D. C. Turk. 1995. "Perspectives of Chronic Pain: An Evaluative Comparison of Restrictive and Comprehensive Models." *Psychological Bulletin* 118:238–47.

Osterweis, M., A., Kleinman, and D. Mechanic. 1987. *Pain and Disability*. Washington, D.C.: National Academy Press.

Percy, W. 1983. *Lost in the Cosmos: The Last Self-Help Book*. New York: Farrar, Straus and Giroux.

Procacci, P. 1974. Discussion of J. J. Bonica, General clinical considerations (including organization and function of a pain clinic). In *Recent Advances on Pain*. J. J. Bonica, P. Procacci, and C. A. Pagni, eds. Springfield, Ill.: C. C. Thomas, 294–98.

Reiser, S. J. 1978. *Medicine and the Reign of Technology*. Cambridge: Cambridge University Press.

van den Berg, J. H. 1974. *Divided Existence and Complex Society*. Pittsburgh: Duquesne University Press.

———. 1978. *Medical Power and Medical Ethics*. New York: Norton. (Original work published 1969.)

Vrancken, M. 1989. "Schools of Thought on Pain. *Social Science and Medicine* 29:435–44.

13

THE EFFECT OF ETHNICITY ON PRESCRIPTIONS FOR PATIENT CONTROLLED ANALGESIA FOR POST-OPERATIVE PAIN

BERNARDO NG,
JOEL E. DIMSDALE,
JENS D. ROLLNIK, AND
HARVEY SHAPIRO

The relationship between ethnicity and pain has been of interest to clinicians and researchers for many years. Since 1960, more than 200 articles have explored this association. Fewer articles have examined ethnicity and post-operative pain (Pferrerbaum et al. 1990; van Aken et al. 1989; Streltzer and Wade 1981; Flannery 1981). Some of the studies found no ethnic differences (Pfefferbaum et al. 1989; van Aken et al. 1989), others did find differences but could not relate them exclusively to ethnicity (Streltzer and Wade 1981; Flannery, 1981). In the area of laboratory-induced pain, ethnic differences have not been demonstrated (Zatzick and Dimsdale 1990).

Recently, a number of well-designed studies have appeared. Despite examining rather different populations, the studies reached similar conclusions—that ethnicity has a large impact on treatment of pain. One study from Los Angeles reported that Hispanic patients were less likely to receive analgesics in an emergency room than were non-Hispanic whites (Todd et al. 1993). Another study from San Diego found ethnic differences in the amount of analgesic received for post-operative pain (Ng et al. 1994). A recent multicenter study found that minority (black and Hispanic) patients were more likely to have inadequate analgesia for treatment of pain associated with metastatic cancer (Cleeland et al. 1994).

One of the intriguing aspects of pain is that pain treatment requires an interaction between patients and staff, and transcultural studies have shown

This chapter is reprinted by permission of the International Asssociation for the Study of Pain and originally appeared in *Pain* 66 (1996), 9–12.

that staff's recognition of patient's suffering is influenced by ethnicity (Davitz et al. 1976). Since the treatment of post-operative pain with PRN ("when necessary") medication requires interaction between patient and staff, it is difficult to establish if ethnic differences in the amount of analgesic received is due to the patient's pain-related behavior, or to the medical staff's perception. In order to address this issue, we studied patients treated with Patient Controlled Analgesia (PCA) for post-operative pain.

Patient Controlled Analgesia, or PCA has been used for post-operative patients since 1970 (Smythe 1992). When patients are prescribed PCA, the interaction between patient and staff is reduced, giving patients more control in the treatment of their pain. With this system, the main interaction between patient and staff is with the physician while the device is being set up.

The main variables on a standard PCA prescription are drug of choice (in most cases Morphine), bolus dose, and lockout interval. The bolus dose is the amount of drug administered with each successful activation of the device. The lockout interval is the period after successful activation of the device during which no additional analgesic can be administered (Smythe 1992). An optional variable is a continuous infusion, automatically delivered by the device independent of patient action (Ferrante and VadeBoncover 1993).

Numerous clinical trials have attempted to standardize the initial PCA regimen, but no consensus has been reached (Smythe 1992). Thus physicians rely on their experience and clinical impression of the patient (e.g., tissues involved in the surgery, narcotics requirement during surgery and in the recovery room, physiologic responses under general anesthesia, pre surgical narcotic use, age, gender) (Ferrante and VadeBoncover 1993). After the initial PCA setting, the physician typically adjusts the device, taking into account the patient's response to the initial treatment settings.

From the perspective of researchers studying pain in different ethnic groups, we realized that PCA offers a novel advantage in studying the ethnicity/pain question. It minimizes and standardizes the patient/staff interaction, which is implicit in all PRN medications.

METHODS

We reviewed 471 consecutive cases of patients treated with PCA for post-operative pain, from January 1993 to June 1993, by the Pain Service of the Anesthesiology Department of UCSD Medical Center. Included were patients who were prescribed PCA for pain control following a surgical procedure. We excluded patients who did not have a surgical procedure prior to the use of the PCA (e.g., sickle cell anemia crisis), or did not use the PCA in the immediate post-operative period (first 8–12 hours). With the authorization of the Human Subjects Committee, the information was gathered through the Anesthesiology Department records and the Hospital computerized database.

Patients' ethnicity was coded in the hospital database as Asian, black, Hispanic, Native American, white, and others. The same database provided information about each patient's age, gender, and insurance status, which we coded as "private" (e.g., HMO, Blue Cross) or "public" (e.g., Medicaid or no insurance).

We examined each patient's use of narcotics before the surgery (medically indicated or not) because we expected this to influence the amount of analgesic required. The type of anesthesia during the surgery (general or regional) and the use of intraoperative narcotics were also tabulated. The pain site (head, neck, torso, extremities, etc.) in relation to the surgery was also considered, since the injury of some tissues can be more painful than others (Ferrante and Vadeboncover 1993).

From the records of the PCA settings, we registered the bolus dose (mgs of morphine equivalents), lock out interval (minutes), continuous infusion (mgs of morphine equivalents per hour), and total narcotic dose in the first 8 to 12 hours after surgery (mgs). The narcotic consumption after the PCA settings were readjusted was not included in our analysis because we focused on the initial PCA prescription. Generally patients remain on the PCA until PO analgesics are tolerated, which is usually 3 to 5 days.

PCA devices allow two very different measures of analgesia—that which was *prescribed by the physician* and that which was *self-administered by the patient*. As dependent variables we studied: the amount of narcotic prescribed (bolus dose×60/lock out period=mgs/hr), and the amount of self-administered narcotic (total dose/period on PCA=mgs/hr). When a continuous infusion was ordered, the amount of narcotic prescribed included the dose per hour (bolus dose × 60/lockout period + [infusion/hr] = mgs/hr), and the amount was also reflected in the total dose of administered narcotic. We used lognormalization where values were not normally distributed. All of the narcotics were calculated as equivalents of morphine using standardized algorithms (Knoben and Anderson 1988; Jaffe and Martin 1990). Patients also completed a visual analog scale (scores 0–10) summarizing their minimum and maximum subjective pain scores during the first 8 to 12 post-operative hours.

Analyses were performed using SPSS (*Statistical Package for the Social Science*) software. Analysis of variance and post hoc LSD-tests (0.05 level of significance) were performed using ethnicity as the independent variable. Pearson's correlations were calculated between selected variables.

RESULTS

After reviewing the information of the 471 originally identified subjects, we excluded 17 because their ethnicity was not identifiable or they formed very small groups for analysis. Four major ethnic groups were identified, Asians (n = 37), blacks (n = 30), Hispanics (n = 73), and whites (n = 314).

The variables that were significantly different among the ethnic groups included: age ($F = 7.352$, $p < 0.001$), insurance status ($F = 13.324$, $p <$ 0.001), and amount of narcotic prescribed ($F = 7.352$, $p < 0.01$) (Table 13.1). A higher amount of narcotic was prescribed for whites than for Hispanics, and for blacks than for Hispanics and Asians (LSD-test, $p < 0.05$) (Figure 13.1). We reanalyzed the sample after excluding those subjects who had received a continuous infusion. Again, we observed a difference in the amount prescribed, with blacks and whites having more analgesic prescribed than Hispanics (LSD-test, $p < -0.05$).

We also examined the amount of narcotics ordered as a function of: age, gender, pre-operative use of narcotics, insurance status, and pain site. Age correlated negatively with self-administered narcotic ($r = -.154$, $p = 0.001$). Men had more analgesic prescribed than women (11.32 mg/hr vs 10.27 mg/hr, $F = 5.374$, $p < 0.03$). Patients with a prior history of narcotic use self-administered more narcotics (59.61 mg/hr vs 28.37 mg/hr, $p < 0.001$). Narcotic prescription was unrelated to health insurance. Patients with more than one pain site had more narcotic prescribed (14.21mg/hr vs 10.49 mg/hr, $F = 3.364$, $p < 0.02$).

We wished to determine if variables such as pain site were accounting for the differences in PCA prescriptions across the ethnic groups. For this reason we performed an ANOVA (Analysis of Variance) with covariates (age, gender, pre-operative use of narcotics, health insurance, pain site), using narcotic prescribed as the dependent variable. Ethnicity persisted as an *independent* predictor of amount of narcotic prescribed even after controlling for these covariates.

The self-administered narcotics, including self-administered and self-administered plus infusion, were not significantly different across the ethnic groups. The proportion of subjects prescribed continuous infusion also did not differ across the ethnic groups (Table 13.1). The self reported pain also did not vary significantly among the groups.

DISCUSSION

During the period reviewed every individual on Patient Controlled Analgesia (PCA) was treated by the Pain Service. The Anesthesiology Department already knew the patient from the pre-operative evaluation, but the physician doing the pre-operative evaluation was not necessarily the same who prescribed the PCA during the post-operative period.

Our results suggest that factors like age, gender, pain site of the surgery, and history of pre-operative narcotic use influence the physician's decision on the initial PCA prescription. However when we statistically controlled for these variables, ethnicity persisted as a significant independent predictor of amount of narcotic prescribed. This suggests that ethnicity itself influences the way the physician perceives and treats patients' pain.

The amount of narcotic prescribed was greater for whites than for His-

Table 13.1
Sample Characteristics

Ethnicity	Whites	Blacks	Hispanics	Asians	Analysis
n	31	30	73	37	Sum = 454
Self-administered narcotics (mg/h)	2.79	2.60	2.16	2.01	$F = 1.58$
Ordered narcotics (mg/h)	11.03	12.13	9.53	10.21	$F = 2.862^*$
Continuous infusion (%)	21.7	30.43	25.86	19.3	Chi-square = 0.881
Minimum pain score	3.11	2.97	3.09	2.94	$F = 0.07$
Maximum pain score	7.36	6.69	7.14	6.27	$F = 2.14$
Private insurance	52.9	40	13.0	46	Chi-square = 37.038**
Gender (%)	64.65	73.33	53.42	51.3	Chi-square = 6.632
Former narcotics use (%)	10.5	13.3	6.85	8.1	Chi-square = 1.421
General anaesthesia	97.09	96.3	10	96.88	Chi-square = 2.124
Intraoperative narcotics (%)	65.02	60.7	74.29	51.3	Chi-square = 5.900
Age	46.85	41.17	37.82	46.19	$F = 7.352^{**}$
Pain site					
Head or neck	3.5	0	1.3	2.7	Chi-square=6.604, df = 9
Torso	63.06	70	64.38	78.38	
Extremities	17.0	20	20.55	8.1	
Site >1	3.82	0	4.1	2.7	

Values in this table are raw data; however some of the statistical procedures employed base-e-log normalization.
*$P < 0.05$.
**$P < 0.001$.

Figure 13.1
Ordered Pain Medication (PCA)

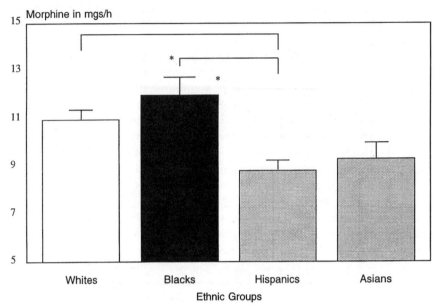

15 Morphine in mgs/h

Whites   Blacks   Hispanics   Asians
Ethnic Groups

Oneway $F = 2.862$, $P < 0.05$ (LSD-test).

panics, and greater for blacks than for Hispanics and Asians, Nonetheless, the subjective pain level (maximum and minimum pain score) and the amount of narcotic self-administered did not differ significantly across ethnic groups. This suggests that the degree of pain control was similar across all ethnic groups, and patients were able to provide themselves with as much analgesic as they felt necessary, especially since all groups were able to achieve minimum pain scores (Cleeland et al. 1994). The finding also supports the idea that the advantages of PCA extend to patients of different ethnic origin. The results suggest no ethnic differences in the patients' expectations of pain control, or the degree of medical knowledge that might influence the use of the PCA device.

It is important to mention that the values of narcotic self-administered and prescribed are taken from the first post-operative period (8–12 hours), before the anesthesiologist has had the chance to see how the treatment is working and then readjust the PCA settings, so they reflect the physician's prediction of the pain the patient will have.

Our sample of 454 patients contained relatively few blacks or Asians. Clearly, replication on a larger sample size is desirable. We lack information on two possible confounding variables—patient size and language. If the Hispanic patients were of generally smaller body size, that may explain why they received smaller prescriptions. It is our impression however this this patient group's size was not disparate. If anything, the Asian patients seemed to have a smaller body size, and yet they received prescription for more medication than did the Hispanics. Similarly, if the Hispanics did not speak English, this might account for their lower prescribed doses, although, here again, one might expect that the Asian patients would have had similar problems. In a basic sense the thesis of this chapter is that in order for pain to be treated effectively, there must be communication between doctor and patient. Cultural factors (certainly including language differences) influence this communication markedly. Even if it could be shown that our Hispanic patients did not speak English, our central observation would remain unchanged—that physicians' appraisal of patients from a different cultural background affects their prescribing practices.

The findings of ethnic differences in prescription pattern of analgesic agents are compatible with an accumulating literature on this topic. The advantage of using a PCA for such studies is that one can begin to disentangle the patient's self-administering behavior from the physician's prescribing behavior. This study suggests that ethnicity exerts a prominent effect on physician's behavior, even when patient behavior is relatively constant across ethnic groups. Although other issues like the effectiveness of communication between physician and patient before the surgery, physician's ethnicity, and prior experience in treating pain still have to be considered, it seems clear that ethnicity has a profound influence on the physician's treatment plan.

ACKNOWLEDGMENTS

The authors thank Kevie Naughton, Mark Wallace, M.D., and Charles Berry, Ph.D., for their assistance.

REFERENCES

Cleeland, C. S., R. Gonin, A. K. Hatfield, J. H. Edmonson, R. H. Blum, J. A. Stewart, and K. J. Pandya. 1994. "Pain and Its Treatment in Outpatients with Metastatic Cancer." *New England Journal of Medicine* 330:592–96.

Davitz, L. J., Y. Sameshima, and J. Davitz. 1976. "Suffering as Viewed in Six Different Cultures." *American Journal of Nursing* 76(8):1296–97.

Ferrante, F. M., and T. R. Vadeboncover, eds. 1993. "Post Operative Pain Management." New York: Churchill Livingstone.

Flannery, R. B. 1981. "Ethnicity as a Factor in the Expression of Pain." *Psychosomatics* 22(1):39–50.

Jaffe, J. H., and W. R. Martin. 1990. "Opioid Analgesics and Antagonists." In *Goodman and Gilman's The Pharmacological Basis of Therapeutics*. 8th ed. A. G. Gilman, T. W. Rall, A. S., Nies and P. Taylor, eds. New York: Pergamon Press, 485–521.

Knoben, J. E., and P. O. Anderson. 1988. *Handbook of Clinical Drug Data*. 6th ed. Hamilton, Ill.: Drug Intelligence Publications.

Ng, B., J. E. Dimsdale, G. P. Schragg, and M. Landys. 1994. "Ethnic Differences in Analgesic Consumption for Post Operative Pain." *Psychosomatic Medicine* 56(2): 179.

Pfefferbaum, B., J. Adams, and J. Aceves. 1990. "The Influence of Culture on Pain in Anglo and Hispanic Children with Cancer." *Journal of the American Academy of Child and Adolescent Psychiatry* 29(4):642–47.

Smythe, M. 1992. "Patient-Controlled Analgesia: A Review." *Pharmacotherapy* 12(2): 132–43.

Streltzer, J., and T. C. Wade, 1981. "The Influence of Cultural Group on the Undertreatment of Postoperative Pain." *Psychosomatic Medicine* 43(5):397–403.

Todd, K. H., N. Samaroo, and J. Hoffman. 1993. "Ethnicity as a Risk Factor for Inadequate Emergency Department Analgesia." *JAMA* 269:1537–39.

van Aken, M. A. G., C. van Lieshout, E. R. Katz, and T. J. Heezen. 1989. "Development of Behavioral Distress in Reaction to Acute Pain in Two Cultures." *Journal of Pediatric Psychology* 14(3):421–32.

Zatzick, D. F., and J. E. Dimsdale, 1990. "Cultural Variations in Response to Pain Stimuli." *Psychosomatic Medicine* 52:544–57.

PART IV

MODERN MEDICAL INQUIRY AND CULTURE CHANGE

Medicine, whether we construe it as a science, a field, a discipline, an art, or a calling, is a part of culture. Like any other aspect of culture, medicine has an element of unrecognized internal logic, and is influenced by non-medical cultural phenomena in a multitude of ways. Discourse in any part of culture organizes what participants think, what they "see." What we "see" is the end point of what we think we see. Medical students learn to solve problems with corpses. They have learned their lessons of cause and effect on static objects, developing a cross-sectional rather than a longitudinal orientation to problem solving. The ethos and mystique of a profession grow out of the transformed shadows of its cultural survivals: corpses are passive and are not colleagues; there is the implicit expectation that the patient will assume the same attributes. Indeed, the most obvious behavioral characteristic of the cadaver is its patience. Whatever is learned from the corpse has to be learned anew from the living body, but the affect and the context of the original lessons are never erased (Romanucci-Ross 1982).

This cross-sectionalizing of the inherently longitudinal is as apparent in larger historical contexts as it is in the biographical. Fleck's *Genesis and Development of a Scientific Fact* (1979) is about a problem in medicine. Whatever we may learn from Fleck, we need to keep constantly in mind his definition of a "fact" as a "stylized signal of resistance in thinking" (1979:98), a road-block in the flow, a cross-sectionalization of the longitudinal. Ways of seeing, or knowing, or doing, or thinking are stylizers of cultural processes in any culture.

Clinical decision-making should be dictated only by what the physician considers good for the patient, but actually many decisions converge at this very point. Much of the decision-making can occur in a hospital where technical aspects of patient care, cost of care (from staff salaries to "empty bed expenses"), and competition with other hospitals mean that these decisions are influenced by business interests. The board of trustees are advocates and surrogates for community interests (Who is bringing money and business into the community? Do we want to go into the health sciences business? Will this attract other business?). This does not mean that the community does not want emergency services and an assurance of quality, as well as decisions consistent with present medical knowledge. It may mean, however, that cost-benefit does not have the same meaning to the patient as it does to other individuals and groups. Policy decisions, then, are products not only of the sum of all individual decisions made by good doctors but also of resources, personnel, and the science and art of the possible.

The field of the art and science of medicine, then, is a culture, an island of cognition, affect, social structure and institutions, codified language; it has boundaries that include members and exclude others. As an information system, the field of medicine is a relatively closed system of knowledge; it has many vested interests in remaining that way. Physicians who stray too far from the properly defined and encoded clinical perspective, or from what is generally deemed to constitute proper basic research, are likely to be shunned, or at least ignored, by peers and superiors. This is a most serious control system since, rhetoric to the contrary, the most lauded work is done not by individual practitioners but by teams: one article in the *New England Journal of Medicine* listed some ninety-six authors. The rewards in this culture are for those who go deeper and deeper into the thesaurus of the medical lexicon, into the most technical aspects of diagnosis. The accomplishments that elicit the most praise are those displaying the finest motor, auditory, and visual skills, or the most ingenious measurement and quantification. That which cannot be measured is deemed, more or less, not to exist; at best it is ignored in any notions of causality. Agonies and ecstasies of scientific meetings center on complex new technologies that require ever more years of training for organ-system specialists. This culture of medicine is organized as much by these implicit structures as it is by its overt functions of easing suffering and curing the sick. And as such, it behooves us to try to understand how these structures influence the whole healing process.

Modern medicine is also characterized by its refiguration of the body image, that is, how the body is represented to the "self" of the members of the culture. Some cultures view the body as a container or a fortress that can be penetrated by substances, such as tiny ghost arrows or sorcery packets that will cause illness and/or death; some see evil substances that have to be sucked out of the container. Some view the body as a house ("container") that appeared to have populations of migrating souls. Soul loss and soul gain as causes of illness characterize many societies throughout the world. Patients and their doctors have "black box" theories about the invisible interior of the "container" body and act upon these theories with ritual and herbal and other natural remedies.

But with the beginnings of modern medicine in Europe, with such simple inventions as the stethoscope, for example, the problem became to bring to the surface that which is layered in depth, to make the invisible visible and to project it on a plane. Daremberg wrote, "As soon as one used the ear or the finger to recognize on the living body what was revealed on the corpse by dissection, the description of diseases and therefore therapeutics took quite a new direction (Daremberg 1865: 1066). Foucault describes this period in European medicine as the beginning of mapping the territory of disease, noting that the "sight/touch/hearing" trinity defines a perceptual configuration in which the inaccessible illness is tracked down by markers, gauged in depth, drawn to the surface, and projected virtually on the dispersed organs of the corpse (Foucault 1973:164).

We have retained this body image in our Western culture, but not without a refiguration by adding new layers to the anatomy based on the study of corpses. This added metaphorical thinking can be especially instanced in the treatment of those "dis-eases" which were formerly considered nuisances or aberrations but are now medicalized. Kugelmann provides his version of the new body image as it is related to the therapy of stress. He notes that we no longer have time for grief work, for unresolved conflicts, and therefore we have adopted an "ideology of adaptation" so that we can reduce the toxic effects of stress while keeping the tension that stress provides for excitement and motivation. Kugelmann suggests that to the anatomical base of our body image we have added new layerings, specifically the "strength of materials" notions from engineering, energy concepts from thermodynamics, and the "information body" of systems thinking. In this provocative chapter he would have us consider the vampire (in a sense our ideal) as the person who thrives on needing and using a system (of people and energy).

The intersection of cultural values with medicine is most pronounced in psychiatry. Because it is concerned with disorders of mood, thought, and behavior, psychiatrists must deal with symbols, images, and metaphors in the culture. We therefore see the pendulum of psychiatric research interests swing to and from "extreme" explanations with cultural emphases in specific time periods, a phenomenon Tancredi addresses in Chapter 15. The rapidly developing field of forensic psychiatry has rendered the relevance of cultural influences on personality (of those labeled and of those who label) compelling. The forensic psychiatrist, through his taxonomy of psychiatric diseases, helps to assess which "deviant behaviors" are the result of "problems," however defined, and which are the result of the willful intention of the perpetrator. Romanucci-Ross examines the beginnings, the trajectory, and the aftermath of one cultural case of "the New Psychiatry."

Medicine cannot be effectively considered in our times without a discussion of ethics and the impact of technology on the structure of behavior. Tancredi and Romanucci-Ross in Chapter 17 explore the cultural dimensions of bioethics as well as one aspect of the now entrenched concept of patients' rights, exemplified in one population, the elderly.

In Chapter 18, Romanucci-Ross and Moerman examine some epistemes in both clinical medicine and scientific medical research, viewed as domains of experience and structured reasoning. Both the discourse of Western medicine and its nondiscursive practices stem from values and ideologies with unrecognized and unexplained consequences. Contemporary paradigms are discussed to illustrate that perceiving always involves applying concepts about "cause" to spatial matter (the body) and the nonspatial (mind). We hold that such a concept is neither useful nor accurate in today's scientific world. (For a basic philosophical analysis of the place of Cartesian dualism today, see Churchland 1986:7–23).

In our final chapter we explore the idea of a medical anthropology, and the possibility of an even more intellectually satisfying future for this necessary discipline.

REFERENCES

Churchland, Paul M. 1986. *Matter and Consciousness: A Contemporary Introduction to the Philosophy of Mind.* Cambridge, Mass.: MIT Press.

Daremberg, Charles. 1865. *La Medicine: Histoire et Doctrines.* 2nd ed. Paris: Didier.

Fleck, Ludwig. 1979. *Genesis and Development of a Scientific Fact.* Thaddeus J. Trenn and Robert K. Merton, eds. Chicago: University of Chicago Press. (First published 1935.)

Foucault, Michael. 1973. *The Birth of the Clinic: An Archaeology of Medical Perspective.* Trans. A. M. Sheridan Smith. New York: Pantheon Books.

Romanucci-Ross, Lola. 1982. "Medicalization and Metaphor: Their Meanings in Culture." In *The Use and Abuse of Medicine.* Martin W. De Vries, Robert L. Berg, and Mack Lipkin, Jr., eds. New York: Praeger.

14

STRESS AND ITS MANAGEMENT: THE CULTURAL CONSTRUCTION OF AN ILLNESS AND ITS TREATMENT

ROBERT KUGELMANN

Stress has become an important topic in health care in recent years, and the management of stress a major way of helping people cope with the stresses of their lives. Whatever stress is—there is much uncertainty on this, despite the certainty with which it is discussed both in scientific and everyday settings—it is as much a "social thing" as it is a "natural thing."[1] In this chapter I set out first of all to describe the social world in which stress feels natural. I then turn attention to stress management, which is a set of techniques to help people be at home in a stress-filled social world. I use a device not often used in this type of essay, namely an extended metaphor.[2] A metaphor asserts an identity between two terms that are otherwise dissimilar. The metaphor I elaborate compares the effects of stress management to the transformation of a human being into a vampire. I mean the metaphor seriously although not literally (the empirical evidence has not yet been collected). The importance of metaphors cannot be overestimated. They are not simply ornamentations; they convey meaning, and types of meaning, that can escape "plain talk." In part, the metaphor of the vampire intends to convey that what at first blush appears good in stress management does not promote well-being. Stress management does not "reduce" stress, it makes stress tolerable. To use a simile: it is like handing out gas masks during a smog alert and proclaiming that the problems of air pollution have been solved.

STRESS AS A SOCIAL PHENOMENON

Stress is an existential condition characteristic of our times. It happens in a world that is constantly changing, and results chiefly from the pressures of technological change and the social dislocations that accompany it. In that technology is as much a mode of consciousness as it is a set of material things, technological innovation at times takes place without new machines. Stress happens in a world that is without form or proportion, a time-space of white noise in which temporal and spatial boundaries collapse. They collapse because time is only quantitative, and hence scarce; the future especially floods the present. Spatial limits disappear, and under stress people find themselves on the go, never dwelling. Speed provides the means to occupy the stressful world. The occupants experience themselves less as flesh and blood than as sources of energy as they consume time, money, and energy, and swim in a flood of information. They find that they desire stress; in controlled amounts it makes them feel alive, productive, important. It promises to transform them into quasi-immortal beings who cope and prosper. They do so at a price: They consume increasing amounts of energy and information to make it through the week. Then they find, some of them, that they cannot take it any more. They make lists. They develop symptoms. Stress takes its toll, since despite their best efforts, their hardiness, their buffers and supports, they have not become pure energy. They are threatened with a realization that the world to which they have adapted does not nurture or sustain their lives without extraordinary effort and resources on their part. The world is alien and hostile, bombarding them with stimuli, demands, and data as if they were astronauts flung adrift in the reaches of outer space. What can they do?

They are doing two things. First, they are getting sick and tired, sick and crazy, and are dying of stress. Stress is a modern demon taking its toll on the freeway of life. It has achieved legal status by becoming the basis for workers[1] compensation claims. In this way and others it proves costly to the American economy. Hence, second, the management of stress has become a profitable enterprise, for stress reduction is good for corporate health. Happy, healthy employees produce better and more efficiently than stressed-out ones. The message has penetrated deep into consciousness as people (primarily the managerial class) take up stress management as a form of self-discipline, as the spiritual exercises of the day. Stress management is a martial art, protecting people from the ravages of being under stress.

In an article in *Insurance Review*, Terry Monroe, the president of a stress management firm, stated, "The single most important cause of stress from our absolute depressed feelings about our inability to change—a sense of lack of control over our lives."[3] His comment is profound, pointing to the dilemma of stress. On the surface, it appears that what he says is false: All we do is change, insofar as we adapt to the new, often eagerly. At the least, even those among us who do not idolize progress seek information to help us cope. But all of this adaptation is not the kind of change that would be needed to slip the yoke of stress. At the heart of stress lies a helplessness, a kind of despair over the incessant series of losses whose rapid succession does not leave room for mourning. Despite the energizing effect of going with the changes and the comforts they offer, people under stress do feel helpless, since they need to be hooked into systems beyond their control or ken. The urge, as the quotation from Monroe suggests, is to change ourselves in order to overcome the lack of control. That is what stress management invites: change by taking charge.

Because stress is the condition of living in constant and unsettling change, it is a form of grief. More specifically, it is a kind of unresolved grief unique to the modern age. Like all grief it has the goal of reconciling past and future by tying them together in the present. Stress, I would hold, is grief in which losses are not mourned but accommodated. Moreover, the implicit dictate to take control, to adapt to the new, and to shed the familiar short-circuits the work of grief. Grief is the "work," as Freud observed, of accepting the reality of lost love. Love dies hard, especially when there are mixed feelings toward the lost object. In the course of the grief work, the bereaved undergoes a transformation. The self that loved the lost love must itself die in order to live again. "Man is but a network of relationships," Saint-Exupery wrote, and when one of those relationships ends, the man changes. Peter Marris sees in grief two opposing impulses that account for the necessity of a moratorium, a period of stilled time, to heal the wound of loss:

Grief, then, is the expression of a profound conflict between contradictory impulses—to consolidate all that is still valuable and important in the past, and preserve it from loss; and at the same time, to re-establish a meaningful pattern of relationships, in which the loss is accepted. Each impulse checks the other, reasserting itself by painful stabs of actuality or remorse, and recalling the bereaved to face the conflict itself. Grieving is therefore a process which must work itself out, as the sufferer swings between these claims, testing what comfort they might bring, and continually being tugged back to the task of reconciling them.[4]

The resolution, Marris continues, rests upon "a sense of continuity . . . restored by detaching the familiar meanings of life from the relationship in which they were embodied, and reestablishing them independently of it."[5] This gradual reformulation of the self and its commitments is fraught with danger. Reconciliation is not guaranteed; the grief may never end, becoming chronic.

Grief is the genus; stress, the species. Stress, like grief, entails loss: loss fundamentally of the familiar (body, self, world). Stress expresses an ambivalence, a particular case of the conflict that Marris describes for all grief. Grief is an existential condition in which one's becoming has been placed into question by loss. Death has gripped what I love, so I must let go in order to live; I am pulled away by my ongoing living, which refuses to stop entirely even for death. But I face nothing when I let go. Like Orpheus, I cannot help but look back; like him, I leave the realm of death for the sunlight. This existential momentum that sweeps me up in the passion of grieving under stress is channeled into what feels like tension, pressure, and energy by demands that leave no place or time to let go and reconcile death with a viable future. Instead, since time is scarce, I divert the passion of grief into productive work and into consumption. These activities appear to fill my neediness and satiate the desire that springs from loss. This diversion is expected and enticed in various ways, not the least of which is the assumption that technologically driven change is natural and inevitable and good.

Grief, intensely personal, is also predictable in its course and resembles a disease or a wound. Cultures ordinarily provide rituals of mourning to give a place for the conflict of grief to work itself out. In the West, mourning has been progressively lost as a public custom. We do not know how to deal with loss in the time-honored ways: moratoriums and social rituals of mourning. Stress reflects and compounds the dilemma. Grief requires time, a specific temporality. Where time is money, grief is expensive. Under stress, time as qualitative, as suitable for an activity, does not exist. One constantly adapts to loss and awaits the next blow, leaving one perpetually poised on the threshold of change, being neither here nor there. Losses accumulate; the grief work is never done. This vitality of grief has been renamed "energy," upon which we feed. Stress, then, is a kind of grief in which the wound of loss is kept bleeding in order to keep the mourner energized for the work of consumption.

"THE IDEOLOGY OF ADAPTATION"

"Stress management" as a term embraces the large majority of means to reckon with stress. Essentially, it represents an ideology of adaptation:[6] By a series of measures, one comes to have the discipline both to accommodate to the inevitability of change, especially that bred by technological progress, and to gain mastery over the process of change in a variety of ways. The approach is clearly holistic, ranging through dietary measures, exercise, mental techniques of self-development, styles of social interaction, and changes in organizational systems. They all have the common end of reducing the toxic effects of stress while maintaining enough tension in the various systems to provide motivation and excitement. In particular, stress management tends to generate special attitudes toward one's own body and self.

The management of stress is a metaphor derived from management, and it implies that stress is one of the things to be administered. The discipline of management dates from an 1886 address, "The Engineer and an Economist," that Henry Towne delivered to the American Society of Mechanical Engineers. Towne later wrote that management's principal task is to "welcome and encourage every influence tending to increase the efficiency of our productive processes."[7] This goal remains true; a more recent author amplifies the purpose of management thus:

As a minimal responsibility, management must balance a multitude of individual efforts and keep peace in the corridors. ... To put it in engineering parlance, a large corporation is a system in dynamic equilibrium; its parts are moving fast, and if they run in gross imbalance, centrifugal force will tear them apart.

The supervisory role is primary, then, but taken alone it is insufficient. ... The manager is expected to be "creative." ... Presumably what it means ... is that management must generate energy as well as channel it.[8]

In the present day, as the scope of management has expanded, the management of employee stress has become part of the mandate. Hence the manifestolike wording of the following:

The rapidly changing nature of work presents an unprecedented challenge for today's managers to create conditions that will release the power of a work force. For too long this group has been constrained by stress associated with change, uncertainty and insecurity. To release this stress, managers must learn to free their employees from such inhibiting forces.[9]

The terms are clear: Change and its anxiety generate stress that binds the power of the workforce. Workers of the world, relax; you have nothing to lose but your stress.

An ideology of adaptation informs stress management, as May and Kruger admit: "As technology continues to alter and depersonalize the world, people will experience a need to interact more frequently and effectively with each other, particularly in the workplace."[10] That people must adapt to such a world is beyond question. That this world is depersonalized does not matter, since "events have no meaning in and of themselves. Meaning comes from how the event is viewed."[11] These frank admissions of the hostility and senselessness of the world and the need to feel comfortable within it ensure that grief over the loss of the familiar and the meaningful will never be resolved. There is yet more change to come.

MANAGING THE BODY

Work on the body is integral to stress management. Typically, the argument for such work is that because of Cartesian dualism, we are out of touch with our bodies. We need to get in touch with them for purposes of health and happiness. Stress long endured makes us ill, but fortunately there are specific things to do to stay or get healthy. Primarily these are life-style changes. The information that moves us to do these things gets us in touch with our bodies. Knowledge about cholesterol, immune systems, coronary arteries, and so forth is common, guiding action toward our bodies.

There are more direct measures to use to get back in touch with the body. They involve relaxation and visualization, and present a body image for a stress-filled world. One such technique is "body scanning," an elaboration of progressive relaxation: "Body scanning uses your inner awareness, rather than your eyes, to examine your body. This kind of scanning involves directing your attention quickly and easily to various parts of your body."[12]

The technique works, insofar as it calms and centers, while teaching its practitioners about the location of stresses in their bodies. As an anxiety-reducing method, scanning and its numerous equivalents act as so many Trojan horses, for along with quietude they ever more securely infiltrate into one's being an alienated image of the body:

When you scan, you will imagine various parts of your body and check to see if they are tense. Some people imagine a picture of their body, others imagine their muscles as they would be drawn in an anatomy book, and still others imagine parts of a stick figure. One individual found it easier to imagine an x-ray machine scanning his muscles.[13]

This activity of dissecting the felt body into its elements of tension and relaxation exemplifies "getting in touch with your body."

If I feel better when I relax and scan, why call it a Trojan horse? But what do I get in touch with? What image or set of images does stress management inculcate? It is, I would suggest, a compound image, a four-layer inscription written into the flesh. The top layer is the "information body" of systems thinking. Hence the appropriateness of the term "scan," which has acquired the meaning of reading or analyzing patterns of lights and shadows and converting them into electrical impulses for the purpose of information processing. Information processing is inseparably linked with control or "purposive influence toward a predetermined goal."[14] Hence what one reads or processes exerts an influence on experience and action. A basic insight of the Information Age is that information, tied theoretically to decision theory and to thermodynamics, is not simply "the facts"; in its current usage it carries an implicit coercive force. As Barry Glassner writes of the fitness movement, so too with body management (which subsumes fitness):

A great advantage of a fit body is that it can be entrusted to perform competently and reliably. . . . The fit body-cum-self is cognized as an information-processing-machine, a machine which can correct and guide itself by means of an internal expert system. When information from the medical and psychological sciences or from health crusaders is received via exercise and diet instructions or the media, the self-qua-information-processor is able to use that information to change its own behavior for the better.[15]

When we get in touch with the "information body," we have the experience of feeling as "self" what is actually fragments of conceptual schemata that are purveyed by health authorities through the media for the purposes of conforming our behavior to what these authorities have decided is our "good." We are told what we need.[16] The information "processed" in body management derives from three scientific pursuits (at least): the science of thermodynamics, the science of the strength of materials, and the science of anatomy (which are inscription layers 2, 3, and 4). Layer 2 exerts influence by directing consciousness to questions such as, How much energy do I have? How can I get more? Since energy is the ability to do work, the questions help us shape our bodies to continue to perform with improved efficiency. Layer 3 asks, How much stress can I take without breaking? How can I strengthen my material? These are engineering questions. Layer 4, the basic text upon which the others are inscribed, is the anatomized body. This layer derives originally from the study of corpses, formerly of criminals; the use of these bodies for dissection was a form of punishment.

This anatomized body is, as phenomenology has taught us, an alienated body, since it is no body—no thinking, feeling, willing body. Through emblems omnipresent today courtesy of X-ray, television, and CAT scan, we have come to accept the corpse as the real body. Stress management is a form of training that further instills in our consciousness this corpse with its layers of inscriptions in order to mold behavior and experience. To what end? To the end of managing stress, that is, living with loss of the familiar without getting sick or going crazy.

Nevertheless, the image of oneself as a living corpse, though we do not usually phrase it thus, calms, reduces anxiety. There are several reasons that the image reduces stress. First, it fosters a sense of control. Since science reveals the inner working of the anatomical image, to the extent that I live with that image, I participate in the power that knowledge brings. I take up the role of an anatomist, of an X-ray machine, of a physician. Second, knowing my body in these terms allies me with the medical community. I become an active member of the health care team when I can describe myself in such terms. Third, the very anonymity of the image provides a measure of community. As stress isolates one in white noise, so this image of the anonymous body makes me feel that I am not alone. This body image is appropriate for a stressful world, since it is not the body as lived through and familiar; it is a body I can have, not be. Finally, the image enables me to stay under stress. In no way does it negate stress and, in fact, it facilitates being under stress. The body is but one of the systems to manage, and in this image it is quite manageable. But at a price: I imagine my flesh as an animated corpse.

SELF-DEVELOPMENT

The distance from which the body is touched implicates the psychological techniques of self-development. Typically they promote an internal locus of control, a sense of self-mastery, effective coping skills, and other measures to offset the sense of helplessness. By taking up crises as challenges to master and as problems to solve, one develops into a person who can thrive in an increasingly depersonalized setting. In a discussion of problem-solving therapy we learn that an inability to solve problems causes stress. The goal of the treatment is as follows: "The client is taught how to think and behave in an autonomous, flexible, and scientific manner. Indeed, Mahoney (1974) metaphorically depicts problem-solving therapy as an educational process whereby the client learns how to function as his or her own 'personal scientist.' "[17] As is true with the body, psychological techniques develop an image of the self: here, autonomous, flexible, scientific. Specifically, this image is of a person capable of recognizing a problem, of finding alternative solutions, of evaluating means and their consequences, and finally of perceiving "cause and effect relations in interpersonal events."[18] This calculative thinking of an autonomous (independent, individualized), flexible (adaptive), scientific (detached enough to see causal networks between people) self is ideally suited to manage stress, for such a self has sufficient distance from the world not to value the familiar too highly merely because it is familiar.

Flexibility and detachment are two goals of stress management. The ability to wield power is another, equal in importance. Power proves therapeutic in two forms. An inner locus of control, that is, the perception that one's own actions make a difference, reduces stress. Since, in this ideology, events mean nothing in themselves, an inner sense that one has power—illusory or not—goes a long way to ease the perception that events are out of control. In limited interpersonal spheres, such confidence is persuasive. But the situation differs when dealing with constant change demanded by technological developments and their social organization. Then an inner locus amounts to an ability to adapt to the inevitable.

Beyond inner locus, real power reduces stress. Here the whole notion of stress as literally a load that one carries collapses. The number of demands and tensions in life does not automatically translate into a level of stress. Despite the picture of the harried executive, underlings suffer from stress more than do their superiors. Not the Richard Corys but the Willy Lomans succumb to distress. As Kets de Vries discovered, a "power effect" helps to keep managers healthy: "Reduction of uncertainty, through control over information and people can be considered a countervailing force to feelings of helplessness."[19] Moreover, in a kind of voodoo operation, stress can be delegated: "Through the abuse of power, managers can induce stress in their subordinates, and for the person in charge, control over subordinates can have a stress-reducing effect. It is responsibility without control that gives rise to stress."[20] Power operates, however, within constraints that are not only organizational.

Without diminishing the possibility of an individual making a positive difference, those who possess of power need also to adapt to the constantly changing world. In a study of computer anxiety among managers, for instance, two researchers investigated how managers responded to increasing expectations that they operate desktop computers. Change enters an organization, they write, "through technology, structure, or people," because an organization is a system that embraces even the top dogs. They concluded that "effective adaptation to computer technology is taking place in these companies," that managers appreciated the "increased efficiency" the computer offered, but that many complained that they had "less face-to-face contact" than previously.[21] Even the powerful decision makers must go with the flow or face loss of position.

Instrumental thinking and the attainment of power are thus two important tools for managing stress. A third, which touches more intimately on the human spirit, deserves attention: the management of stress through self-monitoring and meditation. "Self-observation is the first step in personal stress management," write Quick and Quick, for it helps one to learn the causes of stress in oneself.[22] It is one aspect of the introspection endemic to the control of stress, and a form of "palliative coping," in that when the world cannot be altered, one can change one's self. Meditation, alcohol, drugs, and television are ways to alter self, meditation carrying the implicit promise of doing so without producing sickness.

Meditation in its various forms manages stress by increasing self-governance and discipline. Since change is inevitable, emotional calm makes these disruptions easier to take. While noting that meditation is a "contemplative state as against a calculating or analytic state of mind," Sethi reasons that meditation is also a tool to achieve relaxation and one's goals. Meditation frees one from stress because in realizing the illusory nature of the autonomous ego, one also realizes that "the release from stress lies through and not away from the problem—and the problem is born in, and has its sole existence, in [sic] the mind."[23] The wisdom of ages speaks in these words, yet one may wonder at the ease with which difficult disciplines such as yoga and meditation find acceptance.

Despite the personal well-being that comes from these techniques, they are means to accommodate people to living stressfully without great pain. Stress is accepted as natural. As Ellul asks, "What can limits mean when psychological devices make it possible to push back all limits?"[24] In sum, these practices of stress management have as their goal the infinite remolding of the human being to fit a world of endlessly engineered changes. Ellul captures the essence of such techniques in observing, "It makes men happy in a milieu which normally would have made them unhappy, if they had not been worked on, molded, and formed for just that milieu."[25] This intention of stress management rarely receives overt mention; it is characteristically disguised in an argument such as the following: "Stress is a naturally occurring experience essential to our growth, change, development and performance both at work and at home. Depending on the way in which stress is managed, it may have a detrimental effect on our well-being and health—or it may have a beneficial effect."[26] If one believes that stress is both natural and essential to growth, then of course he will cleave to it as to a lover. But the rhetoric fails when he perceives stress as a product of a blood-sucking quest for efficiency.

THE VAMPIRE IN THE SHADOW OF STRESS MANAGEMENT

Thusfar the discussion has focused on *what* stress management seeks to accomplish, describing it in its own terms and setting these terms into their social and existential contexts. Now I turn to the implications of stress management, by making the argument that the "cure is worse than the disease." The extended metaphor (also called an allegory) of the vampire serves the end of drawing out these implications. The allegory provides a commentary on the "good" that stress management accomplishes.

Stress management intends a good end, the easing of human suffering and pain. In this effort it is not without success. Yet trailing the good intentions like a shadow is a sinister presence that undoes the good by compounding suffering through miring us deeper in stress. Stress management attempts to construct a rational, powerful, creative, calm being whose body is an animated corpse. For this being, suffering, grief, illness, and even death are not inevitable. The changes to which it adapts include medical advances that sustain its life for an increasing length of time and creature comforts that eliminate physical work and the discomforts of nature. The price that the being has to pay for these benefits, however, is enormous. It entails a craving to become the very source of energy that keeps it in the formless, abstract, disembodied realm of stress. It entails, most fundamentally, not living through the work of grief, never resolving the conflict of grief, but rather accepting an endless series of hammer blows of loss as the condition for receiving the benefits of stress.

Where have we met such a being before? Only in our nightmares and in tales of gothic fantasy. Is it any wonder that this being, whose name is universally known, inspires ever new and increasingly sympathetic treatment in films and novels? This being is the vampire.

Vampires occur widely in myth and legend, but it is less to its archetypal than to its cultural manifestation that I make reference. The same famous evening of storytelling that hatched *Frankenstein* conceived John Polidori's novel *The Vampyre* (1819). While Polidori did not create the vampire, his book fascinated western Europe and inspired numerous imitations, the most famous of which is Bram Stoker's *Dracula* (1897). In our own day, countless films have dramatized Stoker's novel and played with the theme. A change in attitude toward the vampire becomes noticeable if we compare the 1979 film *Dracula* with its predecessor of 1933. In the early film, the count is clearly evil despite his cultivated manners and charm, and good triumphs in the end. In the more recent film, Dracula has become a more sympathetic figure, strikingly erotic and the melancholic representative of a vanishing race. In the film's ending, good wins out only temporarily, and we are promised, in the language of mass media, sequels. In another film, *The Hunger* (1983), beautiful male and female vampires lead a life of quiet charm, teach music, and stalk nightclubs. This film's brilliance is in making clear that the vampire is addicted to the blood of life, that it, is hopelessly helpless without getting its needs filled by transient interpersonal relations.

The most striking re-evaluation of the vampire occurs in recent novels, including Fred Saberhagen's *The Dracula Tapes* and Anne Rice's trilogy of novels, *Interview with the Vampire, The Vampire Lestat,* and *Queen of the Damned.* These novels share a common device: The narrators are vampires; we experience the world through their eyes. In Saberhagen's book, the tapes were made by the count, who retells Stoker's novel from his point of view, arguing that Jonathan Harker and the others lied about him (and were certainly mistaken about the climax of the novel). Rice's trilogy also begins with a vampire speaking into a tape recorder; the speaker is Louis, who was initiated into vampirehood by Lestat (hero of the second novel). When Rice was interviewed after the publication of the third book, a reporter asked her if she would like to be a vampire. She answered that she would, in order to go into dangerous parts of cities at night and to fight crime. To be a vampire is to "take back the night," make it possible to live without fear in the alien world that creates stress.

Two things are essential to the nature of the vampire: it cannot die, and it feeds on blood. In both regards, stress management techniques tend to produce vampires.

Its Deathless Body

To become a vampire, a person must undergo a physical transformation. Louis, the interviewee in Rice's first novel on the topic, recalls what happened after he drank the blood that initiated the process: "All my human fluids were being forced out of me. I was dying as a human, yet completely alive as a vampire; and with my awakened senses, I had to preside over the death of my body with a certain discomfort and then, finally, fear."[27] The vampire body, devoid of human flesh, has more acute senses, greater strength and agility, perfect health, and it never ages. In these qualities it approaches the cultural ideal. What is telling in Louis's account are two aspects of the transition: first, at the moment when he should die, he does not. The death of the old self, characteristic of grief, has been bypassed in this transformation. Second, the body becomes an animated corpse; during a process of change, consciousness hovers in discomfort and fear (and then in equanimity, as feeling drains with the fluids).

Let us imagine the scene again, in the quotidian: "I" sit at home, tired and frazzled, exhausted from the pressures of the day, from fighting traffic, from stemming the flow from the checkbook, from watching television in order to unwind. Sleep eludes "me." What "I" realize, in the typical story of salvation from stress, is that "my" life-style must change. Not, mind you, that "I" will refuse to participate in the noisy world. That seems unimaginable. No, "I" take up stress-reducing measures and soon feel better, more relaxed, more in control.

Rather than dying to the stressful world—whatever that could mean at this juncture—"I" have taken it on, on its own terms, becoming disciplined. Rather than give in, at the moment of being drained "I" bite back, becoming the center of the whirlwind, not its victim. Thereby "I" become more in harmony with stress, living on its purchasable substances, energy and information. The desperation that led "me" to embrace stress management is the act that transforms "me" into a vampire. Now stress energizes rather than drains "me"; "I" do not have to die (or get sick), for "I" have transformed stress into my energy.

As Rice depicts it, the critical moment has this form, as the initiator says to Louis:

Be still. I am going to drain you now to the very threshold of death, and I want you to be quiet, so quiet that you can almost hear the flow of blood through your veins, so quiet that you can hear the flow of that same blood through mine. It is your consciousness, your will, which must keep you alive.[28]

When Louis accepts, at the moment of death, the blood from the vampire's wrist, he experiences a wholeness and oneness known only by the infant at the breast. All loss has been overcome in this moment of unity. There is no longer reason to suffer or grieve when "I" become that which would kill "me." The moment does not make the vampire blind to its needs; in fact, the vampire honestly accepts its need for other people, and anyone will do. He thinks in terms of systems.

Its Feeding on Blood

The vampire's grotesque parody of the Christian Eucharist needs to be viewed in the context of the present age. Blood for us has undergone a metamorphosis. Blood used to be the very stuff of our selves, defining us as noble or common. As one of the four humors, blood had powerful psychological and medical properties, to the extent that bloodletting was a necessary practice, as was the building up of blood. Now, however, blood is a commodity to be bought and sold, a chemical soup capable of being shared by many physiological systems. "Give the gift of life" read the ads for blood drives, revealing the symbolic equivalents of blood. Blood is life, blood is energy, the raw material for living.

The vampire is a blood addict. Blood enables it to maintain its animated corpse in the pink of health. Stress is for people what blood is for vampires. Is it any surprise to learn that people are now becoming addicted to the stress of life? The energizing effect of undergoing stress has the potential for compulsive activity, especially when it has power as its accompaniment. "I work best under pressure," or as Waino Suojanen, an authority on human resource management, observes: "There is plenty of anecdotal evidence that some executives deliberately seek out the management life because they get a high out of controlling people."[29] And some "managers become so proud of their ability to stand up under crises that they are always creating crises to stand up under, or are always starting fires in order to put them out."[30] One gets addicted to the experience of transcending normal human life in these instances: Power, a strong medicine that (as noted above) can reduce stress, becomes poison, mastering those who too often find balm for their lives in its exercise.

In recent years the phenomenon of stress addiction has arisen, in part because addiction has become a catchall term and in part because a consumer society pushed to its limits has the addict as its ideal type. The vampire dispenses with trivial commodities, sinking its teeth into the ultimate product. The psychologist and Jungian analyst Linda Leonard concurs in part in her claim that "Dracula as Demon Lover is an archetypal symbol of addiction."[31] The figure of the addict so exercises the contemporary imagination that whereas in the past the addict was an Other, now it appears as a figure of the self. Stress addiction, or "how to turn tension into energy," like the lust of the undead, goes to the source of what addiction desires: the high, that verticality which lifts us above the merely human. We addicts thus share in the vampire's fate, becoming bestial in search of the next hit, the next sublime moment, the next crisis.

Stress management produces vampires, then, to the extent that it aids in the loss of the flesh and in adaptation to a world of relentless change. As "I" lose the flesh, through the recession of limits by human engineering, "I" feel more at home in an abstract, formless, noisy space-time. Stress thus managed promises immortality as human limits are transcended, but it is the deathlessness of the vampire. " 'I've done with grief,' she said, her eyes narrowing as she looked up at me. 'If you knew how I long to have your power; I'm ready for it, I hunger for it.' "[32] So says one vampire to another. Through managing stress we trade grief for power, loss for energy. The conflict that grief would heal becomes harnessed for work.

"THE ABSENCE OF STRESS IS DEATH"

What alternative is there? The phrase that heads this section comes from Selye, and although he did not mean it in quite the way I take it, it indicates the direction. Where death has a place, stress cannot abide. The vampire narratives provide the form: Only when mortals dig up and face in the light of day what they fear becoming, and only when they dispatch the vampire in a ritual of burial, can they lay their fears to rest. The ritual slaughter of the vampire is not simply an act of violence, since the vampire craves rest; its will cannot act on this desire.

The vampire is an appropriate image for the outcome of stress management primarily because a vampire successfully achieves not only empowerment and high self-esteem but also immortality. The vampire stories play with the theme of earthly immortality, which has such great appeal. If the psychoanalysts are correct, at some level of our beings we do not believe that we are mortal, so that we are all tempted to want to become something like vampires.[33] The "cure" for stress management, then, is in part to reconsider the place of death in human life.

In the stories, the primary means to vanquish a vampire is to locate its grave, unearth it, drive a stake through its heart, and bury it again. Then and only then will the undead find release from this life and its soul seek its final reward. Like insomniacs, vampires cannot find peace by themselves: they cannot succumb to passion, cannot be possessed by the elemental force of death that would life the burden of life from their shoulders. What heals the vampire informs us as to the place and the time of the action: the place is the body, the time is the mourning that begins at the graveside.

The Stake in the Heart

> Then comes a sudden jab of red-hot memory.
>
> C. S. Lewis, *A Grief Observed*

A loss that occasions grief is a wound. This is no mere analogy, but the painful reality that the bereaved feel. The location of the wound varies, but typically the heart centers the pain. Since stress is unresolved grief, it is necessary to recover the felt sense of the wound of loss in order to mourn. With stress, however, the sense of being struck is usually diffuse, less focused, given its disembodying nature. Stress bombards; we take flak from all sides. At other times, the experience has precision: "Employees feel like we're the anvil and everybody's beating on us with a hammer."[34] But whether the wounds come as the flak of hurriedness or the hammer of criticism, the first task is to disengage these moments from the engineering mentality that asks, How much can I take? Is my material adaptable enough?

Can I cope? For these moments are not attacks, they are stabs in the heart of the vampire. They contain the potential to bring back to reality an old idea and perception that things that matter have their dwelling in the flesh. The work of grief that this pain facilitates can have the salutary effect of so wounding us that we realize the flesh is no animated corpse but our very selves. Loss wounds the heart (not the pump) because love and commitment dwell in the heart. When the stake is planted in the vampire's chest, blood (energy) rushes out and the corpse decays. These are the effects one seeks in order to escape being under stress. The stab wounds of loss cannot be accounted for by the animated corpse and the knowledge (anatomy, physiology) of it. Only the story of one's particular loves can express the nature of the wounds. The decaying corpse can thus begin to become flesh again.

The flesh is the body of the familiar. This definition is true to the old echoes of "flesh" from Scripture and elsewhere, which bring together the self as somebody and all that belongs with somebody: "flesh of my flesh" (children, kin), "one flesh" (husband and wife), "the flesh is weak" (desire, passion, resistance to excesses of the spirit). Like William James's notion of the "material me," the flesh is also all that is concretely mine: clothes, dwelling, possessions, land. That under stress, dwelling in the body and in places and moments, becomes problematic, means that with stress, the flesh withers, vanishes, is transcended. To bring the flesh back into perception, an antistress meditation may prove helpful. From the *Secretum* of Petrarch comes a meditative exercise from a late medieval tradition. It is particularly graphic, even grotesque, flying in the face of our sanitized images of the healthy, anatomized body. It evokes the flesh in all its materiality. Petrarch provides a guide to the proper meditation on death that is the polar opposite of our command: Relax!

So here is a test which will never play you false: every time you meditate on death without the least sign of motion, know that you have meditated in vain, as about any ordinary topic. But if in the act of meditation you find yourself suddenly grown stiff, if you tremble, turn pale, and feel as if already you endured its pains . . . [and after meditating on the Four Final Things] then you may be assured you have not meditated in vain.[35]

Notice that Petrarch urges the person meditating to feel passionately about death, in contrast with the scanning technique described above, which seeks to eliminate the least "motion" or muscle tension. The passion that Petrarch encourages is fear or dread, which will be resolved in the meditation because the goal is to come to grips with death, not simply be terrified of it. What differentiates Petrarch's meditation from those of stress management is not only the contrast of the religious to the secular context of meditation, which is significant in and of itself, but his insistence on passion. Stress is the absence of the passion of grief, as we have seen above. What Petrarch's meditation reckons with is the necessity of submission to passion in order to grasp the realities that passion is passionate about. Now to the meditation:

Of all tremendous realities Death is the most tremendous. So true is this, that from ever of old its very name is terrible and dreadful to hear. Yet though so it is, it will not do that we hear that name but lightly, or allow the remembrance of it to slip quickly from our mind. No, we must take time to realize it. We must meditate with attention thereon. We must picture to ourselves the effect of death on each several part of our bodily frame, the cold extremities, the breast in the sweat of fever, the side throbbing with pain, the vital spirits running slower and slower as death draws near, the eyes sunken and weeping, every look filled with tears, the forehead pale and drawn, the cheeks hanging and hollow, the teeth staring and discolored, the nostrils shrunk and sharpened, the lips foaming, the tongue foul and motionless, the palate parched and dry, the languid head and panting breast, the hoarse murmur and sorrowful sign, the evil smell of the whole body, the horror of seeing the face utterly unlike itself.[36]

This practice comes from a mentality alien to the modern mind, although in one way at least the late medieval period resembles our own. This type of meditation arose in a time of war and plague, when death was ever present. In our own day, when the term (and concept)"megadeath" has been coined in the wake of two world wars, bureaucratically organized genocide, and the specter of a nuclear winter, the practice of meditation on death may not be entirely foreign to our secular mentality.

I call this practice an "antistress" exercise because it makes us neither more nor less resilient to stress. Its aim is to pierce the "I" that lives under stress and expose it to the losses that stress as a construct makes difficult to mourn. It holds up to the imagination an image of the body as bound to loss and to death: not the anatomized body, fixated by embalming fluids, but the flesh with its feelings and frailties. This vision of the dying flesh, which we are less capable of experiencing today than in Petrarch's time, may move us from stress to a passion for living. As Aries comments:

"We must leave behind our house, our orchards, and our gardens, dishes and vessels which the artisan engraved," wrote Ronsard, reflecting upon death. Which of us faced with death would weep over a house in Florida or a farm in Virginia? In proto-capitalist eras—in other words, in periods when the capitalist and technological mentality was being developed, the process would not be completed until the eighteenth century—man had an unreasoning, visceral love for *temporalia*, which was a blanket word including things, men, and animals.[37]

When we stop for death, we can grieve, and when we grieve, we can love again. To the extent we thus stop, we step out from under stress.

Burying the Dead

Ubi caritas gaudet, ibi est festivitas (Where charity [love] gives
pleasure, there is the festivity).

John Chrysostom

Stress occurs when losses of the familiar, which happen at an accelerating
pace, become problems to solve and challenges to face, when innovation
and progress in efficiency fall upon the earth like manna. This peculiarly
modern form of grief allows for no resolution, for the position of loss keeps
us energized, pining for we know not what, feeling our inferiorities and
helplessness, and hence vulnerable to the demand that we take charge and
flexibly adapt. So we willingly bite back on that which feeds upon us, hungry
for anything to fill the void that white noise creates.

To stop for death is a first step to enable the grief to emerge from the
iron bands of stress. Then to celebrate loss through mourning. But that has
been rendered difficult. Nietzsche, who saw our time of stress on the hori-
zon, observed: "The trick is not to arrange a festival, but to find people who
can *enjoy* it."[38] We are incapable of celebration to the extent that we live
stress as stress. Men under stress live in no-man's land. They cannot, we
cannot, stop for death, take the time to acknowledge the completeness of
things as they are, which affirmation grounds celebration, even the celebrations surrounding death.[39] Vampires, the addicted, the stressed-out, cannot
acclaim the goodness of things as they are.

How to celebrate mourning? How, that is, to lay the vampire to rest, cover
the grave, pray for its soul, walk back to town? Laying the vampire to rest
means in part easing its neediness. The constant need for fresh blood drives
the vampire, and the ambivalence of its grief keeps it so needy. To begin
to celebrate mourning means to celebrate the neediness rather than satiate
it with fixes of energy. Mourning begins when we are exhausted, stressed-
out, frazzled.

I have extended the allegory of the vampire to include what "cures" a
person of the condition. Nevertheless, it is important to recognize that this
so-called cure is not a new prescription about what to do when "stressed-
out." I do not envision support groups beginning, using Petrarchian meditation, for example. Part of our current dilemma is that academics and other
professionals concoct treatments for the illness of being alive. My task is
complete if I can provoke a pause in the automatic function of problem
solving. Something vital happens when the power to solve problems is re-
nounced. Now to conclude.

The rush of stress covers a poverty all the more profound because it is
unrecognized. The energy of stress has its generator in the betwixt-and-
between nature of stress. The alien world, the ambivalence toward loss, the

accommodation to change: A stockpile of emptiness builds up and, not being recognized, not lived through in bereavement, feeds the frantic pace. Then, "wiped out," the cycle begins anew. To refuse energy in the name of poverty makes celebration possible. To be thus impoverished is a condition no commodity can enrich; only the gifts that come freely in celebration can answer such poverty. In this celebration of the loss of the flesh and the familiar we find that we are reflected, not in the chrome and glass of downtown, the coffins of vampires, but in the bums and bag ladies looking in the trash cans or, hands outstretched, asking for a gift.

They teach us how to be poor. Ask for a gift. Gifts are not scarce commodities. They are always essentially plentiful. With arms outstretched, backs turned to the temples of scarcity, we celebrate: "A festival is essentially a phenomenon of wealth; not, to be sure, the wealth of money, but of existential richness. Absence of calculation, in fact lavishness, is one of its elements."[40]

Thus enfleshed and impoverished, we celebrate our losses, not nostalgic for the past, not enthralled with the brave new world. In enacting grief for ourselves and our world, we take up a place, stepping from white noise with its swirling winds and fast lanes. Our place is filled with modern junk, surrounded by noise and speed, with fleshless energized calm vampires, but a place, nonetheless, in which to bury the dead.

NOTES

1. On this distinction, see Alfred Schutz, "The Social World and the Theory of Social Action," in *Collected Papers*, Vol. II: *Studies in Social Theory*, ed. A. Brodersen (The Hague: Martinus Nijhoff, 1971), 9.

2. Actually, all social scientific writing uses metaphors and other rhetorical devices. However, they tend to be masked under an antirhetorical rhetoric, which has been labeled the "rhetoric of objectivity." Greater attention is being given to the rhetoric of science in recent years. See Michael Billig, "Repopulating the Depopulated Pages of Social Psychology," *Theory & Psychology* 4 (1994):307–35; Donald McCluskey, "The Rhetoric of Economics," *Journal of Economic Literature* 21 (1983): 481–517; A. J. Soyland, *Psychology as Metaphor* (London: Sage, 1994).

3. Cited in Susan Banham, "Stress in the Workplace—What Can Be Done about It?" *Insurance Review* (May/June 1985):12.

4. Peter Marris, *Loss and Change* (Garden City; N.Y.: Anchor Books, 1975), 31–32.

5. Ibid., 34.

6. Peter Marris, "The social impact of stress," in *Mental Health and the Economy*, ed. L. A. Ferman and J. P. Gordus (Kalamazoo, Mich.: W. E. Upjohn Institute for Employment Research, 1979), 311.

7. Allen C. Bluedorn, Introduction to "Special Book Review Section on the Classics of Management," *Academy of Management Review* 11(2) (April 1986):443.

8. Carl B. Kaufman, *Man Incorporate: The Individual and His Work in an Organizational Society* (Garden City, N.Y.: Anchor Books, 1969), 140.

9. Gregory D. May and Michael J. Kruger, "The Manager Within," *Personnel Journal* (February 1988):57.

10. Ibid., 65.

11. Ibid., 57.

12. Edward Charlesworth and Ronald Nathan, *A Comprehensive Guide to Wellness* (New York: Atheneum, 1984), 60.

13. Ibid., 62–63.

14. James Beniger, *The Control Revolution: Technological and Economic Origins of the Information Society* (Cambridge, Mass.: Harvard University Press, 1986), 7.

15. Barry Glassner, "Fitness and the Postmodern Self," *Journal of Health and Social Behavior* 30(2) (June 1989):184.

16. Ivan Illich, "Disabling Professions," in *The Disabling Professions* (Boston: Marion Boyars, 1977), 11–40.

17. Donald Meichenbaum, David Henshaw, and Norman Himel, "Coping with Stress as a Problem-Solving Process," in *Achievement, Stress, and Anxiety*, ed. H. Krohne and L. Laux (Washington, D.C.: Hemisphere, 1982), 139–40.

18. Ibid., 138.

19. M. F. R. Kets de Vries, "Organizational Stress Management Audit," in *Handbook of Organizational Stress Coping Strategies*, ed. A. S. Sethi and R. S. Schuler (Cambridge, Mass.: Ballinger, 1984), 267.

20. Ibid., 269.

21. Virginia T. Geurin and Gary F. Kohut, "Dimensions of Computer Anxiety among Managers: A Field Study," *HRMOB Proceedings 1* (Philadelphia: Association of Human Relations Management and Organizational Behavior, 1987), 305–9.

22. James C. Quick and Jonathan D. Quick, *Organizational Stress and Preventive Management* (New York: McGraw-Hill, 1984), 266.

23. Amarjit S. Sethi, "Contemplative Strategies for Technostress Management," in *Strategic Management of Technostress in an Information Society*, ed. A. S. Sethi, D. H. J. Caro, and R. S. Schuler (Toronto: C. J. Hogrefe, 1987), 297.

24. Jacques Ellul, *The Technological Society*, trans. J. Wilkinson (New York: Vintage Books, 1964), 324.

25. Ibid., 348.

26. Jonathan Quick, Rebecca Horn, and James Quick, "Health Consequences of Stress," *Journal of Organizational Behavior Management* 8(2) (1986):19–20.

27. Anne Rice, *Interview with the Vampire* (New York: Ballantine, 1976), 21.

28. Ibid., 18.

29. Quoted in Richard Lyons, "Stress Addiction: 'Life in the Fast Lane' May Have Its Benefits," *New York Times*, July 21, 1983, III, 1:1.

30. Larry Pace and Waino Suojanen, "Addictive Type A Behavior Undermines Employee Involvement," *Personnel Journal* 67(6) (June 1988):40.

31. Linda Leonard, *On the Way to the Wedding* (Boston: Shambhala, 1986), 93.

32. Rice, *Interview with the Vampire*, 270.

33. A classical Greek variant of the vampire image is the figure of Tithonos, the human husband of the immortal Eos, the Dawn. Eos promised to grant Tithonos a wish if he would consent to be her spouse. He asked for immortal life but, alas, he did not ask for eternal youth. So he lived and lived, growing older and older. His fate will be increasingly realized as life expectancy is enhanced.

34. Curtis Austin, "DART's Problems Shake Staff," *Dallas Times-Herald*, April 2, 1989, A-23.

35. Francesco Petrarch, *Petrarch's Secret or the Soul's Conflict with Reason*, trans. W. H. Draper (London: Chatto & Windus, 1911), 34–35.

36. Ibid., 32–33.

37. Philippe Aries, *Western Attitudes toward Death from the Middle Ages to the Present*, trans. P. Ranum (Baltimore, Md.: Johns Hopkins University Press, 1974), 45.

38. Quoted in Joseph Pieper, *In Tune with the World: A Theory of Festivity*, trans. R. Winston and C. Winston (New York: Harcourt, Brace & World, 1965), 10.

39. Ibid., 21–22.

40. Ibid., 15.

15

SCIENCE OF THE MIND IN CONTEXTS OF A CULTURE

LAURENCE R. TANCREDI

Since the mid-1950s there has been a revolution not only in the practice of psychiatry but in the dominant ideology of what occurs in the formation and mediation of behavior. Historically the concepts of man and his behavior have been informed by a view of external influences on man. During the pre-Christian era in Greece (Simon 1978), the identity (psyche) and seat of man's behavior was perceived as midway between the gods and man himself. Homer had no term for "self," nor did he portray the psyche as a reflecting, thinking, feeling center of activity of living persons, certainly not an activity within the person. As Simon suggests, Homer did not perceive of people thinking for themselves (Simon 1978:56). Rather they are engaged in dialogue with a god, another person, or even parts of themselves. Hence concerns of good and evil, though clearly understood within a framework of societal values, did not essentially originate in the individual, nor were they attributable to personal responsibility in the sense in which Western man conceives of that notion. Man was as much a victim as a perpetrator.

Madness was similarly understood in terms of external forces. Some 3,000 or more years ago, before man could write and begin the process of objectifying knowledge, he was led by the impulses of oracles and those who heard voices. These voices were frequently perceived as coming from the gods, who would give advice on how to deal with novelty and stress. It was an era of reliance on subjective experience—often understood as a predominantly right-hemisphere function (Jaynes 1977)—as there was no way to categorize and systematize thinking, a phenomenon which became possible only with the written word.

Plato constructed a model of mental functioning in which the mind was a battlefield where parties within the person fought for dominance and control. During this conflict madness occurs when the impulsive segment of the mind wins out. Hence, as suggested by Simon (1978:71), madness is a consequence of intentionality, that of a part of the individual dominating. Plato, therefore, introduced the concept of "intentionality," which has been central to subsequent psychodynamic theories of human thought and behavior, and certainly of the actions of mental disturbances.

The era of the great conceptual thinkers in psychiatry was also an era of looking at the effects of early external influences on the child. Freud viewed much of what later represented the content of the individual personality and mind to have been laid down during the first five years of life. In keeping with Locke's philosophical notions of the receptive mind, man's brain was seen as born with a clean slate on which the influences of early experiences embedded the characteristics of the personality as well as the basis for behavior, and therefore informed the nature of that person's intentionality. Individualized reactions were seen as essentially shaped by these early experiences, particularly those involving interactions with mother, father, and siblings, as well as others in the community.

Psychoanalysis focuses on understanding the story of the individual. Each story, though different, can be subjected to the scrutiny of Freudian, Adlerian, or Jungian techniques, to name a few. In that way the particular method for analysis, derived by observation and theory, provides the framework for connecting individual patients to an underlying identifying culture and to each other. Psychoanalysis is a method for exploring basic values, influences, thoughts, and behaviors in the context of a culture that shapes and informs personal qualities.

As a scientist Freud did not preclude the importance of biology on individual personality and mental functioning. However, the sophistication of that biology was considerably limited during his lifetime. He found richer territory in literature and the culture of his time for patterns of interrelational experiences that could explain personal characteristics and behavior. His was a pragmatic science, one that allowed the individual to be understood along a clearly articulated metapsychology. This understanding afforded interpretation which, in the hands of a skilled analyst, would lead to psychological change.

Though seen by many until the middle of this century to be the comprehensive tool for understanding human behavior, psychoanalysis—particularly the psychodynamic understanding of personality—was not without its problems. Freud created an analytical structure for comprehending the psychodynamics of feelings and actions that could be applied by experts and understood by the patient. However, it was open to idiosyncratic and even ideological forces. The power of interpretation became the important product of this technique. But unfortunately there were few guidelines for differentiating valid and invalid interpretations. There was no such thing as an empirical study that could be conducted to provide reflection on the merits of a particular analysis, on its overall effectiveness as a method for understanding and treatment. The product presented to the patient often made sense; but although it was drawn from his history and experience, it may not have been relevant or accurate in terms of describing what was actually happening, what was impacting on the patient's thoughts, affect, and/or behavior, and how and why these were different than those experienced by the majority in a culture.

The repercussions of psychodynamic interpretation in psychoanalysis and its less intensive forms of psychotherapy were pervasive. With this tool the psychiatrist until recently was accorded almost untrammeled power over those seen as abnormal and mentally ill. This power extended not only to the treatment environment where the psychiatrist's authority for interpretation and recommendations for therapy were rarely questioned, but also to the realm of social control. The legal system quickly saw the merits of psychodynamics as a way to scientifically establish criminal-mindedness or the nature of an offender's motivation, or more likely as a measure to rationalize its handling of deviant and criminal behavior.

The psychiatrist has been empowered with the right to incarcerate mentally ill patients. Until recently, this right was almost absolute. Psychiatric determinations of serious mental illness, frequently predicated on the practitioner's highly subjective interpretations of a person's behavior, justified commitment for often indeterminant periods of time. In fact it wasn't until the late 1950s and early 1960s that two advancements allowed for the emergence of a patient's rights movement. The first of those developments was the introduction of psychotropic medications, particularly neuroleptics and antidepressants, which were found to be highly effective in treating acutely and chronically ill patients. They brought about positive changes in the thinking processes of seriously disturbed psychotic patients, ameliorated the negative symptoms of conditions such as schizophrenia, calmed and tranquilized potentially violent and agitated patients, and reduced the likelihood of suicide among the seriously depressed. Most important, these medications have rendered patients manageable and therefore receptive to the benefits of psychological and social therapies.

The second major development flowed naturally from the advantages provided by psychotropic medications. That development was the so-called therapeutic community. This community-based method of care allowed for a shift from traditional institutional care. Patients could now be treated in the community through day-care and outpatient programs and thereby live with their families or in residential facilities close to their friends. The major results of these developments were the deinstitutionalization of mentally ill patients and the move toward minimizing the role of psychiatry in social control.

This shift has not been complete, for psychiatrists still have qualified powers to institutionalize seriously ill and dangerous patients. But the grounds for institutionalization have become more narrow and objectively defined and the period of incarceration curtailed considerably since the pre-1960s period of mental health care. Psychiatrists also continue to be frequently invited into the courtroom to provide understanding of criminal and destructive behavior, knowledge which can lead to exculpation of criminal behavior in the extreme or more humane methods of handling these deviant members who are deemed a danger to society.

It was only a few years ago that the Austrian novelist, Thomas Bernhard, wrote *Wittgenstein's Nephew*, which involved his relationship with Paul Wittgenstein, the nephew of the prominent twentieth-century philosopher Ludwig Wittgenstein (Bernhard 1988). Bernhard and Paul Wittgenstein were patients at hospitals located near each other in the suburbs of Vienna. Bernhard was in the Hermann Pavilion of the Baumgartnerhohe for pulmonary patients and Wittgenstein was in the Ludwig Pavilion, a part of an adjacent mental institution, Am Steinhof. Bernhard frequently visited Wittgenstein and observed the circumstances of his detainment and the behavior of psychiatrists and other health professionals toward the mentally ill. As a result of his observations he wrote the following statements, which reflect to some extent the nearly global view of the pervasiveness of psychiatric influences:

Like all other doctors, those who treated Paul continually entrenched themselves behind Latin terms which in due course they built up into an insuperable and impenetrable fortification between themselves and the patient, as their predecessors had done for centuries, solely in order to conceal their incompetence and cloak their charlatanry. From the very start of their treatment, which is known to employ the most inhuman, murderous, and deadly methods, Latin is set up as an invisible but uniquely impenetrable wall between themselves and their victims. Of all medical practitioners, psychiatrists are the most incompetent, having a closer affinity to the sex killer than to their science. All my life I have dreaded nothing so much as falling into the hands of psychiatrists, besides whom all other doctors, disastrous though they may be, are far less dangerous, for in our present-day society psychiatrists are a law unto themselves and enjoy total immunity, and after studying the methods they practiced quite unscrupulously on my friend Paul for so many years, my fear became yet more intense. Psychiatrists are the real demons of our age, going about their business with impunity and constrained by neither law nor conscience. (Bernhard 1988:8)

Bernhard's characterization of psychiatry is perhaps stronger and more critical than justified, certainly with regard to the current environment of psychiatric care. Historically many of the professions—law, the ministry, accounting, to name a few—relied on their own shorthand language for communicating complex notions among one another. In the case of medicine, Latin indeed served as the basis for its own unique language. Initially it was likely that this language, which was fixed in its historical permanence and therefore not vulnerable to changing interpretation, was scientifically expedient. It provided a quick and easy method for distinguishing medical facts and for assuring comprehension of information among caregivers and colleagues. But in time, as in the case of law, where Latin terms remain a major influence, the professions discovered the merits of a unique language for maintaining and augmenting the mystery behind their particular profession.

Bernhard's view of the psychiatrist as the "most incompetent . . . having a closer affinity to the sex killer than to their science" also seems to be a gross exaggeration. Though arguably the content and tools of the science of psychiatry may have been imprecise until relatively recently, it was nonetheless, even in those more primitive days of practice, possible to differentiate competent from incompetent practitioners. And surely the argument is strong that no particular field or profession has a monopoly over competence, or to the contrary, incompetence. On the other hand, when seen from a different perspective, that of the enormity of power that the field exerts over the individual, Bernhard's warning cannot be disregarded. An incompetent psychiatrist by virtue of his focus on the mind can wreak havoc and long-term damage for the patient. Incompetency on a medical level can do likewise, but Bernhard would surely view damaging the mind as a far more serious act than causing a long-term physical disability.

Finally, Bernhard's comment that "psychiatrists are a law unto themselves and enjoy total immunity" is also no longer valid. There has been a progressive paring of psychiatric discretion over individual rights. Furthermore, in the realm of accountability, psychiatrists are increasingly subjected to malpractice suits. The rate of psychiatric malpractice has increased over the past 20 years. In part this has been due to the increased use of medications with concomitant injurious side effects. But malpractice has also increased in non-pharmacologic areas, such as determinations of the proper care of a suicidal patient and infractions in the psychiatrist/patient relationship.

PSYCHIATRY AND THE BIOLOGICAL ERA

The interaction of psychiatry and culture during the twentieth century has entered a new period due to advances in the biological understanding of mental illness. With these advances many of Bernhard's criticisms have undergone reconsideration. There have been two significant developments that have induced shifts in this conceptualization. First, it has been shown that medications—psychotropic drugs—can affect not only the level of agitation of a mentally disturbed patient, but his mood, behavior, and even process of thinking. Until the discovery of Thorazine, the psychiatrist was limited in his armamentarium to psychoanalytical principles and more drastic physical methods such as electroshock therapy and even psychosurgery. Psychoanalytical principles at best provided only a framework for understanding the psychodynamics of psychotic thinking, but they provided little or no benefit for afflicted patients.

The physical treatments have had even more limited applicability. Electroshock has been shown to be most effective for treating profoundly depressed patients, particularly psychotic depressions associated with menopause. For the psychotic, uncontrolled patient electroshock might have had a calming effect, but it does little to ameliorate their underlying condition. Psychosurgery, a procedure that was performed thousands of times between 1945 and 1955, often created more problems than it resolved. The procedure, referred to as a frontal lobotomy, was frequently done blindly through the insertion of metal rods in the supraorbital fissure, and consequently vital blood vessels were not infrequently lacerated, causing strokes and permanent disability or death (Valenstein 1986:144–47). In the treatment of schizophrenia, where this technique was frequently used, there was little evidence that it provided any benefit. Following lobotomies, patients, if not seriously injured, would develop a blunted affect and limitations in cognitive functioning. To this day psychosurgery remains as a treatment, but for only a very narrow group of patients—severely obsessive-compulsive patients refractory to more conventional treatments. During the 1930s and 1940s both electroshock and psychosurgery were used more for "social control" purposes in mental institutions to reduce agitation, violent behavior, and general dissidence than for treatment of seriously disturbed patients.

The mid-1950s revolutionized the ability of psychiatry to treat the seriously mentally ill. Thorazine and its related medications allowed schizophrenics and other psychotic patients to become manageable and therefore amenable to more socializing therapies such as psychotherapy and occupational therapy. These medications impacted on something more basic than the behavioral manifestations of psychosis. They actually affected directly the way the patient thought and the content of that thinking. The illogical, disconnected thinking frequently seen in acutely psychotic schizophrenic patients was readily corrected with these medications. This capacity highlighted the importance of biochemistry on brain function and mental activity.

Second, the focus has moved from emphasizing external influences on mood and behavior to accenting internal factors. The advent of neurophysiology as well as psychotropic medications pointed to the complexity of biochemical reactions occurring in the brain. Enzymes and neurotransmitter substances dominate as the foundation for interaction in the biological model, whereas the psychoanalyst focuses on metaphors, mental content, process of thinking, and the history of the mind. The neurophysiologist sees the synapse of nerve cells as the nidus for demonstrating abnormalities that affect thinking and behavior. Dopamine, serotonin, GABA, and a wide range of other neurotransmitters exert their effect at the synapse and thereby impact on disorders of mood, thought, and behavior.

Most recently serotonin has gained particular attention. Levels of serotonin in specific areas of the brain, especially the limbic section, correlate with as diverse a set of human behaviors and moods as depression, obsessiveness, and suicide, to name a few. If serotonin is low in vulnerable sections of the brain one is likely to find severe depression, possibly coupled with obsessive-compulsive symptoms. Low serotonin has also been shown to be related to self-destructive acts, including suicide. Studies of serotonin levels in the brain have also been correlated to rageful, violent behavior and even murder. In keeping with these correlations, it is important to note that some of the most successful treatments of obsessive-compulsive disorders and violence include the administration of medications such as Prozac, Paxil, and Zoloft, as well as other medications that are targeted to increase the level of serotonin in the synapse of nerve connections. In the case of the most recent antidepressants, such as Prozac, this increase in serotonin is achieved by the medication's blocking the re-uptake of serotonin at the pre-synaptic site. These re-uptake blockers alter not only the biophysiology of the cell but, on the broader level, personality characteristics and cognitive functioning in the recipient.

An amazing group of diagnostic technologies has coincidentally been developed over the past 20 years that in recent years have assisted considerably in research into biochemical functions in the brain. These imaging technologies, such as positron emission tomography (PET), magnetic resonance imaging (MRI), and single photon emission tomography (SPECT), have provided a "window" into the biochemistry of the brain, most specifically the kinetics of enzyme and neurotransmitter actions, much as psychoanalysis has provided a "window" into the psychodynamics of the mind. PET and MRI offer the unique opportunity of studying biochemical brain processes as they relate to specific mental activities (Volkow and Tancredi 1991). The brain-mind relationship, long recognized since the time of Descartes as representing two separate spheres or a dichotomy of human activity, has been bridged in recent years through neurophysiology and the use of these imaging techniques. With MRI it is now possible to observe brain activity concurrent with the performance of specific mental acts. For example, MRI allows the observer to see connections in the brain when a subject is asked to consider an image, conceive of a word, and/or associate that word with other words or thoughts.

The accumulation of biochemical and biophysiological understanding of the brain/mind parallels in some respects, though years later, the evolution of the understanding of psychodynamics. The difference rests mainly on the fact that psychobiology has not yet offered a broad-based theory concerning the nature of man. In contrast, Freudian analysis relies on the existence of such a broad framework, whereby sexual development and differentiation is central in both the theoretical level and its empirical application.

The shift to a biochemical framework for comprehending human emotions and thought has been stimulated by pragmatic exigencies. It is easier and more efficient to treat depression and schizophrenia, for example, with appropriate medications than to subject patients to hours of psychoanalysis with steady, though very slow and minimal, progress toward amelioration of their condition. The relationship between action (the giving of medications) and outcome (change in mood, thinking, and behavior) is not only temporally more connected with medications, but the extent of change can be calibrated along an axis of dose/result. Nothing comparable exists for psychotherapy, even though for patients it may make more sense to understand their feelings in the light of certain events in their life history than in the light of brain biology, which may be influenced by both genetics and early environment.

GENETICS AND THE MIND: TOWARD IMMUTABILITY

A major turning point substantially reinforcing the critical role of biology in mental processes, and particularly mental illness, has been the rapidly occurring discoveries since the late 1980s in behavioral genetics. Psychopharmacology and basic neurophysiology had indeed effectively introduced the merits of biology in understanding mental processes, but there remained many analytical questions regarding how essential this biology is in explaining complex human conditions. Many have been unconvinced of its validity. How could an enzyme or neurotransmitter initiate a thought or image? Is this biological process not merely the machinations of biochemical activity after the mind formulates its intentions? In other words, could biological events merely be the physical equations that bring about the superordinate mental intentions of the subject? In this case the biological only elucidates how a series of equations fall in line to produce a psychological response, but by no means does it initiate, nor direct, the intentions of that response.

Behavioral genetics has begun to influence our ideas about the "basic" cause of human behavior toward the biological rather than the psychological. The notion behind behavioral genetics is that genetics is essential in determining behavior. Though not a new notion—it has been considered by many thinkers from the time that Mendel did his groundbreaking research on genetic transmission—we now have the tools to identify behavior, or at the very least predispositions to behavior that may be linked to specific DNA or biological substrates. On the most conspicuous level we have seen diseases like Huntington's Disease and Charcot-Marie-Tooth Disease, where specific genetic abnormalities are associated with distinctive behavioral manifestations. Less exacting, major psychotic illnesses such as schizophrenia and manic depressive disease, though not yet identified by a specific gene defect—these complex behaviors may never be shown to be the result of a single gene defect, though some preliminary data suggests that manic depressive illness may be a defect in the eighteenth chromosome—they nonetheless have been shown to have strong familial and genetic antecedents.

Epidemiological studies of families and relatives suffering from these diseases have established the presence of powerful familial and genetic correlations. On a less pathological level, recent research has supported the presence of a "risk-taking" gene as well as one that may be responsible for accident proneness. The risk-taking gene seems closely related to the ability of an individual to take risks in all aspects of life—career, sports, human relationships—in contrast to many who are incapable of taking even reasonable risks. Studies of twins have revealed similar close associations of personality traits with genetics. In cases of identical twins separated at birth and reared in totally different families, when examined years later, similarities are striking—to the behavioral point of comparable academic careers and occupational choices, similarities in taste, and similarities even in selection of life partners. Since Seymour Kety's work on twins in Denmark, identical twin studies have long been the basis for asserting the familial and genetic loading of schizophrenia.

The implications of combining knowledge of behavior genetics, which sets a deterministic thread as well as a claim of immutability to individual destiny, with biological studies of neurochemical substrates of behavior that may operate at any specific period in a person's life are staggering. The concept of determinism through inheritance alters the individual's sense of his own identity. With genetic information it will be possible to profile the potential for individual development, comparing capacities with opportunities. In addition, behavioral genetics is coming at a time when there is a growing fragility in the relationship between social controls (interests, needs, prerogatives) and individual rights (autonomy, self-determination, individual interests and prerogatives). The delicate balance may be severely affected, resulting in a slanting of power in favor of preserving social identity over that of the individual.

Economic realities alone are pushing toward affirming the need to defend the greater social good (i.e., communitarian values and the like). When fueled by behavioral genetics and biological understanding of correlates of behavior, the possibility has arisen of effectively manipulating the types of individuals who will people a society. Psychological tests and therapy are now powerful enough to provide for this degree of profiling. Genetics allows for the early identification, and if need be elimination, of undesirable genes, or the possibility of attenuating these predispositions through manipulation of the gene, that is, gene "therapy." Hence behavioral genetics and biological substrates that cover the range of biological influences from the family history as well as individual differences from environmental factors operating at any point in time create many tensions for the field of psychiatry and culture as well as for the individual trying to develop himself. First, genetics creates existential limitations on individual development and fate. Second, the possibility now exists for genetic categorizations of families and even broader social groups, especially where intermarriage prevails. And third, it is likely that notions of hierarchy or architectonics based on genetics and behavior will emerge. It will be possible to determine the superiority of certain genetic configurations based on their ability to adapt to central core values in society.

Finally, there are the complex societal requirements of establishing responsibility and guilt where appropriate. With knowledge provided by behavioral genetics, it may be difficult to justify attributing responsibility and guilt to offenders. Will society elect to avoid designating individuals as "guilty" per se, but see them instead as operating under deterministic influences? What about in the case of collective criminal actions, will these be seen as also secondary to genetic factors? For example, should the collective guilt associated with the Nazi atrocities during World War II, or the "hanging" atrocities against the blacks in the south be seen as genetically mediated? If so, how does one deal with restitution or rehabilitation to societal norms? In other words, how will biological processes augmented by behavioral genetics change our notions of how correction should occur among those engaging in deviant behavior? Might such correction include genetic counseling, or more active methods to prevent the formation of certain gene configurations, or the requirements for genetic therapy to eliminate the aberrant gene? Assuming behavioral genetics negates the value of personal guilt or responsibility (what does this mean with regards to free will?) and instead shifts such responsibility to the family or larger social unit, which may have been in the position to prevent the transmission, does this shift not empower the larger social unit to impose even greater control over the individual?

RECONCILING BIOLOGY AND PERSONALITY

As with all findings in as complex a field as psychiatry, things are never clear cut or fixed. The movement for validating psychoanalysis, the analysis of the individual in the backdrop of cultural symbols to establish abnormality, was one extreme motion of the pendulum. Similarly, the effort toward emphasizing the power of biological and genetic substrates in producing such behavior has involved a pendular swing in the opposite direction. Truth inevitably lies somewhere between these extremes.

The brain is a magnificent, flexible organ of the body. It is a system whereby limitations are not determined by the brain's own physical boundaries (Tancredi and Volkow 1992). Instead, the brain is capable of extending into the external as well as the internal world to which it experiences stimuli, responds, and incorporates in an integrative manner. The brain essentially contains the capacity for *openness*, which includes the power of incorporation. It incorporates symbols and representations in an ever-expanding process. As a physical phenomenon, incorporation relates to the concept of "ordering." It is through the incorporation of symbol stimuli that the brain can incorporate, interpret, and differentiate more complex stimuli. This allows the capacity of the brain to expand in terms of its ability to incorporate increasingly complex concepts and images.

Empirical examples of this capacity for incorporation can be seen in a wide variety of experiments that have been conducted on animals. When subjected to stressful circumstances, changes occur in the concentration of norepinephrine (Dunn 1988) and adrenergic receptors (Pavcovich, Cancela, Volosin et al. 1990) in the brain. These changes not only affect the ability of the animals to have specific behavioral reactions, but such exposures to stress eventually change the animals sensitivity to other stresses. (Antelman, Eichler, Black et al. 1980).

Not all interactions that affect the brain lead to permanent physical changes in the brain. Some interactions may have no response, others an immediate response with no long-term changes, and still others may lead to permanent or long-term changes. When openness lead to morphological changes in the brain, we talk of openness including the principle of *plasticity*. By this notion we refer to the brain's capacity to alter itself through the process of learning (Rose 1981). Under particular conditions, therefore, segments of the brain may be activated, resulting in a temporary or permanent transformation of the neuronal environment. For example studies with PET covering an over four-month period following detoxification from cocaine have disclosed that cocaine abusers show a significant decrease in dopamine D-2 receptor availability (Volkow et al. 1994). This decrease persists for at least 3 to 4 months after detoxification (and in some studies these changes have been long term and perhaps permanent) (Volkow et al. 1992). Concomitantly, there was an associated decrease in metabolism in several regions of the frontal lobes, especially the orbito-frontal cortex and cingulate gyri. Dopamine dysregulation of these brain areas, which involve channeling of drive and effect, could lead to loss of control resulting in compulsive behavior. This essentially renders the brain in a different space, possessing different potentialities for reactions to external stimuli.

The combination of brain openness and plasticity introduces the possibilities of the history of the person feeding into and affecting the brain. A purely genetic and biological view of human behavior, mood and thinking therefore being highly limited. The individual is not merely a product of the internal physical brain playing out its own genetically determined evolution. Without positing the presence of mind separate from brain, openness and plasticity nonetheless allow for the brain to be a product as much of the outside world as of internal forces (see also Chapter 19). Genetics may narrow the range of possible responses for the brain, but it does not limit development to one or even a few courses. Hence the brain biology as measured by enzyme assays or imaging technologies is a factor of not only genetics, but environment, altering biochemical reactions. Essentially genetics provides the core thrust of the individual. But learning interrupts the stable stream so that the physical brain and personality are altered in very small gradients.

Hence we have come around nearly full circle in our travels through psychiatry and culture. Initially culture, or the history of the person experiencing early relationships and social values, was seen as most dominant in shaping and informing the personality of that individual. Then the biological age, the discovery of psychotropic medications and the nature of neurotransmission, introduced the importance of seeing the brain as a chemical factory, a series of chemical reactions dictating the impulse through nerve endings and, on the broader scale, specific characteristics of the individual. Genetics introduced a notion of immutability by suggesting that DNA sets the stage, and very narrowly, for how a specific person would develop. This fortified the notion of the brain as not only a chemical factory but one with very strict and rigid rules in its functioning.

But more intensive investigations of brain functioning have once again altered our notions of the human condition. Openness and plasticity reintroduce the importance of environment and history in human development. In doing so, these discoveries expand our ideas of how personalities are created. They also alter our notions of the origins of mental illness. DNA transmission is insufficient to explain how mental illness develops. There is more to the story—a combination of genes, psychological conditioning, and more direct environmental insults, all of which operate to affect the biophysiology of the brain. Recognition of the complexity of interaction of biology with family and society supports the importance of prevention and treatment through biology, in particular psychopharmacology, as well as psychological and social therapies.

CONCLUSION

It is interesting to note that the biological revolution in psychiatry is very recent. It is at best 50 years old, a brief period of time when viewed against the backdrop of centuries of reliance on psychohistory and verbal therapies for treating psychiatric disorders. When it became scientifically evident that studies of the biophysiology of the brain yielded an extraordinary understanding of human thinking and behavior, it was natural that in time psychiatrists would embrace these discoveries. Hence we have seen extraordinary strides in research in brain biophysiology and in psychopharmacology for the treatment of a wide range of psychiatric disorders. These developments brought about a dramatic shift in the nature of psychiatric practice. Psychopharmacology has dominated in the 1990s as the primary treatment method for most psychiatric disorders. Psychoanalysis has been a dying discipline, and psychotherapy, a less intensive form of analysis, left to the domain of psychiatric social workers and clinical psychologists.

However, as discussed above, the pendulum seems to be swinging once again. Research on brain processes has confirmed the openness and plasticity of the brain, which means that external stimuli can bring about changes in the biophysiology of the brain, and therefore mental processes. Once again the impact of environment and early conditioning on the formation of personality must be considered. This will inevitably affect not only our concept of human development but the nature of psychiatric practice, which must actively encompass the psychological and social therapies.

REFERENCES

Antelman, S. M., A. J. Eichler, and C. A. Black et al. 1980. "Interchangeability of Stress and Amphetamine in Sensitization." *Science* 207:329–31.

Bernhard, Thomas. 1988. *Wittgenstein's Nephew: A Friendship*. Chicago: University of Chicago Press.

Dunn, A. J. 1988. "Stress-related Activation of Cerebral Dopaminergic Systems." *Annals of the New York Academy of Science* 37:188–205.

Jaynes, Julian. 1977. *The Origin of Consciousness in the Breakdown of the Bicameral Mind*. Boston: Houghton Mifflin Co.

Pavcovich, L. A., L. M. Cancela, and M. Volosin et al. 1990. "Chronic Stress-Induced Changes in Locus Ceruleus Neuronal Activity." *Brain Research Bulletin* 24(2): 293–96.

Rose, S. P. R. 1981. "What Should a Biochemistry of Learning and Memory Be About?" *Neuroscience* 6:811–12.

Simon, Bennett. 1978. *Mind and Madness in Ancient Greece: The Classical Roots of Modern Psychiatry*. Ithaca, N.Y.: Cornell University Press.

Tancredi, L., N. Volkow. 1992. "A Theory of the Mind/Brain Dichotomy with Special Reference to the Contribution of Positron Emission Tomography." *Perspectives in Biology and Medicine* 35:549–71.

Valenstein, Elliot. 1986. *Great and Desperate Cures*. New York: Basic Books.

Volkow, N. D., J. S. Fowler, and G. Wang et al. 1994. "Decrease Dopamine D-2 Receptor Availability Is Associated with Reduced Frontal Metabolism in Cocaine Abusers." *Synapse* 13:197–203.

Volkow, N. D., R. Hitzemann, and G. Wang et al. 1992. "Long-Term Frontal Brain Metabolic Changes in Cocaine Abusers." *Synapse* 11:184–90.

Volkow, N. and L. Tancredi. 1991."Biological Correlates of Mental Activity, Studies with PET." *American Journal of Psychiatry* 148:4–10.

16

THE "NEW PSYCHIATRY": FROM IDEOLOGY TO CULTURAL ERROR

LOLA ROMANUCCI-ROSS

Many roads led to the "new psychiatry," but perhaps the most compelling path was to be found in the logic of its forensics. Although the forensic aspect of psychiatry was originally limited to advising the courts with respect to personal responsibility for criminal acts, later in the twentieth century it evolved into a process of assessing whether such deviant behaviors were due to specific mental disturbances over which the individual had no control or whether they were the result of deliberate intent.

After many years of professional training in which he or she learned a new language, professional rules about causality, and a new way of relating to self and others, the psychiatrist was guided in such assessments by a taxonomy of mental illnesses (*Diagnostics and Statistical Manual* 1994). He later learns the meaning of concensus or difference of opinion with other professionals. Professional notions of causality may or may not coincide with beliefs of other members of the society; professional ideologies and lay ideologies may influence one another, or perhaps they may become confrontational—a phenomenon that is pertinent to the current discussion.

In time the psychiatrist assisted the courts in deciding whether a criminal offender should go to prison or to a mental hospital. Was the defendant competent to be tried in a court of law, that is, did he understand the charges? The expert made judgments on the possible reversibility of disordered states, on the effectiveness of therapies or medications, and on possible determinable side effects. In short, the expert in psychiatry decided on "dangerousness" to self and others and on the place of madness and/or deviance in society.

Questions about "the place" of behaviors and persons in any society depend on cultural expectations and attitudes; in a sense they are stipulated explicitly or implicitly in contractual arrangements among the members of the society. The function of psychiatry is also that of establishing that an individual's deviance is evidence of true pathology contrastive to other forms of deviance in which criminal or offensive acts come from calculated intentions of a mind that knows the difference. As the agency of this, forensic psychiatry must also refer to the mediating role that the psychiatrist plays between the prosecution and the defense (he may work for one or the other) and the determinant role in the sentencing process.

But where, external to this mediated process, is the objective proof of "criminal intent"? Such constructs have appeared from statistical data, giving us distributions of deviations; is it this concept that informs the psychiatrist in the personal face-to-face doctor-patient relationship?

Tancredi (1983) has effectively argued that a conflict of interest does indeed exist in the situation in which the psychiatrist is hired by the court to establish certain facts while, at the same time, he makes judgments about doctor-patient relationships (e.g., whether or not it is fair to obtain information "legally" against the patient when a patient's defenses are "down"). In such a role he may indeed be the final arbiter of the death sentence.

The intersection of cultural values and medicine is most pronounced in psychiatry because it is concerned with disorders of mood, thought, and behavior that the psychiatrist necessarily must extrapolate from everyday life. The disturbance he examines "involve an infusion of symbols, imageries, and metaphors of the culture into the context of specific patterns of behavior" (Romanucci-Ross, Moerman, and Tancredi 1983:262). Whether behaviors indicative of mental disturbances are biochemically induced or willfully intended, it must be acknowledged that the data on mental illness are always and everywhere products of observations, analyses, and theoretical explanations of the (professional) observers of mental illness. Deviance is not something to be discovered, it is a cultural construct resulting from a concensus of value-laden opinions coming from the experience and judgment of a cultural group. The definition is re-enforced by statistical occurrence; the rate of occurrence is shaped by the negative evaluation of and disincentives provided for its manifestations (Romanucci-Ross and Tancredi 1986). Quick upon the heels of the "deviance label" we see a "moral" culpability in some societies or within certain groups.

Finally, we note that madness is, in any culture, a negotiable and negotiated event. It is frequently in the interest of a family, a tribe, or a complex society to put some individuals away from the traffic of everyday interactions—to avoid expense and trouble, or to facilitate new beginnings for the survivors of this negotiated event. Mappings of structured behavior tell individuals or groups-within-groups where the boundaries are and which behaviors will be acceptable.

THE "NEW PSYCHIATRY"

The "deinstitutionalization" movement was activated in the United States, and in European countries as well, because the institutions (literally, the buildings) were deteriorating. In the same time period we saw the advent of psychotropic medications, which were making it possible for many mentally ill to live outside such buildings. The confluence of events that made the time ripe for an innovative approach included the civil rights cause, that is, the abuse (intentional or unintentional) of various groups by the needs of the majority.

In Italy, the psychiatrist Dr. Franco Basaglia and his group planned their own version of a deinstitutionalization program (see Lovell & Scheper-Hughes 1986). Basaglia wanted to syncretize the social psychology of George Herbert Mead and other symbolic interactionists, so he put into motion what I would call a modelic psychiatric critical theory to alter consciousness in his society, and that was his forensic—*his* persuasive discourse. His goal was (incredibly) this: a unified social and cultural effort to restructure the entire Italian society so that all of their collective frustrations might be addressed. He reasoned that men are not shaped by their environment but by their interpretation of their environments; "repressive institutions" would never permit change to occur, so change must be imposed.

We shall look at the dissonance of the Basaglia movement and its aftermath in one ethnographic context to briefly illustrate that the ideological substrata of beliefs about mind/body function and dysfunction have deep historical (and religious) roots. This appears to perdure despite information from the media and insights of pioneers seeking to interpret the sources of illness. There is much creativity in many cultures in what is absorbed or rejected.

In the area in central Italy in which I began this research in 1970, people did not consider themselves healthy or even happy, even though observing them at festivals, ceremonies, or family gatherings, one would not have that impression. Most conversations involved an excursus into the conditions, past and present, of the heart, kidneys, liver, stomach, and certainly blood pressure. They did consider themselves anxious, annoyed, repressed, and frustrated. Waiting rooms of physicians and healers featured discussions of symptoms, signs, and remedies, which were taken as seriously by other patients as whatever the doctor or healer might have to say. They combined Western medical and traditional folk healing with much skill (Romanucci-Ross 1986), from diagnosis to pharmacognosy.

By 1990, not much had changed, and, in fact, combining elements of scientific medicine and folk beliefs became even a bit more sophisticated. To follow, I quote a "case" from my ethnography (see Romanucci-Ross 1991).

Carina told me I simply had to go to a monastery in a nearby town in the high hills; there I would see a painting called "the face of Christ," where many of the afflicted came to pray and, as one example:

A woman of Ascoli, who had a bladder tumor, went to this sanctuary to pray, taking her X-rays with her. She went because she had a dream of the Madonna who told her to go to this shrine and to pray long and hard. This woman, while in prayer, felt an excruciating, lancinating pain. Well, the next time she went to the hospital for X-rays, the tumor was gone! She returned to the shrine with both X-rays to place them underneath the painting of the face of Christ. A light from above broke on the X-rays! After this, on the X-ray that had shown the tumor she saw the face of Christ and the image of the Madonna of Loreto. On the X-ray that did not show the tumor there was an image of a bunch of roses. Now, *everyone* saw these images, for the woman pointed them out as she wept over the grace (*grazia*) that had been given her. She is now a *miracolata* (miracled one) and occasionally rents a bus to drive people—almost all of whom are women—to this shrine. That's how I got to go. I must go there for help, as I want to remain here in my apartment, self-sufficient; I want to cook meals for my relatives as I always have on Sundays and *festas*. (From Romanucci-Ross 1991:135–36)

In another instance, Maria needed an eye operation for what she described as "three months of darkness," which occurred shortly after the birth of her son. When I asked what her doctor called it, she said "detached retinas," but that had little to do with her explanation to herself about the experience.

The doctors "took out the eyes and sewed them" and Santa Lucia gave her the "gift of sight." She was consumed by the fear that she was too thin, that her husband would tire of her. It had taken her such a long time to conceive but neither she nor her husband wanted doctors to see her about that because "the uterus is the most important part of a woman," and second in importance were the eyes. The uterus, eyes, and brain were all connected—that is why she became blind and then hysterical, as she was told. She now takes tranquilizers to "keep" her husband. She was very concerned about what this small madness, blindness, and 16 years of sterility meant. She had always cared for others, always gone to mass. What did I think she had done to deserve this?

The above is but a footnote to what could be noted generally, that the experiencing of the world, particularly by women, was in large part a narrative of what the body experienced and how it was interpreted. The discourse was that of emotions and selected body parts along with feelings attributed to them. In some cases, organs have analogues in mystical bodies in the Catholic religion. Anger and hopelessness are to be found in states of liver and lung. Heart and eyes express divine and sometimes sexual feelings.

SOCIO-MORAL MYTHOPHYSIOLOGY: A MODEL

The psychosomatic drama is culturally informed with certain precepts. Above all, a balance must be maintained, which means an avoidance of extremes of temperature, extremes of emotions, with an eye kept on *balance* in food types and activities—heavy foods, light foods, foods that cleanse, foods that fortify, and those that target certain organs in distress. The purpose of all of this is to keep the blood cleansed—one must be vigilant about system balance, and remedies can be found in nature itself. If possible, this route to cure is preferable. Some might call this a folk explanatory model.

But preventive medicine goes further than just counseling about following natural laws to avoid excess, it tells you to obey certain rules in social relationships. To keep one's place, to be modest, this is necessary to avoid *invidia*, or envy (*'mmidia* in the dialect).

The introduction of psychotherapy and psychoanalysis in the Piceno area, from the 1970s, was of great moment to some young professionals and their clients, but among many others it had a curious effect. Some went to a new type of folk healer that emerged about that time to seek help in finding former "selves" in previous lives in ancient cultures. They were then told how these problems should have been resolved. Somehow it was very "natural" at some cognitive/affective level to apply that solution to the current problem that had directed client to the healer in the first place. (These healers "improved" in time, as we shall see.)

Other therapists use the Frommian/Freudian approach, but in conjunction with "family therapy," not as we know it, but with an interesting cultural inflection. Knowing the generations and the specific dates and outcomes of significant events, particularly illness, disaster, and death, gives one important avoidance clues and qualifies as psychotherapeutic preventive medicine. Numerology, always an important aspect of dreams for other decision making moments, is called into play also. As I have noted in another work (Romanucci-Ross 1986), creativity in the combinatorial arts in this area applies to illness, cure, and healing with some quite original effects.

The years of the deinstitutionalization movement for the mentally ill in the United States, from the late 1950s through the 1970s, saw a similar movement in Italy, but with a very different approach. As indicated earlier, Dr. Basaglia, together with a small group of his colleagues and some health care workers, began what was later formally known as "democratic psychiatry." As in the United States, costs of care were escalating, buildings for such care were deteriorating, and psychotropic medications made living outside of the asylum feasible for many patients, as we indicated earlier.

The political climate in the more communist-oriented northern parts of Italy provided a receptive attitude in many voters; the movement turned into an indictment of the state and psychiatrists as state agents. "Madness," Dr. Basaglia held, was a label placed on behavior that had been caused by poverty and frustration. Such societal neglect was nothing less than institutionalized violence. Furthermore, the socially approved state therapeutics in themselves were just another aspect of violence by the state. What this meant specifically was that "madness" had to be removed from the medical context.

Basaglia's goal was to expose power structures, within psychiatry, in medicine, in the asylum, and in the larger society. He and his group were the force behind the passage of Law 180 in 1978, which, among its other effects, attacked the notion of "dangerousness to self and other" that permitted psychiatrists to put a patient into the *manicomio*. Because of the law, the number of *manicomi* in Italy was reduced by half (Lovell and Scheper-Hughes 1986:377). The movement had more success in the north than in the politically conservative south of the country. Journalists everywhere, however, seldom let pass the opportunity to point out that once set free, many former inmates did indeed indulge in arson, mayhem, and murder, as they had verbally threatened while inmates in the *manicomi*.

Of interest to me in my fieldwork episodes over the years in both the north and south, was that this "alternative psychiatry" or "democratic psychiatry" was most often discussed in terms of the goals of those who held political power. Many expressed their expectations, fully met, that city and provincial administrators would do anything, irresponsible as it might be, to save money (for their own later harvesting of it, of course), and that the political liberals and radicals would embrace any irresponsible doctrine to break up the current power structure to rebuild their *own* power structure (after which repression would be even worse).

Most people in the area I studied seemed to believe that there is a moment when the presentation of the self in any context "can cease to be an artifact in communication or an artistic performance and can become, instead, an act of madness in the eyes of the beholder" (Romanucci-Ross 1991: 146). Therefore, it is thought that what is observed can be a case of labeling and *possibly* a case of deviant behavior, and that it is very difficult to bracket off one from the other. The question then becomes, What should be the primary social concern addressed? In this part of the world the safety of the child takes precedence over the rights of the "deviant," and the belief is very strong that the order of things is as it is for good historical reasons and should not be lightly discarded.

This is not to suggest that the "lay" or folk modelic is not open to new ideas, but rather that when they are accepted, several operant conditions are present. First, that the elements of what is being borrowed have an appeal that resonates with meaning to those who will absorb the new ideas. At the same time elements must find a "fit" somewhere in the grammar of the folk or lay experience so that it is amenable to the acceptable combinatorial rules. For example, would assumptions about illness simply exclude other causal explanations? Does it fit into notions of responsibility or duties and obligation in the family structure? Folk healers in this area have personalities that do conform to what is called a "sensitive" person and have other mystic qualities as those found among saintly *personae* in the Roman Catholic religion.

The mid-1980s marked the beginning of the rise of psychoanalysis as therapy in the region. This, although adopted more or less by the *literati* in the city, nevertheless had the curious effect of providing more clients to the recognized folk healers. Such therapies with these healers focused on "former lives," women had lived in exotic places such as Egypt, the Himalayas, or India. In great detail the client was told of her past life, yet was given the appropriate psychological terminology for the reasons and the meanings of past acts and their consequences. The methods of these healers pleased the clients because they did not call into question the virtues of the social structure called "the family" in its present existential form. No one here and now is at fault. Not unlike the psychoanalyst, the healer provides a framework (even if hypothetical or a fantasy) within which the client can formulate or resolve problems. A new borrowed discourse is (partially created) around events, providing space for furtherance of innovation, perhaps at a later time, or, in some instances, arousing a reactive contradictory response.

Dealing with mental illness or defining "mental health" translates, in any culture, into a confluence of political systems, the law, moral codes, ideology, and beliefs about illness and health. An Italian commentator noted that one "could drown" in the ink spilled over the Basaglia movement in psychiatry. Though highly informed, most of it is polemical. Rightly so, as psychotherapy is an interactional process between therapist and patient, the goal of which is to effect changes in thinking, feeling, and behavior in the patient, which in itself would pose a problem in some cultures.

FROM BODY TO BODY POLITIC

The Italian Mental Health Law (Law 180) was included in the general health law passed by the parliament in December 1978. It accorded priority to voluntary over compulsory psychiatric treatment, promotion of comprehensive treatment, eliminated the concept of "dangerousness," and stipulated that community health services (SPTs) were to be an alternative, not complementary to mental health hospitals. Community-based services were to be provided for geographically defined catchment areas. Necessary short-term psychiatric hospitalizations were to occur in 15-bed diagnostic and treatment units (SPDCs) in general hospitals. All admissions to asylums were to cease after 1982.

Before 1978 the practice of psychiatry in Italy was governed by statues and regulations from 1904 and 1909. Some of the salient features of these declared voluntary admission impossible and commitment became a matter of court records, counting as a criminal conviction. The reform law (Law 431) of 1968 sanctioned voluntary admissions and permitted outpatient care, though this was not actualized to any degree (Maj 1985). Law 180 surpassed in scope and intent other similar laws in other countries. Dr. Franco Basaglia and a group of health workers who agreed with his views on mental illness were instrumental in the passage of the 1978 law. In the early sixties, Basaglia counted himself among the "existential psychiatrists" (see Basaglia).

"Critical theory," whose adepts were seekers of codes and messages and the application of semiotics to political structures to decode and deconstruct, were another source of innovation for some reflective psychiatrists. They pondered (quite rightly one might assert) the concept of patients' rights, the very concept of normalcy and of medical discourse itself, and these notions were seen as being imposed by forces in the culture at large. (Nor was it the first time psychiatry pursued reformist thinking; for example, the 1930s in the United States was a period of pause and reflection on treatment and outcome—the "mental hygiene movement." This movement, too, meant to redefine mental health issues as social problems, but it was a failure [Goldman and Morrissey 1985].) But Basaglia's ideas of reform in the 1960s became a social movement and soon allied itself with left-wing political parties. By lobbying, and with three quarters of a million signatures, they pushed the parliament to pass the law. It was said at the time that the government wanted to avoid confrontations, that there were the customary number of resignations and then its passage was assured.

During the years of the same movement in the United States (the late 1950s and into the 1970s), we also saw professional scrutiny occurring within psychiatry, but with a different cultural accent and without open political affiliations (though one could note political affinities), and certainly it did not have the Italian intensity. In Italy the professional movement turned into an indictment of the state regarding the cause and treatment of mental illness, and the majority of psychiatrists stood accused of being state agents.

Basaglia turned this into praxis in northern Italy at Gorizia, where he had been appointed director of a 600-bed public asylum. He asserted (as had some others in other countries) that madness was a label placed on behavior, but that the real causes of madness were poverty and frustration over lack of opportunities. Such neglect by society was violence institutionalized. Furthermore, he maintained that the therapeutic approaches in vogue were in and of themselves a further violence, perpetrated and legitimized by the state (Basaglia 1981). In other words the state had a medical pretense that allowed it to isolate and incarcerate those who could not fit into proper patterns of production/consumption behavior. Even the use of psychotropic drugs was a furtherance of the tyranny of the state by lulling *both* the patient and the psychiatrist into believing that therapy was occurring, that something was being done. Moreover, the state had put into place what Basaglia called "circuits of control," that is to say, the loci and linkages that included asylum, boarding house, halfway house, and other medical or quasi-medical

spaces in which a person is defined as sick and treated by control and repression.

Reform, having been introduced in Gorizia, was also taken on in Arezzo,
Ferrara, Perugia, Emilia, Naples, and some cities in central Italy as well.
Basaglia had his colleagues and helpers literally open doors and windows of
asylums urging timid and fearful patients "to be free." When they hesitated,
asylums were sometimes dismantled physically so that they would have pal-
pable visible symbols of freedom. Artists and students were invited to live
in asylums. Patients, those who "wished to remain," were offered the concept of "the assembly"; these were scheduled frequently so that patients
could voice complaints.

In retrospect, Basaglia's goal may or may not, in many instances, have
been therapeutic, but it was unquestionably political: to expose the power
structure both outside the asylum and within it. Together with the component of existential psychoanalysis and the politicization of normal and
abnormal, Basaglia's new democratic psychiatry was turned into theater. In
a two-pronged attack plan, academic and clinical psychiatry remained concerned with deterministic explanations, while the people were quite receptive to the theatrical aspects that helped bring about his reforms. In some
cities "street scenes" were incorporated into parades to illustrate how a psychiatrist would condemn an individual to confinement by pronouncing him
or her insane. Children in schools were shown mini-plays in which a child
was marginalized simply because of the opinion of others. Workers in factories were exposed to dramatized concepts of deviance.

While theatricalization of psychosocial concepts was helping recruit a
larger constituency for greater political force, "teams" were forging new political ties or strengthening those already existing with political (liberal to
left) neighborhood groups or labor unions. Democratic psychiatry was also a
formal organization of workers in the mental health fields.

Psychiatric tasks were not separated from welfare work. The same staff
that treated patients in the hospital wards was responsible for following them
in the city, and those who were too frail or too elderly to find a place in the
city remained as "guests." Some of the vacated wards were converted into
apartments for this purpose. As noted earlier, some of these apartments already housed needy artists who could contribute to the political movement
by painting murals or posters with a message. They were expected to use
their talents to deconstruct madness.

About ten years ago the Basaglia experience came to an end because
despite the spread of economic depression in many areas of the country, the
leaders and followers of democratic psychiatry had continued to press local
governments for more and more entitlements for former patients. In this
pursuit they had more success in the cities of the north, which were more
heavily governed by the Communist Party (PCI).

Although Dr. Franco Basaglia had raised questions of fundamental importance about how any society constructs madness (Romanucci-Ross 1983), the movement unfortunately became intertwined with more trenchant and overinvested public issues of governance and distribution of national resources.

A BACKWARD LOOK AT SEA CHANGE

In retrospect, it usually takes longer to know what occurred than the length of time occupied by actual occurrence, most of the time being needed to "close the parallax error" of different points of view, or, indeed, even to define the parallax (Romanucci-Ross 1991:9). But some events, indisputable, can be known about this period of innovative psychiatry in Italy.

The number of beds and residents in asylums has declined steadily since 1963 (i.e., they were already in decline before 1978 and Law 180). Between 1963 and 1968 the average decrement was 1,390 beds per year, from 1973 to 1978 the average decrement was 3,305 beds per year, and postreform it was 4,140 beds per year. (However, it is not known whether ex-patients who came back as "guests" were counted as patients.) Furthermore, *admissions* to these places continued to increase even after they were declared illegal as of 1982, while private hospital admissions did not increase (Tansella 1987). In 1984, provisions for "alternative structures" had been found inadequate (Centro Studi Investimenti Sociali 1984; see also De Salvia and Crepet 1982). Identifying and triaging chronic patients was made difficult by variability in their clinical condition due to functional disabilities within the population and across time, and quite simply by fundamental differences in the concept of chronicity for a wide variety of clinical diagnoses including substance abuse, personality disorders, and so forth. Fifty-four percent were treated outside the hospital. Importantly, diagnosis was not a significant predictor of outcomes, nor was it a predictor of use of services (Calabrese et al, 1990).

There has been a rapid expansion of certain mental disorders in Italy, evidenced by a significant increase in the sales of psychoactive drugs (+40.5% between 1981 and 1987) (Farmindustria 1988). The suicide rate has risen by 56.5 percent between 1980 and 1987 (Istat 1989). The death rate due to psychological causes has risen by 63.5 percent between 1981 and 1984 (Crepet 1990). What does it mean, therefore, if we learn that admissions of psychiatric cases fell by 11.1 percent or that there was a decrement in the number of inpatients in forensic hospitals (−36.5% between 1970 and 1985)? Inpatient mortality is greater than that of the general reference population (Bacigalupi et al. 1988). The reform of psychiatry left important therapeutic categories to the discretion of individual services; these defined for themselves what would be included in their assignments and what would be excluded. Alcoholism, drug abuse, vagrancies, hopelessness, and so on might or might not be involved (Williams and Tansella 1990: 51). Still, in

regions where more general hospital psychiatric beds (SPDCs) were provided, there was less of an increase or even a decrease in suicide rates *(An-
nuari delle Statistiche, Sanitarie)*. It must be noted that there are great
differences between regions and within regions, including urban/rural differences, in addition to variability in the resources given to various places,
so that the number of SPDCs cannot be considered an independent variable.

A study was arranged to look at two treatment environments set up according to the reform, an SPDC and an SPT (community service center).
The investigators wanted to demonstrate that characteristics of the therapeutic setting influence both the emergence of symptoms and patient outcomes. They found, through a true/false questionnaire (translated from
English to Italian), that the SPT workers were more "involved" with the
patient (Burti, Glick, and Tansella 1990). These patients returned home
in the evenings, so it is obvious one could get more "involved" in conversation, and knowing the family was part of the treatment. These authors did not consider their study definitive and concluded that there is
still a need for such a study as well as for a study instrument than can be
used in Italy.

A multicenter study (Barbato et al. 1992a) wanted to access six-month
outcomes for patients discharged from 21 general hospitals after short-term
inpatient treatment in an SPDC. Using two outcome measures—relapses
and community tenure—they found that 43 percent relapsed at least once.
Those who volunteered to be studied were of lower social status and poor
social network. The investigators experienced a high loss rate due to the
failure of many services to trace a high proportion of their patients for follow-
up assessment. At face value the relapse rate is rather high when compared
to samples of similar psychiatric patients. A high rate of recidivism associated
with good community tenure meant, to the investigators, a largely unsatis-
factory degree of implementation of reform. They conclude of their study,
"it demonstrates that quality of care assessment in terms of patient outcomes
is not routine in a significant proportion of the services involved in the care
of psychiatric patients in Italy" (Barbato et al. 1992b:195). Nevertheless, the
best predictor of rehospitalization within six month was previous contact
with psychiatric services. The highest risk was a previous admission, rather
than diagnosis, which failed to show significant association with either end-
point. These findings support Calabrese's view that standard sociodemo-
graghic or clinical variables are inadequate in shaping new community
services (Calabrese et al. 1990).

Researchers on the reform in Italian psychiatry leave us their "controlled"
studies with which they themselves were not too satisfied for reasons beyond
their control (e.g., more studies should be randomized), but they do give us
insights in their commentaries, which in the Italian case are more to the
point and more valuable than the study conclusions themselves.

As in many other aspects of the distribution of resources in Italy, there is an inequity between the north and the south, between regions, and between large cities and smaller towns within regions (and most professionals and planners feel this issue must be legally addressed). Then there is the question of implementation of the integration model. Williams and Tansella (1990) correctly state that some centers and hospitals in some ways implement the law, some are very slow in accomplishing it, and some simply ignore it. Integration has been found much more likely to occur for patients with severe disorders and a previous history of psychiatric treatment. This was not what was intended for SPT integrated care, which meant to address appropriate intervention at every level of psychiatric need.

The reorganization has benefited hospitals and outpatient services, but community care facilities are inadequate (particularly those intermediate services crucial for continuity of care). Home visits and rehabilitation are increasingly being abandoned. There is a "chronic shortage" of up-to-date empirical data and little data on conditions of discharged patients. The quality of care of hospitalized patients is not at an acceptable level (Crepet 1988; Glick 1990), nor are any mechanisms in place to ensure improvement in quality of care. The abrupt ordered cessation of admittance to state mental hospitals did not occur, and these hospitals still care for chronic patients (Calabrese et al. 1990). Mental health of the general population does not appear to have been affected by the transformation of psychiatric care. Some do not feel that reform has made major changes in the general picture of care, and point to the fact that modernization had begun before the reform. Lacking has been the coordination, the control, the necessary financing, and the trained staff for the new kind of care (Crepet 1988).

More lamentably for the epistemological bases of democratic psychiatry, it has been noted by some researchers that when associations were described in a study, they were not with incidence and prevalence of mental disorder but with service uptake variables—suggesting that "the social environment itself does not strongly affect the onset of illness, but does powerfully shape the extent to which individuals initiate and sustain contacts with services when unwell" (Thornicroft, Bisoffi, De Salvia, and Tansella 1993). Patients without families or informal caregivers place a disproportionate burden on psychiatric services.

Some Americans who have observed the reform in Italy (at close range, in a short period), have speculated on what we, in the United States, might learn from the experiment. One view expresses the desirability of combining our "medical model" in psychiatry with the community service part of the Basaglia model, though admitting the data to assess the latter properly do not exist (Glick 1990). Some have said that American society prevented an anti-institutional movement because it had no radical conjuncture, but that the Italian experiment has produced "new knowledge that will nevertheless be useful to understand the 'sciences of deviance' " (Lovell and Scheper-Hughes 1986:380). But this new knowledge was not specified.

In the American experience, however, we note that the medical model does not deal with the very definition of madness (Romanucci-Ross and Tancredi 1986). If American reforms did not have a radical conjuncture, they were pushed along by other larger inclusive movements such as the campaigns for civil rights and the rights of defendants in criminal trials. Legal challenges then resulted in an accretion of law;[1] the protagonists of which come to be known as "the mental health lobby." We, too, appear to be in a phase of discussing our failures in mental health reform, and we appear to be asking the same questions that were raised before our experiment: Who needs to be hospitalized? Who is dangerous and therefore must be hospitalized? Where are the cost/benefits in inpatient and outpatient community care? What is a reasonable fiscal policy on insurance-based care? And, once more, even after judicial decisions, shall we discuss right to treatment (of, say, the homeless) and right to refuse treatment (of, say, the "really" mentally ill)? In the American context, we have collected a great deal of quantitative data, but its relevance in a new context has yet to be determined.

The Italian experiment must be seen in its own cultural context, however, since its uniqueness may make the experiment relevant to no other cultures. One Italian writer summarized the post experience attitude in his city, and I find it reflects that of many other cities and locals: "The place of alternative psychiatry in Naples is now a pagoda submerged in a green, translucent swamp . . . a pagoda that has known frustration, deceit, unveiling of opportunity, the hubris of the offended medical establishment, bourgeois rules in deinstitutionalizing and misery" (Piro 1980:10). Even the most ardent supporters of the democratic "new" psychiatry recognize that what is needed now is a totally new set of health services, a new set of "circuits of control" with a new emphasis on rehabilitation and prevention (De Leonardis 1981).

Those in the area in central Italy in which I conducted research[2] do not feel culturally or politically allied to the north or south and, therefore, claim a certain objectivity. In this area, too, the effects of the Basaglia experiments were felt; for example, ex-patients (some seriously disturbed) were liberated from asylums and housed in homes for the elderly. This was resented by all; some local judges kept assuring me that this was contrary to any Italian law, yet it continued. The general assessment of Law 180 was that it was a political ploy on the part of the Communists of the north to use professionalism (in this case psychiatry) to further their political goals. Others went along, hoping to save money as asylums were closed and to gain money for all the new services financed by the national government. And further, regional competition fueled it along. True or not, this was a perception shared by many, not only in the region in which I worked but in other parts of the country where I sojourned.

All illness is a constantly negotiable event, and the psychosomatic drama is always and everywhere culturally informed. To describe such attitudes in Italy would take much more space than available here (Romanucci-Ross

1986). Syncretic approaches to diagnosis and cures take advantage of current medical models but always also go outside them. Preventive medicine contains a large repertory of what natural *and* social laws are to be obeyed to have the body/mind remain in balance. In Italy there is a great interest in emotional states, and the language of emotions is also the language of the body. Stages of ecstasy, dreams, hysteria, and meditation are very relevant to the practical life. They are central to meaning and may tell one of his/her personal destiny—not unlike the vision quests of certain American Indian tribes. It is not likely, in such a belief system, that one explanation (the socioeconomic frustration model) would ever win the day for long. A school of psychiatry may presume it has found the truth, but, for Italians, it would be no different than any other truth, which is open to constant renegotiation.

Another important area that undoubtedly affected the movement is the attitude of Italians toward the law (this should not have been unforseen). Obeying the law strictly is often impossible, for the legislature adds new laws and regulations as a matter of course, but does not remove existing laws (Di Muccio 1994:32). For that reason public administrators are hesitant to make administrative decisions that might have legal repercussions. Many feel that since it is impossible to strictly obey the law, one need not bother. Instead of being guaranteed by law, privileges are distributed by political parties. Given all of this, individuals make their own justice through "deals" (Sgroi 1992).

A MOMENT OF CULTURAL ERROR

Self-conscious self-perception and an awareness of the influence of culture on behavior is a highly developed skill in most Italians. Unquestionably due to the painful fashioning of a nation over the millennia by conglomerates of ethnic groups, most are able to describe their cultural constraints or the liberating features of their way of living. It is therefore quite remarkable that Dr. Basaglia and his followers appear not to have shared that awareness, or chose to ignore what they should have known.

The moment of great cultural error occurred when the psychiatric testimony of Basaglia and his followers transcended the evidence and, through political praxis, influenced substantive issues of law. This was considered by many throughout the country (but particularly in the non-Communist cities and areas) as having gone beyond acceptable limits. In many contexts (in a manner of reasoning that can be equated with some aspects of the Federal Evidence Rule 704(b) in the United States) I was told that an expert witness can testify with respect to a mental condition as an expert, but he is not an expert on the ultimate issue, the legal one of freedom or restraint, which should be decided by the "Trier of the Fact."

If the Basaglia experiment had not gone too far, it might have helped public attitudes toward mental illness. Its almost total politicization hardened earlier positions against the movement (with endless accounts of those re-leased who committed crimes), perhaps overdetermining all strategies for once again isolating the sick person.

Those who were never Basaglia believers do not completely reject his arguments about madness. All appear to agree (in interviews—structured or unstructured) that some people are unjustly asylumed—that some are put away by spouses or other family members for reasons of convenience or profit. There are very strong reservations, however, about this problem lead-ing to a national policy of liberation for *all* considered "mad"; the general position seems to be that observed behavior can be *both* a result of labeling and abnormality and that it may indeed be difficult to determine which is which. There is a sense that protection of others, particularly children, from the insane should come first that is, how many and who will be at risk? And, principally, *any* cause favored by those in Italian Communist strongholds is highly suspected—sure to be an opening for an eventual frontal attack on family, church, and the concept of private property (Romanucci-Ross 1991: 27–29).

Between the political ideology (acquired from another culture) of the Bas-aglia movement, which called for an abrupt political solution and imple-mentation to a problem, stood "the culture" of Italian provenance. In this particular case, the culture-bearers, ever-cynical of governmental solutions, saw problems of interpretation of mental illness, regional factionalism, "ac-commodations," and lack of evaluative procedures all through the lens of a long historical experience with imposed solutions that merely compounded the original problem. As with any other people with a long history of Hu-manism, there is a distrust of systems. And because of all this, party affili-ations do not have the same meanings they have in the United States. Social rules, rather than ideology, characterize Italian party membership; many card-carrying Communists are mass-attending Catholics (Pizzorno 1966). The strategy of the individual in any politically innovative situation is dif-ferent than that of institutions involved in the game—the individual strives for "the best of both worlds" (Kertzer 1980:259).

THE COMPASS OF CRITICAL THEORY

Those of "right-wing" persuasion can also attract semioticians able to de-code and deconstruct the messages of those in power who may have dia-metrically opposing political views and notions of empowerment. Silvio Berlusconi, then new prime minister, was greatly aided in his victory through his vast holdings and television networks, and his knowledge of control through advertising. He was able to build a new coalition and defeat the ex-Communist PDS. The "activist" magistrates who finally incarcerated scores of politicians and businessmen for corruption pleased everyone immensely at the start. But a generalized reaction was not long forthcoming. Large numbers had been privileged by party memberships that had brought them positions, jobs, and even sickness and disability benefits as rewards for party service (an example of making one's own justice). Berlusconi emphasized he was for the respectable people who "pass exams" in school and in work— in other words, those who don't *need* community services.

Reality changes quickly in Italy, and, as Italians like to say, "When the reality is different, we are different." Whoever designs the next and new model of "circuits of control" for the care of the mentally ill might be well admonished not to ignore the nature of Italian culture and the modal personality that is its distillate.

NOTES

1. On prediction of future dangerousness: *Barefoot v. Estelle*, 463 U.S. 880 (1983); on competency to stand trial: *Dusky v. U.S.*, 362 U.S. 402 (1966); on criminal responsibility because of mental disease or defect: *Durham v. U.S.*, 214 F. 2d 862 (O.C. Cir. 1954); on right to refuse treatment: *Rennie v. Klein*, 476 F. Supp. 1294 (D.N.J. 1979) and *Rogers v. Okin*, 478 F. Supp. 1342 (E.D. Mass 1979), among others.

2. Anthropological field research was begun in 1970 and has continued into the present; it was conducted in periods of time corresponding with sabbatical leave years and portions of summers. The focus was on ethnographic data collection and medical anthropology over an area in central Italy (see Romanucci-Ross 1983, 1986, 1991).

REFERENCES

Bacigalupi, M., F. Cecere, and M. Arca et al. 1988. "La Mortalità dei ricoverati negli ospedali psichiatrici nella regione Lazio: primi resultati." *Epidemiologie e Prevenzione* 34:36–43.

Barbagli, N., and P. Corbetta. 1978. "Partito e movimento: aspetti del rinnovamento del PCI." *Inchiesta* 7(31):3–46.

Barbato, A., E. Terzian, and B. Saraceno et al. 1992a. "Patterns of Aftercare for Psychiatric Patients Discharged after Short Inpatient Treatment: An Italian Collaborative Study." *Social Psychiatry and Psychiatric Epidemiology* 27(1):46–52.

Barbato, A., E. Terzian, and B. Saraceno et al. 1992b. "Outcome of Discharged Psychiatric Patients after Short Inpatient Treatment: An Italian Collaborative Study." *Social Psychiatry and Psychiatric Epidemiology* 27(4):192–97.

Basaglia, F. 1981. "La distruzione dell' ospedale psichiatrico come luogo di istituzionalizzazione." In F. Basaglia, *Scritti I. Dalla psichiatria fenomenologica all' esperienza di Gorizia*. Torino: Einaudi.

———. 1980. "Breaking the Circuit of Control." In *Critical Psychiatry*. D. Engleby, ed. New York: Pantheon.

Basaglia, F., ed. 1968. *L'Istituzione Negata*. Torino: Einaudi.

Burti, L., I. D. Glick, and M. Tansella. 1990. "Measuring the Treatment Environment of a Psychiatric Ward and a Community Mental Health Center after the Italian Reform." *Community Mental Health Journal* 26(2):193–204.

Burti, L., N. Garzotto, and O. Siciliani et al. 1986. "South Verona's Psychiatric Service and Integrated System of Community Care." *Hospital and Community Psychiatry* 37:809–13.

Caciagli, M. 1993. "Tra internazionalismo e localismo: l'area rossa." *Meridiana; Questione Settentrionale* 16:81–98.

Calabrese, L. V., R. Micciolo, and M. Tansella. 1990. "Patterns of Care for Chronic Patients after the Italian Psychiatric Reform: A Longitudinal Case Register Study." *Social Science and Medicine* 31(7):815–22.

Centro Studi Investimenti Sociali. 1984. *Le Politiche Psichiatriche Regionali nel Doporiforma e lo Stato Attuale dei Servizi.* Roma: Censis.

Crepet, Paolo. 1990. "A Transition Period in Psychiatric Care in Italy Ten Years after the Reform." *British Journal of Psychiatry* 156:27–36.

————. 1988. "The Italian Mental Health Reform, Nine Years On." *Acta Psichiatrica Scandinavica* 77:515–23.

De Leonardis, O. 1981. *Dopo il Manicomio: l'esperienza Psichiatria di Arezzo.* Rome: Consiglio Nazionale delle Ricerche, Il Pensiero Scientifico.

De Salvia, D., and P. Crepet, eds. 1982. *Psichiatria Senza Manicomi.* Milano: Feltrinelli.

De Salvia, D., and V. Calleri. 1980. *Streghe, Stregoni, Stregate: Psichiatria e animazione.* Padova: Tencarola.

Diagnostics and Statistical Manual of Mental Disorders. 4th ed. 1994. Washington, DC: American Psychiatric Association.

Di Muccio, P. 1994. "E adesso salvateci dalle leggi incivili." *Il Giornale*, April 25, 36.

Farmindustria. 1988. *Indicatori Farmaceutici.* Roma: Nuove Dimensioni.

Glick, I. D. 1990. "Improving Treatment for the Severely Mentally Ill: Implications of the Decade-Long Italian Psychiatric Reform." *Psychiatry* 53(3):316–23. (Published erratum appears in *Psychiatry* 53[4]:424.)

Goldman, H. H., and J. P. Morrissey. 1985. "The Alchemy of Mental Health Policy: Homelessness and the Fourth Cycle of Reform." *American Journal of Public Health* 75(7):727–31.

ISTAT. 1989. *Statistiche Statali Italiane.* Rome: n.p.

Kertzer, D. I. 1980. *Comrades and Christians: Religion and Political Struggle in Communist Italy.* Cambridge: Cambridge University Press.

Lancet. Editorial 1985. 1:731–32.

Lovell, A. M., and N. Scheper-Hughes, 1986. "Deinstitutionalization and Psychiatric Expertise (Italy and the U.S.)." *International Journal of Law and Psychiatry.* (Special Issue: Anthropological Reflections on Forensic Psychiatry). Lola Romanucci-Ross and Laurence Tancredi, eds. 9:3.

Maj, M. 1985. "Brief History of Italian Psychiatric Legislation from 1904 to the 1978 Reform Act." *Acta Psichiatrica Scandinavica* 316 (suppl.):15–25.

Moos, R. H. 1974. *Evaluating Treatment Environments: A Social Ecological Approach.* New York: Wiley.

Mosher, L. R. 1983. "Recent Developments in the Care, Treatment, and Rehabilitation of the Chronic Mentally Ill in Italy." *Hospital and Community Psychiatry* 34:947–50.

Piro, S. 1980. *La Scacchiera Maladetta: Esercitazione Critica su Psicologia, Psichiatria, Psicoanalisi.* Napoli: Tempi Moderni Edizione.

Pizzorno, A. 1966. "Introduzione alle studio della partecipazione politica." *Quaderni di Sociologia* 15:235–71.

Romanucci-Ross, L. 1983. "Madness, Deviance and Culture." In *The Anthropology of Medicine: From Culture to Method*. Lola Romanucci-Ross, Daniel Moerman and Laurence Tancredi, eds. South Hadley, Mass.: Bergin & Garvey, 267–83.

———. 1985. "L'eloquenza del cogito: Sciamanno e Antropologo tra terapia e politica." *Materiali Filosofici* 14:46–56. Milano: Tipomonza.

———. 1986. "Creativity in Illness: Methodological Linkages to the Logic and Language of Science in Folk Pursuit of Health in Central Italy." *Social Science and Medicine: An International Journal* 23(1):1–7.

———. 1991. *One Hundred Towers: An Italian Odyssey of Cultural Survival*. New York: Bergin and Garvey.

Romanucci-Ross, L., and L. Tancredi. 1986. "Psychiatry: The Law and Cultural Determinants of Behavior." *International Journal of Law and Psychiatry* 9(3): 265–94. (New York: Pergammon Press.)

Romanucci-Ross, L., L. R. Tancredi, and D. Moerman. 1983. *The Antropology of Medicine: From Culture to Method*. South Hadley, Mass.: Bergin & Garvey.

Sgroi, E. 1992. "Farsi giustizia da se: strategie di sopravivenza e crisi della legalità." In L'illegalità diffusa in Italia, *Quaderni di Sociologia* 32(4).

Tancredi, L. R. 1983. "Psychiatry and Social Control." In *The Anthropology of Medicine: From Culture to Method*. Lola Romanucci-Ross, Daniel Moerman and Laurence Tancredi, eds. South Hadley, Mass.: Bergin & Garvey, 284–97.

Tansella, M., D. De Salvia, and P. Williams. 1987. "The Italian Psychiatric Reform: Some quantitative evidence." *Social Psychiatry* 22:37–48.

Thornicroft, G., G. Bisoffi, D. DeSalvia, and M. Tansella. 1993. "Urban-Rural Differences in the Associations between Social Deprivation and Psychiatric Service Utilization in Schizophrenia and All Diagnoses: A Case-register Study in Northern Italy." *Psychological Medicine* 23(2):487–96.

Williams, P., and M. Tansella. 1990. "Italian Psychiatric Care." (Letter; comment.) *Journal of the Royal Society of Medicine* 83(7):476.

17

THE AGING: LEGAL AND ETHICAL PERSONHOOD IN CULTURE CHANGE

LAURENCE R. TANCREDI AND LOLA ROMANUCCI-ROSS

AGING, BIOLOGICAL THEORIES, AND CULTURE

"Aging" in recent years has become a source of fascination to medical and social science researchers. Therefore, we now have some theories on the aging process. Currently, leading schools of thought focus on biological events, one of which is the "Hayflick limit" of cell division, which is that there are finite and determined programmed intracellular events under genetic control. Others are the "defective enzymes due to faulty messages" theory, the accumulation of "metabolic-waste-in cells" theory, and the theory of "free radicals"—electrically charged unbalanced forms of oxygen that can be chemically destructive. Whether old age is the cause of disease or its characteristics are caused by disease is a question whose answer still eludes us. Yet we have made some progress since the early part of the twentieth century, when some distinguished physicians (such as Nobel Prize–winner Elie Metch-nikoff) proposed that disabilities in old age were caused by syphilis, alcoholism, or a poison produced by the bacteria of the large intestine. Biological theories, however, address neither the existential problematic role of the elderly nor bioethics and its legal implications.

In technologically simple societies, the elderly were and are highly respected, and growing old, an accomplishment, is the achievement of a status. The aged are keepers of the lore, the reference libraries for celestial navigation, weather prediction, migratory patterns of birds and fish, and arbiters of disputes who know the ancient laws. They know the healing powers of plants and animals and the spirits. They are the repositories of the knowledge of what sustains the culture. Their counsel is constantly sought, by tribal people as well as by anthropologists. It can be good to be old in an age-ranked society. In harsh climates, with poor resources, the infirm aged were in collusion with the others to acquiesce in death-hastening behavior (cutting food and water, encouraging suicide).

In peasant cultures, much of this obtains, but one must not outlive the social definition of one's usefulness. In recent research by one of us in Italy, a high suicide rate was found among the aged. This was puzzling until it was determined that suicide occurred only among those elderly people who were poor, owned nothing, had no resources that might allow them to remain in the exchange system (Romanucci-Ross 1982b:214–15). They were those who had no family, who could not command respect because there was nothing they could contribute in any way. In Mediterranean rural culture one usually goes into old age not only with one's networks, kin, and childhood friends but also in a cultural "emotional tone" that does not make one feel apart. Young people do not jest about the gait, infirmities, memory slips, or peculiarities of the aged. In technologically simple cultures that are very dependent on their immediate ecological resources, there is certainly a concept of optimum population, but the control of numbers is at the beginning of life, some of it natural (infections, infant mortality, etc.), and some of it cultural (abortion under certain circumstances and even infanticide). Such societies do not have as heavy a cultural investment in the fetus or infant as in the aged person.

As is well recognized, in American society we accent the importance of youth. See this as a metaphor for tearing away from our maternal or paternal European cultures as a young upstart nation, or see it as the desire (again as a trope) for the need for energy and hard work to build a new nation from the wilderness, we give all importance to young bodies and young minds. This American attitude culminated in a book by Margaret Mead entitled *Culture and Commitment* (Mead 1970), in which her main thesis is that now is the time for the old and middle-aged and mature to learn from the young.

We are, in fact, a child-centered culture in contrast with many other cultures of the world. In many countries, the child looks to adults for cues as to how to behave. In the United States, we have adults gazing at children in wonder. Here, the adults are the audience, providers of toys, watchers of children. Becoming old, then, we emphasize in every context, is to become totally obsolete: we align culture against the aged. The culture has strategies for dealing with the aged. Advertising impresarios decide *how* the old are to be made visible. Advertising in medical journals usually features aged models posing as candidates for medication, often for psychotropic drugs or for drugs to control dysfunction, both mental and physical.

We have our warehouses for the old. Private, public, or affluent, they are all characterized by impersonality and infantilization of inmates or boarders, many of them in a confused state caused by overmedication or the synergistic results of multiple medications. Owners and managers of such institutions explain that they try to abide by rules "set by the county board."

But the observer can see that the liveliness of the aged annoys and expressions of their sexuality offend. Such patients are put into "noisy" sections so that they do not subvert the "good" patients. Their reminiscences appear to bore the unwilling listeners. (In many cultures it is precisely the reminiscing that makes the elderly social or national treasures, so to speak.) But we medicate them back to rationality or we silence them.

The anthropologist and psychiatrist Jules Henry, in his field study of nursing homes in the late 1950s (nor can one describe them differently now), made some interesting observations that will not be unfamiliar.

Social conscience was appeased by attending to things with high visibility, such as clean floors, freshly painted walls, the smell of disinfectants, and the like. Neglected were those items of low visibility, such as personal involvement with patients, attention, and communication. The patient who gave up hope "improved" as she/he became easier to manage. Jules Henry wrote with much feeling about the data he gathered over his years of research in old age homes for the poor, the middle class, and the rich. In colorful language he describes some old people eating in a home:

Dogs, too, eat hungrily and silently, beg for food, eat leavings, lick their bowls. Pathogenic institutions cannot handle a human being, for humanness is a threat. For a cruel institution to function within its cruelties it has to redefine its inmates ... as retarded children, as animals, as pets. (Henry 1965:416–17)

Nor is Henry without understanding for the "help" he found there: "Ignorant, poorly paid, working in a human junkyard ... they are nevertheless sound people who withdraw from distorted people." He found instances of petty conflict and spitefulness among the patients in the ever-diminishing number of frames of reference.

We are socialized, in American culture, to feel that we must not accept being cared for unless it is absolutely necessary. Those who are confined long for communion, but nothing in the culture has taught them to achieve it, for loneliness in American culture has generally been associated with deviance. Even our architecture discourages solitude. The center of a house is ideally the family room, of public buildings it is university halls, the conference centers.

By contrast, Japanese house architecture exalts loneliness and pronounces togetherness as a necessity only to continue the practical life. The Japanese tea ceremony exalts poverty, inner wealth, and true life. The tea room is stripped and its main characteristic is emptiness. It is to be filled only with movement, harmony, and tranquillity. The meaning of this is that living is an art (Okakura 1956). Poverty means not deficiency but a state that liberates you from external concerns. During the tea ceremony the mind is cleansed. It is an emptying of oneself of social norms. The art of life includes bringing the outside *in* by way of the garden. The simple and commonplace in its most trivial aspect becomes art, an art that is understood only by cultivating one's own senses through solitude and *not* mediated by "the other." Seclusion expressed in architecture is distantiation from the environment of one's fellow creatures (Engel 1987). In such an unobstructed environment your presence develops its own meaning.

A society creates the kind of personality it needs to maintain itself and accomplish its economic goals. Our mercantilist, industrialist, exchange-oriented society (Fromm 1947:70–75) needs people who will move to new locations, who will not be bound by family ties, who can repress deep needs, knowing or believing they can be satisfied later with credit cards and money. The older America that Tocqueville described was created by men and women who had values such as thrift, hard work, living in one place, monogamy, and family orientation, including the extended family (Tocqueville 1946). But our current "marketing personality" is freer with money, friendly, unsure of himself, needs sex and adventure to "feel alive." Our contemporary American looks to his contemporaries for direction, responds to signals from wider circles outside the family. We are driven by and for technology, and all of this is rewarded. This kind of personality makes possible the suggestibility of advertising—our philosophy in a new key in which the message determines the structure of response.

Old persons not only remind us we are going to get old and noncompetitive, they also remind us of certain death. Their very presence arouses anxiety—an anxiety that permeates all the "methodology" (see Devereux 1967) we employ in studying them: us-and-them, their-problems, them-as-our problem.

MEDICINE AND THE AGING

Most of us are familiar with the demographic trends: In 1980, 11 percent of the U.S. population was over 65. By 2030, 25 percent will be over 65. Between 1980 and 2000, the 85 and older group will experience a 129.3 percent increase; the 75 to 84, a 57.9 percent increase; the 65 and over, a 37.1 percent increase; and the 21 to 64 group, a 24.45 percent increase (Siegel and Taeuber 1986:102–7).

In our society, we have medicalized many a behavior and state. A host of behaviors are called depression, alcoholism is a disease, inappropriateness is a sickness, and cultural marginality may get you into therapeutic hands.

In a society such as ours, old age is treated as a disease for which one can be, and does eventually become, institutionalized. Mood changes will be subject to medication, and any memory loss now makes one a likely candidate for a diagnosis of Alzheimer's disease. Acting young brings accusations of trying to deny one's age. Taking your problems (medical, financial, social, or occupational) seriously will have you labeled a depressed patient, soon treated with a course of polypharmacy bringing on disorientation and confusion.

An aspect of the physician-elder encounter for which the physician might not be prepared is countertransference. A patient in transference endows the therapist with the persona of a significant other in his/her life. A patient may suddenly react to the doctor as a child to a parent, or vice versa, and bring that affect into the encounter. The doctor often relates to the patient as though the patient were someone else in his (the doctor's life), thus blocking his own medical effectiveness. The physician sees his own senescence, relives conflicts with parents, and also, not believing he can really be of help, denies his own failure by denying the validity of the patient's complaints.

Developing an old body takes your personality, your spirit, your "self" into a ghetto. Many behaviors formerly labeled interesting, or "madcap," or stimulating will now be labeled senile. This does not mean that there is no such thing as the real physiological changes which sometimes do accompany aging and, in some individuals, sometimes do affect behavior. But aging in itself does not *necessarily* involve a significant loss of function at defined ages.

What it does mean is that what occurs is the categorizing and labeling of all elderly people as incompetent, which generates public policy decisions (such as retirement at a certain age), which influences medical practices (such as inappropriate medication), which promotes social and cultural patterns of interaction (such as the isolation of the elderly)—all of which render them incompetent.

In Western societies, physicians have a public policy mandate. With access to the most intimate aspects of personal lives and powers of intervention, they are powerful agents for culture change. Their awareness of a few well-known concepts in the psychological and social sciences would lead far beyond good patient care, to really effective patient care, far into the future.

LAW AND THE AGING

The (almost) bloodless revolution of the 1960s made us notice the young and the black and the disenfranchised. This revolution has by now included the insane, the old, and the dying—that is, in the sense that these persons have rights.

Progressive as the revolutions of the mid-twentieth century have been with regard to the elderly, the articulation of legal rights actually lags well behind cultural perceptions and bioethical principles. The rights of the mentally ill, for example, so effectively delineated since the 1970s, are not paralleled in legal development in the treatment of the elderly. The mentally ill have gained a wide range of rights in the way they are treated both within and outside of the mental health system. There has been an articulation, for example, of the right to privacy for the mentally ill; a right to institutional prerogatives, such as communicating with the outside world; rights to treatment; and most recently, in a series of cases, the right to refuse treatment. The case law on the right to refuse treatment has addressed one of the most fundamental issues regarding patients' rights, and that has to do with the capacity or competency of mental patients to make decisions. The landmark case *Rogers v. Okin* and the many cases following that decision affirm the right of competent institutionalized mental patients to have important input into treatment decisions and to refuse treatment except in cases of emergency (*Rogers v. Okin* 1979).

Even for those deemed incompetent, the courts have provided protection through such devices as substitute decision making, the use of guardians *ad litem*, and, in some cases, leaving the judge to make the final decision. Perhaps the only deviation from the strong move in the direction of asserting the rights of a vulnerable group such as the mentally ill was the Supreme Court case that did not require the same level of procedural due process for the right to refuse treatment in the case of those imprisoned and mentally disturbed (*Washington et al. v. Harper* 1990).

But arguably there is some ambivalence even on this issue, as in 1992 the Supreme Court, in another case involving those imprisoned, created some limits on what a state could impose (*Reggins v. Nevada* 1992). In this case the Court held that a state could not force antipsychotic drugs on an unwilling criminal defendant for the sole purpose of rendering the defendant competent to stand trial. However, the state's rights are broad, whereas there is a showing that the drugs were medically necessary for the safety of the defendant or others and no other effective drugs were available that had minimal or no side effects.

Application of these important rights to the growing and increasingly vulnerable geriatric group in our population has only begun to occur. It is generally presumed that the elderly are incompetent (along with minors), and this is used as justification for denying them choices in a variety of medical and health circumstances. It is simply assumed that this segment of society is more likely than "the average" to suffer from some forms of mental disturbance or deficiency. Even applying the criteria, predicated strongly on cognitive capacities, used for young adults in determining competency, the elderly do not uniformly meet the criteria of incompetency.

More important, bases for the test of competency (assuming that such tests are valid for ascertaining cognitive capacity) are perhaps not so relevant in the elderly population as they are in young adults more actively functioning in society. Is it, for example, so important that a senior citizen, who is perhaps retired from his job, is not able to add or subtract as quickly as a young adult or that he or she is not as facile with verbal skills or memory? Possibly the criteria for the determination of competency in later life should place more emphasis on the history of the elderly person, the expression of preferences, the capacity to maintain himself or herself in a suitable ambiance and to sustain life with some sociability and personal satisfaction (Tancredi 1987).

Perusing the statistics on the mental condition of the elderly, we find that the picture is not at all bleak as many would presume. A study in 1985 of nearly 3,500 adults in a community in Baltimore found that only 6.1 percent of those over 65 years of age actually had some form of dementia (Folstein et al. 1985). Furthermore, less than 12 percent of those over 75 years of age had dementia—in fact, only 2 percent of those between 65 and 75 ever suffered from this condition. As to the prevalence of depression, anxiety, and distress, some researchers have shown that age is not a major factor in the prevalence of these conditions (Feinson 1985).

Of course not all of the studies have given us reason for unbridled optimism, but even those were not pessimistic. In a study conducted by Myrna Weissman and other researchers involving over 2,500 seniors living in New Haven, Connecticut, 11 percent of those studied suffered from a DSM-III disorder or cognitive impairment at some time during the study. The picture is even less bleak when one further differentiates the age groups. For example, severe cognitive impairment was shown in nearly 17 percent of all individuals over 85 years of age, but in only 1.1 percent of those between 65 and 74 years of age (Weissman et al. 1985).

More significant than her conclusions on the mental disorders is the fact that Weissman found that 9 percent of those studied indicated they could benefit from some assistance with their personal care and over 30 percent said they needed help in mobility. More recent studies have shown comparable rates of "disability" to those of Weissman, and that the prevalence of disability increases with age. Around 10.5 percent of individuals between sixty-five and seventy-four require assistance with activities of daily living (ADLs). This percentage increases to slightly over 51 percent for those persons 85 years old and over (Kapp 1995). Weissman's findings indicate that the majority of individuals labeled "elderly" in nearly every age category demonstrate a capacity to make their own decisions. These studies, of course, do not focus on the institutionalized elderly, a group that by definition is more likely to be marginal in capacity than the general population. Simply being in an institution for a long period of time creates a dependency and induces infantilization of the individual (Goffman 1961). It may be useful to consider that in 1985 only 5 percent of the elderly population resided in nursing homes or institutions (see U.S Department of Health and Human Services 1987).

Discussion of capacity (described perhaps more accurately as "decisional capacity") is important with regard to the elderly because it is this issue that has justified what appears to be a clear disinterest in advancing the legal rights of this group. We find, for example, that in many jurisdictions the elderly can be placed in long-term care with no consideration of their legal rights (Cole 1987). In contrast, during the 1960s and 1970s we saw an upheaval because of the neglect of the rights of mental patients to due process and other constitutional powers. In fact, the laws were changed so drastically that is has become virtually impossible to commit an individual for an indeterminate period of time or to justify commitment on grounds other than the presence of a serious mental disease or defect and the threat of danger to self and others.

In contrast, the elderly are routinely placed in long-term care facilities, nursing homes, and convalescent homes with no regard for their individual rights. Often informally, family members with no malevolent intention conspire, essentially, to have an elderly person placed in an institution. The elderly individual may refuse this incarceration, but such refusal frequently lacks sanctioning power and legal assistance. Being placed in an institution may be an irreversible condition for the elderly patient. There are no lawyers, for example, for nursing homes or long-term care facilities as there are for mental institutions (Cole 1987). In fact, many jurisdictions, such as New York City, require the availability of legal assistance to patients in mental institutions. But this is not the case with the elderly, who can be placed in these institutions and have no true advocate's presence to assure that continuing confinement is justified, or that the incarceration is justified to begin with.

However, developments during the early 1990s such as the passage of the Americans with Disabilities Act and the Patient Self-Determination Act (1991), are beginning to address a wide range of medical treatment concerns for the elderly as well as the disabled. Issues such as advance directives, surrogate medical decisionmaking, and the due process protections of the medical interest of vulnerable individuals have become increasingly important (see Avila 1993). Health Care Financing Administrative rules flowing from these changes have included closer overview of long-term care facilities and agencies involved in home care services, including the institution of surveillance systems to inspect the presence of immediate and serious threats to the health and safety of residents. These rules also include monitoring not only physical dangers but human rights violations. The impact of these developments have not been thoroughly assessed, nor do they rectify in principle all the areas for possible abuse of the elderly, but they are clearly an important step in the right direction.

Furthermore, on even more important issues, such as the right to refuse treatment, the elderly are not provided with the same kinds of resources legally and in terms of advocacy that exist for mental patients. The law, in myriad ways, supports the cultural perceptions of the elderly as dependent, infantile, and incompetent and therefore in need of the assistance of more competent adults to assure that the proper decisions are made in the medical care context (Tancredi 1987). But what is needed is a sensitization to the particularly vulnerable position of the elderly and affirming and maintaining the rights of those who are not institutionalized and do not desire to be (Moody 1987).

On the other hand, one aspect of the rights of the elderly has already become the focus of much attention from the legal community—namely the right of the terminally ill to elect to discontinue a life-saving treatment, with the inevitable consequence of death. The whole issue of the right to die has undergone considerable legal change since the mid-1970s. There has been an essential demystification of the right to die (Weinberg 1988), particularly through cases such as those of Karen Quinlan (*In re Quinlan* 1976) and Saikewicz (*Superintendent of Belchertown State School v. Saikewicz* 1977), and more recently in New Jersey, cases such as *In re Conroy* (1985). A series of such cases has articulated the right to terminate nutritional supports in those who are terminally ill or irreversibly seriously incapacitated (see *In Matter of Jobes* 1987). Because this group for the most part involves the elderly, the right to discontinue treatment is a cornerstone of the rights of the elderly that is gaining acceptance in most states (see Report of the President's Commission 1983).

A 1992 Supreme Court case, *Planned Parenthood of Southeastern Pennsylvania v. Casey*, may have major implications for further empowering the elderly to make their own medical choices. Although this case involved the review of Pennsylvania abortion laws, it nonetheless dealt with broader based concerns such as a competent individual's informed consent to, or refusal of, medical treatment and care. The court essentially recognized a "liberty" interest in accepting or rejecting medical treatment. Such an interest, according to the decision, has as its critical element the "right to define one's own concept of existence." Though not developed, such a theory may be far more enhancing of individual prerogatives. It essentially shifts from the "privacy" notions (which were rooted in case law acknowledging the primacy of familial relations) that served as the basis for the "right to die" decisions in the past to a "liberty" rationale that extols the individual interests of medically dependent persons.

At the same time that these cases are providing increasing self-determination and autonomy for the elderly, they offer the opportunity to empower community goals over those of the individual (Pollack 1989). This is not an issue where one is dealing with a competent elderly patient who is opting for withdrawal of life support, but it can be a problem when one is dealing with the incompetent elderly patient and determinations are made by family or others to withdraw life support. The laws in this regard are also changing. In the Karen Quinlan case the patient was unconscious and unable to voice an opinion; the court therefore allowed a putative decision maker, the father, to attest to the preferences of his daughter were she alive to make the decision. Such intellectual game strategies offer an opportunity for family and community members to impose upon the incompetent patient values and preferences that may not, in fact, reflect the patient's true disposition.

There is increasing interest, as we have seen in the work of ethicists such as Daniel Callahan (see Callahan 1987), in reconsidering the distribution of resources when one is dealing with the aged, and necessarily emphasizing a kind of utilitarian ethic of the greatest good for the greatest number. At the same time, the expression of such interests, often characterized as within the "intergenerational equity" movement, has stimulated its own group of opponents, who warn of the dangers of categorical discrimination by pointing out that many elderly individuals are healthy, vital, and members who contribute to society and to their own lives (see Osgood 1995). Conflicts imposed by the assertion of individual rights and preferences and the potential for the superimposition of a social-utility standard are just beginning to unravel individual and social values grouped around best interests, social autonomy, and community benefit (Dworkin 1977).

"BIOETHICS" CONSIDERS THE ELDERLY

Jay Katz has suggested "conversation" to overcome the pitfalls of "the Silent World of Doctor and Patient," which he maintains consists of medical arrogance and patient ignorance and submissiveness (Katz 1984). But we suggest that is not enough. Conversations with old paradigms will not necessarily provide information. Conversation sometimes permits the appearance of points of real communication, but it very frequently allows for many points of mismatch of codes and messages. The physician has a body of information constantly, if minimally, transformed while going from patient to patient, and interprets this information cross-sectionally. The patient has a longitudinal experiential history of an illness and a personal calculus of mishaps and optimization strategies for resolution of the problem. The physician/patient encounter is certainly a locus for the exercise of power, but not for a symmetrical exchange of it (Romanucci-Ross 1982a:179).

We have discussed the plight of the elderly in light of social change and indicated that early Americans and modern Americans are not culturally the same. We have made some crosscultural comparisons to illustrate different possibilities in interpersonal relations and worldview, the human condition, and the individual's place in the universe and in the group. Our culture prefers, in our times, segmental and impersonal relations. Our knowledge configurations in medical science train us to think of causation as temporal and reductionistic. We are very good at working with small circuits of control in small arcs of cause and effect. Where does bioethics fit in all of this?

There is little agreement on what "ethics" is, but apparently we can agree that it is about "What should we do? What should we hope for or seek? How should we treat others?"

In philosophy, ethicists work at setting forth principles of morality (excellence in behavior) and justifying them. But most people don't want to be told what is good or bad, nor do they want to be told how to think about it. Like the herpes simplex virus, preprogrammed ethical thought has been all around us all the time, in the special institutions of our culture (homes, churches, schools, clubs, etc.), or it is acquired from the last kiss of a dying grandparent. It disappears into the nooks and crannies of a nerve sheath until a crisis calls it forth to erupt and be seen and heard and noted by all, and to be disseminated to others.

Since there is no objective way to know what the correct view of the world is, societies take no chances. We are immediately socialized to view "reality" as it benefits our culture, so that it may sustain itself. To look at all the societies and cultures of the world is to be stunned by the array of possible solutions to moral dilemmas. Yet we can all recall being told to "listen to your conscience," as though it were not ready-made for you the minute you appeared on this planet.

A prevailing cultural ideology is instilled in the child before anyone is aware of it. An ideology is the way the world is viewed, and one's place within it, the future of mankind, and one's place in the present and future grounded in the past. It is about attitudes toward authority, about interpersonal relationships, the goal of an individual or of a society. These values create a "second reality" more real than what is really "there." A society has a problem when it *recognizes* that it does. And it says a great deal about our values that we now feel that that group known as the elderly pose a "problem" for us.

If we listen to our bioethicists as regards "the problem of the elderly," we can learn some very interesting things, even if we don't learn much about solving the problem. Some, such as Albert Jonson and Daniel Callahan, appear to have evolved from posing the problem as "What is our obligation to help the elderly?" They are the coiners of the phrase "intergenerational justice." (Since our culture differs from most others by placing more emphasis on "within-a-generation" relationships rather than "between-generation" relationships, we have the problem of "justice" rather than altruistic motivation.) Callahan concludes that society should desist from medical goals to benefit the elderly, who should shift their interest to the young rather than themselves. They should accept death, he says, for the sake of others (see Callahan 1987).

The format for discussing the elderly and medical care in our culture is for established groups to ask our bioethicists to frame a series of questions and to answer them. The frames and the questions are highly stylized and cluster around issues such as life support, living space, cost/benefit, and "is there *room* for our elderly." Implicit in the question frame is the belief that we have to make some "terrible choices."

Ethical decisions are also about what we do to ourselves as we make such decisions. It is about whether we have the courage to look at ourselves. It is about accepting the constraints of life—lives of those other than ourselves, including wildlife, and our place in the plant and animal world. There are those who proclaim or gladly acquiesce in the infinite expansion of human activity and unchecked human proliferation at the cost of the space of other forms of life—*all* other forms of life and matter.

One does not hear the bioethicists asking these or other related questions, such as, What is the relationship of person to family, family to group, and of group to ecology? Should one make decisions about who should survive and who should come into being without being accountable for the consequences? (Native healers *are* held accountable for life and death and the consequences of their shamanic rites.)

The existential philosophers, beginning with Nietzsche and followed by Kierkegaard, Heidegger, Sartre, and others, maintained that ethics *is* about values, and that people create their own values. This means, of course, that values are not handed out on stone tablets nor diffused through gamma rays during enlightenment under a bo tree. We summarize the general stance of these thinkers, for they used very different terms in their descriptions.

The world is unintelligible, man's lot is absurd. We begin with the dark night of the soul, which leads to crisis, to our making a choice—to becoming engaged. We thus create and adhere to *values*. The existentialist wants a rich texture in moral reasoning, one that transcends cost accounting (see Nietzsche 1966; Kierkegaard 1975; Sartre 1957; Heidegger 1927).

But one does not hear the bioethicists asking "What should be our ultimate values, such as the place of art in life?" or "What of the role of solitude?" or "What will making 'terrible choices' do to us?"

The basic requirement being able to think ethically is not so much always to "understand the viewpoint of the other," which is nonetheless emphasized, but to recognize that events are framed and placed within other event frames in changing times and with changing facts. The problem of the elderly cannot be solved within our current frames.

Absolute answers are pitifully inadequate, and some questions are obsolete. John Rawls in his *Theory of Justice* (1971) suggests we approach every problem (ethically or morally) not knowing our place in society, our age, our rank, our financial or social status. Only *then* can we consider how to distribute justice or resources fairly. An interesting view, because it is very characteristic of less developed societies to approach ethical problems in exactly this fashion. One is *never* an individual but only part of a collectivity. The goal—the survival of the group values.

CONCLUSION

This chapter has attempted to examine some bioethical, legal, and cultural problems relevant to the elderly. Many of these concerns are applicable to all of us who experience the health care system. What these concerns once more emphasize is that medicine, although based in science, can be, and often is, used for social objectives. Conflicting values then come into play in decisions that can be beneficial or harmful to those affected. We have the law to shore up individual rights through due process, through the asseveration of autonomy and self-determination regarding principles of privacy, and we have a body of bioethical literature that likewise addresses individual rights (Rawls 1971; Walzer 1983). On the other hand, both the law and bioethics are susceptible to interpretation; and this interpretation, based on cultural values, may easily shift at any point from emphasis on community or societal values to emphasis on individual values.

Since the mid-1970s the increasing concern about the cost of health care has indicated that economic factors are pivotal in generating social and political decisions in health care. The crisis of economics in health care is being felt on all levels—the care of children, the care of adults, the care of the mentally ill, and the care of the elderly. But it is this last group that is open to the most potential for abuse. They are a growing number in our society, and they are perceived increasingly as consumers of societal goods rather than as producers. Such factors weigh heavily in the interpretation of constitutional, legal, and bioethical principles regarding self-determination, autonomy, due process, and conflicts between the individual and society. They will continue to do so unless we ask the pertinent *ethical* questions: What kind of life do we want? What kind of world do we want? What must we do, or refrain from doing, to attain it?

REFERENCES

Avila, D. 1993. "Medical Treatment Rights of Older Persons and Persons with Disabilities: 1992 Developments." *Clearinghouse Review*:1267–76.

Callahan, Daniel. 1987. *Setting Limits: Medical Goals in an Aging Society*. New York: Simon and Schuster.

Cole, T. R. 1987. "Class, Culture and Coercion: A Historical Perspective on Long Term Care." *Generations* 11:9–15.

Devereux, George. 1967. *From Anxiety to Method in the Behavioral Sciences*. Paris and The Hague: Ecole Pratique des Hautes Etudes and Mouton.

Dworkin, R. 1977. *Taking Rights Seriously*. Cambridge, Mass.: Harvard University Press.

Engel, Heinrich. 1987. *The Japanese House: A Tradition for Contemporary Architecture*. Rutland, Vt., and Tokyo: Chas. E. Tuttle.

Feinson, M. 1985. "Aging and Mental Health: Distinguishing Myth from Reality." *Research on Aging* 7:155.

Folstein, N., J. D. Anthony, I. Parhad, B. Duffy, and E. Gruenberg. 1985. "The Meaning of Cognitive Impairment in the Elderly." *Journal of the American Geriatrics Society* 33:228.

Fromm, Erich. 1947. *Man for Himself: An Inquiry into the Psychology of Ethics*. New York: Holt, Rinehart and Winston.

Goffman, E. 1961. *Asylums: Essays on the Social Situation of Mental Patients and Other Inmates.* Garden City, N.Y.: Doubleday.

Heidegger, Martin. 1927. *Sein and Zeit.* Trans. J. Macquarrie and E. S. Robinson as *Being and Time.* New York: 1962; Frankfurt am Main: Klosterman.

Henry, Jules. 1965. *Culture against Man.* New York: Vintage Books-Random House.

Kapp, M. B. 1995. "Family Caregiving for Older Persons in the Home." *Journal of Legal Medicine* 16:1–31.

Katz, Jay. 1984. *The Silent World of Doctor and Patient.* New York: The Free Press.

Kierkegaard, Soren. 1975. *Entwerder-Order* (Trans. George L. Stregen as *Either/Or.* Munich: Deutscher Taschenbuchen Verlag).

In Matter of Jobes. 1987. 108 N.J. 394, 529 A.2d 434.

Mead, Margaret. 1970. *Culture and Commitment: A Study of the Generation Gap.* Garden City, N.Y.: Doubleday.

Moody, H. R. 1987. "Ethical Dilemmas in Nursing Home Placement." *Generations* 11:16–23.

Nietzsche, Friedrich. 1966. *Beyond Good and Evil: Prelude to a Philosophy of the Future.* Trans. Walter Kaufman. New York: Vintage Books.

Okakura, Kakuso. 1956. *The Book of Tea.* Rutland, Vt., and Tokyo: Chas. E. Tuttle.

Osgood, N. J. 1995. "Assisted Suicide and Older People—A Deadly Combination: Ethical Problems in Permitting Assisted Suicide." *Issues in Law and Medicine* 10(4):415–35.

Patient Self-Determination Act. PL 101–508, Sections 4206, 4751, 014 Stat. 1388–115 to –117, –204 to –206 (1991).

Planned Parenthood of Southeastern Pennsylvania v. Casey, 120 L. Rd. 2d 674 (1992).

Pollock, S. G. 1989. "Life and Death Decisions: Who Makes Them and by What Standards?" *Rutgers Law Review* 41:505–40.

Rawls, J. 1971. *A Theory of Justice.* Cambridge, Mass.: Harvard University Press.

In re Conroy. 1985. 98 N.J. 321, 486 A.2d 1209.

In re Quinlan. 1976. 70 N.J. 10, 355 A.2d 647, *Cert. Denied*, 429 U.S. 922.

Report of the President's Commission for the Study of Ethical Problems in Medicine and Biomedical and Behavioral Research. 1983. *Deciding to Forego Life-Sustaining Treatment.* Washington, D.C.: U.S. Government Printing Office.

Reggins v. Nevada, 118 L. Ed. 2d 479, 489 (1992).

Rogers v. Okin. 1979. 478 F. Supp 1342 (Ed. Mass.), 1979, *Cert. granted* and case argued sub nom *Mills v. Rogers*, 457 U.S. 291, 102 S.Ct. 2442 (1983). See also *Rogers v. Okin* 738 F.2d 1 (1984).

Rolle, Andrew F. 1968. *The Immigrant Upraised; Italian Adventures and Colonists in an Expanding America.* Norman: University of Oklahoma Press.

Romanucci-Ross, Lola. 1982a. "Medicalization and Metaphor." In *The Use and Abuse of Medicine.* Martin W. deVries, R. L. Berg, and Mack Lipkin, Jr., eds. New York: Praeger.

———. 1982b. "The Italian Identity and Its Transformation." In *Ethnic Identity: Cultural Continuities and Change.* George de Vos and Lola Romanucci-Ross, eds. Chicago: University of Chicago Press, 198–227.

Sartre, Jean-Paul. 1957. *L'Etre et le Néant: Essai d'Ontologie Phénoménologique.* Paris: Gallimard (Trans. Hazel Barnes as *Being and Nothingness.* New York: Philosophical Library).

Siegel, J. S. and C. M. Taeuber. 1986. Demographic Dimensions of an Aging Population. In *Our Aging Society: Paradox and Promise.* A. Pifer and L. Bronte, eds. New York: W. W. Norton.

Superintendent of Belchertown State School v. Saikewicz. 1977. 373 Mass. 728, 370 N.E. 2d 417.

Tancredi, L. R. 1987. "The Mental Status Examination." *Generations* 11:24–31.

Tocqueville, Alexis de. 1946. *Democracy in America.* Trans. Henry Reeve. London: Oxford University Press. (First published as *De la Democratie en Amérique.* Paris: Libraire de Charles Gosselin, 1835–1840.)

U.S. Department of Health and Human Services. 1987. *Fact Sheet on Long Term Care.* September 21, pp. 66–71.

Walzer, M. 1983. *Spheres of Justice: A Defense of Pluralism and Equality.* New York: Basic Books.

Washington et al. v. Harper. 1990. 110 S.Ct. 1028.

Weinberg, J. K. 1988. "Demystifying the Right to Die: The New Jersey Experience." *Medicine and Law* 7:323–45.

Weissman, M., J. K. Myers, G. L. Tischler, C. Holzer, III, P. Leaf, and J. Brody. 1985. "Psychiatric Disorders (DSM-III) and Cognitive Impairment among the Elderly in a U.S. Urban Community." *Acta Psychiatrica Scandinavica* 71:336.

18

The Extraneous Factor in Western Medicine

LOLA ROMANUCCI-ROSS AND DANIEL E. MOERMAN

It has been noted by philosophers of science that the successes of "method" in the physical sciences were contingent upon a division of "physical" and "mental," with the relegation of the latter "to the limbo of a sort of secondary or epiphenomenal existence" (Feigl 1953:612) and the existence of the physical accepted as a fundamental empirical fact. This mind-body problem particularly concerned Descartes, who tried to puzzle out how something nonspatial (thinking) could be causally related to spatial matter. With the enunciation of this problem in the seventeenth century we find the roots of modern science and medicine.

Descartes's influence is considered especially notable on the empiricist philosophers who insisted that epistemology should be the starting point of philosophy. Later, the logical positivists asserted that the meaning of scientific statements cannot be identified with their confirming evidence and that the meaning of a statement is the method of its verification (Schlick 1925). In other words, a new concept is synonymous with the set of operations that determines its applications (Bridgman 1927).

Logical empiricism developed into a phase that provided "logical" tools for reconsideration of the mind-body problem. As Feigl has pointed out, it is true that relations between indicators that can be evidenced (such as language, behavior, and neurophysiological data) must be interpreted in terms of "laws," and this would then make explanation and predication possible in a mind-body identity (Feigl 1953:615). Postempiricists such as Husserl also tried to recapture the Cartesian mode; in the words of Williams, "the problems posed by Descartes' dualism remain at the heart of much contemporary philosophical inquiry (the work of Gilbert Ryle and Ludwig Wittgenstein, for example) being aimed directly against what are still very powerful Cartesian conceptions" (1967:354).

In recent times, the philosophical school popularly known as "Kuhnian" has granted a more significant role to thought itself in the process of knowing. According to Kuhn (1970), one searches for the new paradigm that will revolutionize the manner in which a problem is phrased as well as "solved." Once introduced and accepted, however, the paradigm tends to stabilize thought and reinforces the architectonic of the belief system that will remain unexamined.

The philosophical "school" that focused on the thinking process was formed by scholars in a variety of disciplines. Ludwig Fleck in his analysis of the Wasserman reaction wrote that a "fact" is a "stylized signal of resistance in thinking" (1979 [1935]:98). Just a few years earlier, Gödel proved his "inconsistency" theorem, demonstrating that in mathematics no formal system of axioms could be simultaneously consistent and complete. A consistent system includes undecidable propositions, while a complete system can prove everything, for example "p is not p." (Wilder 1952:256–61). Truth, then, is a function of knowledge that is necessarily either incomplete or illogical. Such a truth is of little value and so one is forced to turn from "truth" to "belief," grounding knowledge in experience, as did Descartes.

To contrast the two views germane to our discussion, in the seventeenth century Descartes could affirm the possibility of knowing the "truth" without a single doubt, based on his own *experience*. He "knew," for example, that blood was pumped through the body because the heart was hot, which caused the blood to expand and to course out through the arteries.[1] Similar properties caused similar behaviors regardless of context, an inference constituting a sort of naïve realism. For Kuhn, the paradigm or "disciplinary matrix" made up of categories, relationships, and decisive examples structures the view of truth that the scientist discovers. When the paradigm changes it is "rather as if the professional community had been suddenly transported to another planet where familiar objects are seen in a different light and are joined by unfamiliar ones as well . . . nothing changes but the view" (Kuhn 1970:111). Thus the Kuhnian view emphasizes the changing nature of knowledge as viewed through new paradigms, whereas the Cartesian view simply builds on past perceptions.

Where is contemporary biomedicine in all of this? In some cases, men and women in medicine have achieved a Kuhnian view of their profession, but most share a greater affinity with Descartes. We attempt here a Fleck/Gödelian view of the "realism" in contemporary medicine, an exercise in a psychological anthropology of medicine assessing values, ideology and paradigms. We indicate and comment on what we perceive to be major developments of present-day scientific inquiry in medicine—randomized clinical trials, animal models, the psychiatric model, the chemical intervention model, and diagnosis—and consider how these "styles" of investigation not only reflect values and ideologies but affect our knowledge of disease and cure.

VALUES AND IDEOLOGY

Physicians learn the wisdom of the body by dissecting cadaver; they focus their attention by "draping" body parts not under immediate scrutiny. They seek order through classification although both order *and* classifications thereof are "mentifacts" (Bidney 1953); both are constructs imposed on the "real world" even though we tend to think that the order is real and the classification describes it. The physician's order (read classification) is the basis for his general procedure: to measure, to compare, to predict.

Generally these values of mastery, order, and power are axiomatic; they need not be considered or thought about. They precede thought; they provide the scaffolding for it. They are good in and of themselves, moral virtues. When these issues *are* considered, they are transformed into virtues of the highest sort as they were for the ancient Romans who equated knowledge and virtue. Consider this text, culled from the ruminations of the surgeon Selzer in his aptly titled collection *Mortal Lessons*:

The priestliness of my profession has ever been impressed upon me. In the beginning there are vows taken with all solemnity. Then there is the endless harsh novitiate of training, much fatigue, much sacrifice. At last one emerges as celebrant, standing close to the truth lying curtained in the Ark of the body. Not surplice and cassock but mask and gown are your regalia. You hold no chalice, but a knife. There is no wine, no wafer. There are only the facts of blood and flesh. (Selzer 1976:94)

By ideology we mean that body of notions that transforms fundamental values into social action. An ideology, or belief system, is a condition of learning and knowledge. It is not fragmented into "religious," "political," "social," or even "scientific" beliefs. A belief system encompasses attitudes in all these aspects of a personal "field" and more often than not contains inconsistencies or is incomplete; but believers live with these inconsistencies and accentuate differences with other belief systems. Contemporary ideology in biomedicine includes the following values: first, causation is temporal, reductionist, and essentially metonymic, that is, the part represents the whole and/or cause is taken for effect and effect is taken for cause. In general, a part, construed as "prior" and "lower," is taken to account for the whole. Occasionally, the equation is reversed. This is related to another "value": that of measurement, comparison, and prediction. It yields action in a variety of forms:

1. "Myocardial infarction is usually produced by thrombotic occlusion of one of the larger branches of the coronary arteries" (Halvey 1972:376). In this case, the part causes the whole.

2. Rheumatoid arthritis is "a chronic syndrome characterized by nonspecific inflam-
   mation of the peripheral joints. . . . The etiology is unknown" (Halvey 1972:1209).
   In this case, the part that causes the whole is unknown, but assumed to exist.

3. "Anorexia Nervosa . . . food aversion, self-induced, which is a manifestation of
   psychiatric illness" (Halvey 1972:1423). Here, the whole causes the part.

The metonymic style looms in importance as it forms the primary structure
for treatment. One "treats" the "cause" of illness, not the "symptoms" of
illness. This treatment is usually conceived to be allopathic; one imagines
that even pediatricians (whose daily practice includes vaccinations) would
vigorously deny being homeopaths. This allopathy is generally the consequence of another major belief in biomedicine: disease is natural while, in
general, healing is cultural.

A general corollary to this second belief is that disease *must* be treated,
even if effective treatment is not available. Culture must at least contest
with nature, even if the game is already lost. Moreover, patients who do *not*
respond to standard treatments (morphine for pain) were not sick in the first
place; they may be classified as "hypochondriacs." Similarly, people who *do*
respond to *inert* treatments (placebos) were not really sick, either. Occasionally, these two processes can interact. A study carried out in a Texas hospital
showed that house officers and nurses considered some patients to be "problem cases." These patients were those who did not respond to standard
treatments, leading to the hypothesis that they were not really sick. Frequently, such patients were then treated with placebos. When they responded favorably to such treatment, this was considered verification of the
hypothesis (Goodwin et al. 1979:106–10).

Similarly, there is a standard reaction to the occasional cases of "spontaneous remission" in patients who have been refractory to treatment; often
enough, this is explained by saying that the condition was probably misdi-
agnosed in the first place. These sorts of phenomena—ineffective drugs,
effective placebos, spontaneous remissions—are generally "impossible"
given the ideological principles under discussion; these fall into the category
of "anomalies." It is a measure of the tenacity of this ideology that a phenomenon (placebos) that can account for as much as 90 percent of ulcer
healing (Moerman 1983:14–16) can be considered an "anomaly."

The placebo or biomedically inert substance that produces relief also
helps eliminate bias in a research protocol. It does not fit the Western master
paradigm:

Many papers have demonstrated the importance and magnitude of the placebo effect
in every therapeutic area. Placebos can be more powerful than, and reverse the action
of, potent active drugs. The incidence of placebo reactions approaches 100 percent
in some studies. Placebos can have profound effects on organic illnesses including
incurable malignancies. Placebos can often mimic the effects of active drugs. Un-

controlled studies of drug efficacy are reported effective four to five times more frequently than controlled studies. Placebo effects are so omnipresent that if they are not reported in controlled studies it is commonly accepted that the studies are unreliable. (Shapiro 1968:58)

Brody argues that the physician of our time cannot deny the placebo data, "but he can adopt an attitude towards it of exclusion, that is, labeling the placebo effect so that it can be readily recognized and thus excluded from research" (Brody 1980:27).

SOME CONTEMPORARY RESEARCH PARADIGMS

We began with mention of Descartes and it is appropriate to refer again to the man and his period, the seventeenth century, since in the times and in the man we recognize the foundations of modern scientific thought. Descartes respected his teachers but stated that only mathematics had ever given him "certain knowledge" (Williams 1967:344). He stressed quantitative measurement and experimentation as well as taxonomy and calculable order.

Descartes accepted the notion of circulatory movement of the blood but not the independent contraction of the heart as the driving force of the system. More inclined to mathematics and deductive thinking, he looked for another mechanical cause of blood displacement: its "heating" and subsequent expansion as it entered the heart (Snellen 1984:22).

William Harvey took up and retained the mistaken idea of "heat" but also *calculated* the total volume of blood in the circulation and estimated the output of the pumping chamber of the heart per beat and per minute. He therefore was able to conclude that the blood must recirculate, driven by the heart (Harvey 1978).

This ideology, with its commitment to observation, measurement, and experiments, led not only to some false starts (through Descartes), but also to productive work (through Harvey) that led to later "knowledge explosions." However, important for our purposes, unexplained ideology still thrives in the research paradigms of our day. We have typified the much valued canons of correct "scientific" behavior and give several examples.

The *randomized clinical trial* is the study of the effects of an intervention in a sizable population expected to experience abnormal events with a given frequency. Patients are assigned to treatment, no treatment, or "ordinary care." The goal is to determine whether or not a specific intervention over a period of time will reduce the abnormal event rate in a statistically significant manner. As an example we refer to the "Coronary Artery Surgery Study" known as CASS (CASS 1983). In this large study, patients were randomly assigned to either customary medical treatment of their mild to moderate angina pectoris, or to coronary artery bypass surgery. After a (mean) six-year follow-up, the groups were compared to see if the surgical procedure extended life. No significant difference was found between medical and surgical treatment. This trial was a corrective response to the emergent "ideal" of having coronary bypass surgery performed.

But such trials can have their pitfalls, as shown in another recent study, for although the randomized clinical trial is the ideal method for assessing treatment allocations, there are dangers in such trials. Even when everything from the complete, carefully collected baseline data and all statistical pitfalls is taken into account, there is still a likelihood of "chance" differences achieving statistical significance when multiple subgroups are analyzed. In a study carried out at Duke University, 1,073 coronary artery disease patients were randomly sorted into two groups; there were no differences in treatment between the two groups of patients. There was no overall difference in survival between the two groups, as one would expect. However, in a subgroup of 397 patients with three-vessel disease and abnormal left ventricular contraction, survival was significantly different in the two randomly sorted groups. Multivariable adjustment procedures attributed the difference to the combined effect of small differences in the distribution of several prognostic factors. On a univariate basis, the "treatment" (that is, randomization) might appear to be a significant factor in the survival of this subgroup ($x^2 = 5.4$; p .025). When the variables were considered jointly, the "treatment" effect became nonsignificant ($x^2 = 2.4$; $p = NS$). In addition, in another subgroup a significant survival difference was not explainable even by multivariate methods. In this case of patients with three-vessel disease, abnormal left ventricular contraction pattern, and no history of congestive heart failure, the respective three-year survival rates of the two randomly differentiated groups were 60 percent and 80 percent ($x^2 = 10.0$; $p = .01$). The authors of this study caution that clinicians must exercise careful judgment in attributing results to efficacious therapy, as they may be due to chance or to inadequate baseline comparability of groups (Lee et al. 1980:508–15).

Indeed, physicians inevitably use "judgment" when they prescribe treatments, this is to say that "science" (the clinical trial) is tempered by "knowledge grounded in experience" (what we have called "belief")—these are combined into what physicians call "clinical judgment."

Some interesting clinical judgments went into the design and analysis of another recent and widely publicized clinical trial. This study used a double-blind method to test the efficacy of lowering blood cholesterol levels in reducing the risk of heart disease in 3,806 middle-aged men. The treatment group received cholestyramine resin (a drug that inhibits absorption of lipids from the intestines) while the control group received a placebo; the subjects were followed for an average of 7.4 years. The drug group was reported to have experienced a 19 percent reduction in risk of death due to coronary heart disease (CHD) and/or definite myocardial infarction, significant at the .05 level, one-sided.

This study was interesting for the fact that in these very well matched groups, all causes and rates of mortality were similar for the two groups, with two exceptions. In addition to modest differences in death due to coronary heart disease, the drug-treated group had a larger number of accidental and violent deaths. Because of this, there was only a 7 percent reduction of all-cause mortality in the drug group (LRCP 1984:351–64).[2] The report of the study notes that "since no plausible connection could be established between cholestyramine treatment and violent and accidental death, it is difficult to conclude that this could be anything but a chance occurrence" (LRCP 1984:359).

The drug-treated group reported a substantially higher rate of gastrointestinal discomfort. While severe gastrointestinal discomforts might reduce awareness (for accidents) or predispose one to abnormal behavior, the possibility of such effects was not considered. It is well known that "many commonly used drugs can cause serious mental symptoms, including depression and disorders in thinking that may resemble schizophrenia" (*Medical Letter on Drugs and Therapeutics* 1981). The drug was being tested for one purpose (which is why the authors took the liberty of using one-tailed statistics; in two-tailed tests, the differences found in this study are not statistically significant); no need to "confound" the picture with other extraneous possibilities.

The randomized clinical trial has had an important effect in medicine. But the design of trials necessarily reflects the assumptions and expectations of the investigators and may provide convincing demonstrations of "obvious" but incorrect notions (cf. Descartes [1637] 1960:68). Statistical significance is no assurance against design error.

Chemical intervention models are a triumph of allopathic medicine. One finds what there is too much or too little of and supplies it or changes the balance. In many instances this has caused great relief to the patient, but often at the expense of long-term effects that are noxious or lethal. Many asthma sufferers have ended up with hypertension (generally treatable) after eight to ten years of treatment with steroids. Those taking the phenothiazines (such as thorazine) have acquired irreversible tardive dyskinesias. In such cases, the effects of drugs on biological systems through time are not taken into account. There are other examples: use of diuretics can lead to elevated uric acid levels and development of gout; radioactive phosphorus used to treat polycythemia vera can lead to leukemia; cyclosporin used to prevent rejection of a transplanted organ may cause cancer.

Adverse interactions of drugs given at the same time or in close sequence (often by different physicians unaware of or unconcerned with one another's treatments) again illustrate ignorance of the time factor, of the patient's biography, and of the synergistic effect of drugs affecting or influencing one another. The effect can also occur by combining drugs with certain foods (*Medical Letter on Drugs and Therapeutics* 1979).

Part of the problem here results from some curious notions that physicians have regarding drugs. Particularly intriguing is the classification of drug effects into "action" and "side effect." Consider the case of the antihistamine Benadryl (diphenhydramine) which, when prescribed for allergies, is said to have the side effect of causing drowsiness. When it is used as a sedative for insomnia, its antihistaminic qualities are side effects ("dry mouth").

Although Withering described the therapeutic values of foxglove extracts 200 years ago, it is only recently that some studies have provided a demonstration of mechanisms of important extracardiac effects of digitalis glycosides, such as slowed heart rate, rise in blood pressure, and other effects mediated by the central and peripheral nervous systems (Longhurst and Ross 1985:99A–105A). Extracardiac "side effects" had long been disturbing to patients who experienced nausea and vomiting, abdominal pain, gynecomastia in men and breast enlargement in women, vision disturbances, headaches, seizures, and coma. Studies such as these that reveal the mechanisms of "drug action" should lead physicians to a revisionist view of the simplistic notion that such actions can be considered in terms of "primary" and "secondary" effects, as is currently the case.

At times, the distinction between "action" and "side effect" can have strange and untoward consequences; this confusion is a result of seeing patients only partially, seeing only the "organ system" that is sick and not the whole person—a kind of tunnel vision. Consider the case of ventricular premature ectopic beats on an electrocardiogram (ECG). The parsing of patients leads professionals in both clinical and research contexts to ignore evidence that lies outside of their expertise and their prejudgment of normalcy. Gordon Moe, a well-known physiologist, noted that if you looked closely at some ECG tracings, you would see a rhythmicity allowing you to predict the sequence of the occurrence of ectopic beats, and to predict that beats could appear, disappear, or become fix-coupled (bigeminal) every other beat with either slight increases or slight decreases in the heart rate alone. He compared his observations with a recently published paper that "demonstrated" the disappearance of premature beats "due to" digitalis. But Moe had shown that what was attributed to digitalis as a direct anti-arrhythmic effect could have been the concealment of a parasystolic focus by a slight decrease in heart rate. The same effect on heart rate could have been produced by "going down an elevator." The international professional audience at this lecture (in Florence, Italy, in 1978) laughed with embarrassed amusement, not wanting to recognize Moe's conclusion that hypotheses need to be enlarged to include factors generally excluded from research paradigms. It seems unlikely that this will occur generally as it requires observing and measuring behavior. Behavior, like a "side effect," is extrinsic to the action expected from the drug.

We consider here more briefly a few other aspects of contemporary medical research and practice where extrinsic factors play an important role limiting and constricting understanding: the use of *animal models*, the *psychiatric model*, and *diagnosis*.

The use of *animal models* is a particularly interesting case of the use of metaphor in medicine. Similarly, it is a case that indicates the (not surprising) difficulties that can occur when people take metaphors literally. Dogs, pigs, and baboons (among others) are widely used in cardiovascular research. The pig is at times a better representation of humans, for, unlike the dog, it has a large right coronary artery and few coronary collateral vessels located primarily on the inner heart wall. The dog, however, is sometimes a good model because it has more collaterals, most on the outer wall, and a number of people with coronary heart disease develop significant collaterals on the outer walls as well as on the inner walls. The baboon is a better hemodynamic model of humans due to its more upright posture than the other animals. One must, then, match the animal to the problem at hand; although these problems have been noted in the scientific literature (Crozatier et al. 1978:H413–21; Sanders et al. 1977:365–70; Tomoike et al. 1981:H519–24), they have been generally ignored as investigators go through the ritual of scientific presentation, confusing the metaphorical model for the object of their ultimate concern.

Attachment to the animal model of disease transmission has long impeded careful inquiry and more correct epidemiological explanations of the spread of certain diseases. A study of historical records with modern research techniques and current medical knowledge can yield surprising results. For example, the transmission of "the plague" was attributed to the abandonment of the infected and dying *Rattus rattus* by its resident flea, *Xenopsylla cheopis*, which regurgitated the plague bacillus, *Yersinia pestis*, into its human victim. But a consideration of such factors as seasonal occurrences of the disease, the number of cases per household, comparisons with the presence of the black house rat in other parts of the world, and the sudden disappearance of the plague in Europe has led to a broader hypothesis. (Medieval physicians knew the plague quite well and described variations in great detail.) Recent research (Ell 1980:497–510) has emphasized interhuman transmission as well as several varieties of "the plague." Those who wrote treatises and texts on the exploration of the occurrence of the plague had rested comfortably on the rat-flea-human mode of transmission, which, though correct part of the time, stifled further investigation for a long period of time.

The *psychiatric model* typifies the procedures by which states and behaviors have been medicalized, traditionally rendering patients helpless as their caretakers decide on medical and surgical interventions. The nature of communication and emotional states are crucial in the diagnosis of mental illnesses. But these were not part of the general ideology of the biomedical practitioners and were considered extraneous factors. It was only after the legal battles of the civil rights era—the 1950s to the 1970s—that such sick persons were given a "say" over their patient status (Tancredi 1983:284–

97). Indeed, many health professionals now *see* these factors but still consider them extraneous, indeed intrusive and destructive (Radine 1983:366–87).

The confluence of the psychiatric model with some features of the general diagnostic process can provide us with an interesting field for the compounding of errors. In the Soviet Union a system was developed during the 1960s for psychiatric diagnosis. Many of the most talented psychiatrists in that country were disciples of a central theory of schizophrenia, developing a definition so exceedingly broad as to include much of whatever else might be included in psychopathology. According to this definition, schizophrenia had three possible course forms: continuous, periodic, and shiftlike. Patients of the continuous type experienced early onset and did not improve; the "periodics" had periods of remission during illness; and the shift like type patient was a combination of the continuous and periodic types. This was further complicated by the additional diagnostic criterion of "severe" or "mild" for any type.

What was (or should have been) troublesome, of course, is that many became "patients" of the "mild" type who would perhaps not be seen—in another milieu—by any psychiatrist at all. There have been studies attesting to this (Hite 1974; Rollins 1972). Interestingly, however, the International Pilot Study on Schizophrenia of the late 1960s and early 1970s noted that two of the nine centers reviewed for diagnostic activities did poorly: Washington and Moscow (World Health Organization 1973).

The goal of the computer program was to rediagnose patients originally diagnosed as schizophrenic at various centers, using the centers' own data on the patients. Moscow's Institute of Psychiatry and Washington did poorly for very different reasons, however; a large percentage of Moscow's diagnosed schizophrenics were reassigned by the computer to neurotic and depressive categories rather than the psychoses. The Washington center had many of its patients reassigned to the psychotic categories. Obviously one center "over diagnosed" and the other "underdiagnosed."

Some have argued that psychiatric diagnoses can be a solution to human (that is, "political" writ small—or writ large) problems (Basaglia 1980, 1981). Reich has noted that such diagnoses are also used to *reassure* all of us; he gives the example of a researcher, Dr. Summerlin, who inked the skins of his mice to make it appear that grafted skin had been "taken," when others could not repeat his experiment with his dramatic results. It was important that the public not be led to think that research in general was a fraudulent activity, for great sums are donated to the research enterprise. The investigating committee "found" that Summerlin's behavior involved self-deception and aberration. Even Dr. Lewis Thomas, president of the Sloan-Kettering Cancer Center, informed reporters that "the fraud in this work was the result of mental illness" (Reich 1981:76–77). The same explanation was put forth by those surrounding Dr. John Darsee's fraudulent research in a Harvard Medical School laboratory (Knox 1983).

Such diagnoses appear to be self-validating in the same manner that it is reasoned (with the benefit of elaborate diagnostic procedures) that a criminal "must be" insane to have committed the act for which he is undergoing psychiatric appraisal (Romanucci-Ross and Tancredi 1986).

Diagnosis (included in the example above) similarly has a variety of extraneous factors that shape and form it, making it far less than the scientific procedure it might be. Studies have consistently shown that medical problem solving is a hypothetico-deductive activity in which early problem formulations partly guide subsequent data collection (Elstein 1978:299). In a review of 50 clinicopathologic conferences, the process of achieving a diagnosis was shown to have determinable steps. First, there is an aggregation of groups of findings into patterns followed by the selection of a "pivot" or key finding (that is, the problem is metonymized). From this is generated a "cause" list that is pruned to a set of differential diagnoses—a listing of diagnostic possibilities—from which one is selected and then validated (Eddy and Clanton 1982:1263–68). The problem, of course, is in the amount of information to be considered; one can only interpret signs and symptoms to diagnose disease, but one's medical training was learned the other way around—from disease. This medical decision-making chain has an effect on the physician's "intuitive" uses of the principle of discriminant analysis, that is, how much weight is given to clinical versus statistical factors, or how knowledge is grounded in experience.

The diagnostic process is further constrained because the "facts" are, of necessity, selected and evaluated in a temporal ordering. Decisions have to be made within a time frame and the presenting symptom does not always indicate that the patient suffers from several afflictions. As indicated earlier in this discussion, one measures what is measurable and classifies those concepts or entities for which there are categories, while masses of information slip through the cracks of elegant analytics. The diagnostic "method" is especially vulnerable to the weaknesses in such an approach.

IDEOLOGY AND REFLEXIVITY

Seventeenth-century science valued "measurement," the relating of things not to ourselves but to each other. The end of the eighteenth century saw the birth of Romanticism, the "transcendental," and a serious consideration of subject-object relations. But in the nineteenth century, what was central to medicine was clinical investigation and experimentation, critical working hypotheses, and structure, both organic and physiological. These were epitomized in the works of Claude Bernard and Rudolph Virchow. And, as Foucault pointed out in *The Birth of the Clinic* (Foucault 1975), we had the establishment of faculties of medicine and the transmission of medical knowledge into social privilege. There was a strong beginning during this period in the exercises of looking at probabilities in diagnoses and, presumably, becoming aware of "extraneous factors." Although Morgagni still specified diseases by points of origin, he began to find cells, nervous tissues in different organs, fibrous lesions, and lesions of serous and mucous membranes (Morgagni 1761). This began the search for "principles" about tissues. It appears to have been a period of exciting theoretical modeling and synthesis in clinical experience as well as research. And yet, Italian anatomists had already made essentially the same transition, from form to function, in the sixteenth century (Castiglioni 1934). This historical fact demonstrates that innovation does not always overcome ideology and affect mainstream science as soon as it should and in the manner it might. Principles are rediscovered centuries later because they then fit the new paradigms. Morgagni founded pathology, and in his classic work on the causes of disease, *De Sedibus et Causis Morborum per Anatomen Indagatis* (1761), he employed the best canons of inductive research. But he was in no hurry to publish his work, fearing criticism and rejection.

Most of the values of the classical period of the seventeenth century have remained with medical science to the current day: to make one's contribution to the total body of knowledge without inspecting the interstices and intersects of the content of that body of knowledge, to dig deeper into "nature's secrets" with little regard for the consequences, to look for causality in relatively isolated systems. In biophysics and bioengineering we find elaborate metaphors from hydraulics or plumbing (when speaking of the circulatory system) or electrical circuitry (when discussing the nervous system). While one can speak of neural "charges" or "discharges," one cannot go so far as to imagine the system as a phone system or computer. Like all metaphors, these can provide insight, and they can facilitate communication. But metaphors provide only the form for understanding; they do not imply isomorphic correspondences, that is, identical formal structures or identical relations between points.

Medical science frequently structures its research around linked propositions in which two or more concepts are reciprocally defined. We investigate the validity of linkages and, of course, usually find them. The case mentioned earlier of an effective placebo verifying a diagnosis of malingering is a good example. Similarly, we are told that early diagnosis improves survival. Of course, if mean patient survival time after contracting an illness is ten years, and if mean time at diagnosis is five years, "five-year survival" statistics will be dismal. If mean time at diagnosis can be reduced to three years, the five-year survival statistics will be dramatically improved. This change, of course, has no relationship to either the effectiveness of treatment or the course of the disease for any of the patients. Aggregates of linked concepts can be made as complex as you like, but, as Bateson has indicated, "the links are provided not by the data but by you" (1979).

BEYOND KUHN?

As for the scientific method, the same processes that have led us to truth have led us to error. We have been numbed by Kuhn into believing that new paradigms will be ever self-correcting in the scientific endeavor. But it is not "yet another paradigm" that will bring us into contact with the "extraneous factors." Kant, long before Kuhn, had noted that experience itself is a species of knowledge that involves understanding (1933:22). Since medical science does and must include behavior, one must apply Devereux's dictum that "the scientific study of man is impeded by an anxiety-arousing over-lap between subject and observer" (1967:xvi); therefore, perception and interpretation of data are distorted, producing "countertransference masquerading as methodology" causing even more distortion. Devereux meant that such structural "anxiety" exacerbates individual vulnerability, revives more idiosyncratic anxieties, threatens to undermine major defenses or sublimations, and exacerbates current problems (Devereux 1967:45).

An example might be provided by a patient with an illness that causes the physician to react to his patient as though he were an early significant figure in the physician's life. Even more pertinent to our present discussion, however, are recently documented professional practices of certain medical scientists who publish inaccurate statements either knowingly or unconsciously and unknowingly, who describe procedures that were not followed or followed in other experiments at other times, who "lose" primary data and/or have little direct involvement with the research leading to the articles of which they are "co-authors" (see Broad and Wade 1982; Knox 1983). "Anxiety," apparently, can be detrimental to medical as well as social scientists, nor is social science the only "science" in which one may confront the occupational risk—as noted by Weston La Barre—of "feeding multiply contaminated data into . . . truth machines" (Devereux 1967:viii).

Indeed the "progress" of science is highly dependent on peer recognition and disbursement of funds by the lay converted. It is a grievous oversimplification to contrast methodology in science with methodology in the social sciences. The development of either is highly dependent on interpersonal interactions, influence, and negotiation of "truth."

Some recent studies have focused on the field of medicine as socially constructed; an interesting collection of essays focuses on certain medical events as part of the social, political, economic, and cultural processes surrounding such events (Wright and Treacher 1982). Other social constructionists have researched the interactions among researches researchers in a laboratory (Salk Institute in La Jolla, California) to observe and analyze daily routine work. These investigators have demonstrated that, among other things, scientists create order out of disorder, impelled greatly if not exclusively by a thirst for credit and credibility (Latour and Woolgar 1979:189–

97). Personal goals notwithstanding, scientists do have an ideal about their "mission":

The myth of science as a purely logical process, constantly reaffirmed in every textbook, article and lecture, has an overwhelming influence on scientists' perception of what they do. Even though scientists are aware of non-logical elements of their work, they tend to suppress them or at least dismiss them as being of little consequence. A major element of the scientific process is thus denied existence or significance. (Broad and Wade 1982:126)

As a result of this, scientific textbooks are nonhistorical, in fact antihistorical. Any reference to the subjective experience is strictly forbidden in scientific literature, and "considered as a literary form, a scientific paper is as stylized as a sonnet. If it fails to obey the rigid rules of composition, it will simply not be published" (Broad and Wade 1982). Physicist Paul Feyerabend, in his book *Against Method* (1975), holds that not only are there nonrational elements in the scientific process, but that such elements are dominant, and that success in science depends not only on rational argument but on subterfuge, rhetoric, and propaganda. Authors Broad and Wade, who have made careers of investigating fraud in medical and scientific research, hold that fraud can flourish in such enterprises precisely because scientists are unaware of their ideologies and the wide ocean between such ideologies and praxis in their endeavors (1982:212–24).

CONCLUSION

We have examined how research paradigms in Western allopathic medicine rest on the ideology that the structure of science is unassailable as the researcher moves through better and better paradigms to "complete description" of "how things really work." We have categorized most of current medical scientific research into models (randomized clinical trials, chemical intervention, animal models, psychiatric models and diagnosis) to show how Western modes of thought expressed in philosophical systems provide the ideological linchpins for these models. We have also examined values and ideological system for its believers. For scientists, any "facts" (in the guise of extraneous factors) that do not validate the ideology are ignored or explained away as irrelevant to the "method." Epistemological flaws in the major research models to which we have alluded point to the more serious problem of how "science" really works and how we *think* it works. How we think it works is a "mentifact" distilled from centuries of philosophers and historians writing about science, with raw materials on "method" provided by the scientists themselves with themselves as appreciative critics (Goodfield 1975:218). Faking data (either consciously or unconsciously), unintentional bias, the "observer effect," and the question of whether one can make a justifiable distinction between science and other modes of thought are questions that have been addressed only recently—not only in medicine, but in anthropology as well (Broad and Wade 1982; Brush 1974; Feyerabend 1975; Goodfield 1975).

Like many other disciplines, medical science and practice have been affected by two twentieth-century movements, existentialism and phenomenology. Both have had similar concerns, stressing the relationship between the individual and systems, between freedom and choice, with anxiety, and with truth and belief as aspects of experience. Resonating to such concepts, there is an emergent contemporary disillusionment with incessant pressure built into the reward system constantly to produce "astounding scientific data." There is also an emergent demand for a new kind of accountability. There is a growing awareness of the lack of those virtues that generations of scientists have declared inherent in the scientific endeavor. Few are offended by Kuhn when he sees the "transfer of attachment form one paradigm to another" as "not the sort of battle that can be resolved by proofs," but rather as a "conversion experience." Confidence has been replaced by mistrust as the new fields of medical ethics and malpractice law prosper, and as a growing literature testifies to the new criticism of scientific research and its protocols.

The real challenge here is to recognize that even though science is not all that some scientists say it is, this does *not* mean that it is *none* of the things they say it is; one does not wish to throw out the baby with the bath. But scientists must recognize the extraneous factors that will define the new medical imperatives in our future cultural transformations.

It is possible that medical scientific pursuits, given world enough and time to incorporate eighteenth- and nineteenth-century philosophical trends (Burtt 1954), as well as some recent attempts to apply the phenomenological method (Spiegelberg 1960), might be able to stand outside a paradigm of all paradigms. We mean by this that consciousness of models, of process, and of the involved self—a constant vigilance against the arrogance of naive realism—will help to keep "ideologies" and "values" as generators of social action, but deprive them of their power to maim the intellect.

ACKNOWLEDGMENTS

We express special thanks to John Ross, Jr., M.D., Professor of Medicine, School of Medicine, University of California, San Diego, who provided valuable counsel on many aspects of contemporary medicine.

NOTES

1. Descartes warns his readers against casual criticism of his work: "I would like to warn [critics] that this movement [of the blood] that I have just explained follows

as necessarily from the mere disposition of the organs which may be observed in the heart by the eye alone, and from the heat which one can feel there with one's fingers, and from the nature of the blood which can be known by experience, as does that of a clock from the power, the position and the shape of its counterweights and its wheels" ([1637] 1960:68).

2. Reduction of risk, based on the published results, is only 4.5 percent; the 7 percent figure is reportedly "adjusted" by a technique not described in the study.

REFERENCES

Basaglia, Franco. 1980. "Breaking the Circuit of Control." *In Critical Psychiatry*. D. Ingleby, ed. New York: Pantheon.

———. 1981. *Scritti I: Dalla Psichiatria Fenomenologica all'Esperienza di Gorizia*. Turin: Einaudi.

Bateson, Gregory. 1979. *Mind and Nature: A Necessary Unity*. New York: Duggon.

Bidney, David. 1953. *Theoretical Anthropology*. New York: Columbia University Press.

Bridgman, P. W. 1927. *The Logic of Modern Physics*. New York: Macmillan.

Board, William, and Nicholas Wade. 1982. *Betrayers of the Truth: Fraud and Deceit in the Halls of Science*. New York: Simon and Schuster.

Brody, Howard. 1980. *Placebos and the Philosophy of Medicine: Clinical, Conceptual and Ethical Issues*. Chicago: University of Chicago Press.

Brush, S. G. 1974. "Should the History of Science Be X-Rated?" *Science* 183:1164–72.

Burtt, E. A. 1954. *The Metaphysical Foundations of Modern Science*. Rev. ed. Garden City, N.Y.: Doubleday.

CASS (Coronary Artery Surgery Study) Principal Investigators and Their Associates. 1983. "A Randomized Trial of Coronary Artery Bypass Surgery: Survival Data." *Circulation* 68:939–50.

Castiglioni, Arturo. 1934. *The Renaissance of Medicine in Europe*.

Crozatier, B. J., D. Franklin, John Ross, Jr., C. Bloor, F. C. White, H. Tomoike, and D. P. McKown. 1978. "Myocardial Infarction in the Baboon: Regional Function and the Collateral Circulation." *American Journal of Physiology: Heart Circulation Physiology* 235:H413–21.

Descartes, René. 1960. *Discourse on Method and the Meditations*. Trans. L. J. Lafleur. Indianapolis: Bobbs-Merrill. (First published 1637, Leyden.)

Devereux, George. 1967. *From Anxiety to Method in the Behavioral Sciences*. Paris and the Hague: Ecole Pratique des Hautes Etudes and Mouton.

Eddy, D. M., and C. H. Clanton. 1982. "The Art of Diagnosis: Solving the Clinicopathological Exercise." *New England Journal of Medicine* 306:1263–68.

Ell, Stephen R. 1980. "Interhuman Transmission of Medieval Plague." *Bulletin of the History of Medicine* 54:497–510.

Elstein, A S. 1978. *Medical Problem Solving: An Analysis of Clinical Reasoning*. Cambridge, Mass.: Harvard University Press.

Feigl, Herbert. 1953. "The Mind-Body Problem in the Development of Logical Empiricism." In *Readings in the Philosophy of Science*. H. Feigl and M. Brodbeck, eds. New York: Appleton-Century-Crofts, 612–26.

Feyerabend, Paul, ed. 1975. *Against Method*. London: Verso.

Fleck, Ludwig. 1979 [1935]. *Genesis and development of a Scientific Fact.* Thaddeus J. Trenn and Robert K. Merton, eds. Chicago: University of Chicago Press.

Foucault, Michel. 1975. *The Birth of the Clinic.* Trans. A. M. Sheridan Smith. New York: Vintage.

Goodfield, June. 1975. *Cancer under Siege.* London: Hutchinson.

Goodwin, J. S., J. M. Goodwin, and A. V. Vogel. 1979. "Knowledge and Use of Placebos by House Officers and Nurses." *Annals of Internal Medicine* 91:106–10.

Halvey, David N., ed. 1972. *The Merck Manual of Diagnosis and Therapy.* Rahway, N.J.: Merck Sharp and Dohme.

Harvey, William. 1978. *Exercitatio Anatomica de Motu Cordis et Sanguinis in Animalibus* (facsimile of 1628 Francofurti ed., Keynes English translation of 1928). Birmingham: Classics of Medicine Library.

Hite, C. 1974. "Bridging the U.S.-Soviet Psychiatric Gap." *Psychiatric News* 9 (part 1):6–17; 9 (part 2):30–32, 40.

Kant, Immanuel. 1933. *The Critique of Pure Reason.* 2nd ed. Trans. N. Kemp Smith. Chicago: University of Chicago Press. (First published 1781.)

Knox, Richard. 1983. "The Harvard Fraud Case: Where Does the Problem Lie?" *Journal of the American Medical Association* 249(14):1797–1803.

Kuhn, Thomas. 1970. *The Structure of Scientific Revolutions.* 2nd ed. Chicago: University of Chicago Press.

Latour, Bruno, and Steve Woolgar. 1979. *Laboratory Life: The Social Construction of Scientific Facts.* Sage Library of Social Research, vol. 80. London: Sage Publications.

Lee, K. L., F. McNeer, C. F. Starmet, P. Harris, and R. Rosati. 1980. "Clinical Judgement and Statistics: Lessons from a Simulated Randomized Trial in Coronary Artery Disease." *Circulation* 61:508–15.

Longhurst, John C., and John Ross, Jr. 1985. "Extracardiac and Coronary Vascular Effects of Digitalis. Symposium on William Withering and the Foxglove: The 200th Anniversary of His First Report." *Journal of the American College of Cardiology* 5(5):99A–105A.

LRCP (Lipid Research Clinics Program). 1984. "The Lipid Research Clinics Coronary Primary Prevention Trial Results; 1. Reduction of incidence of coronary heart disease." *Journal of the American Medical Association* 251:351–64.

Medical Letter on Drugs and Therapeutics. 1979. 21(2).

———. 1981. 23(3):9.

Moerman, Daniel E. 1983. "General Medical Effectiveness and Human Biology: Placebo Effects in the Treatment of Ulcer Disease." *Medical Anthropology Quarterly* 14(3):14–16.

Morgagni, Giovanni Battista. 1761. *De Sedibus et Causis Morborum per Anatomen Indagatis.* (Often reprinted; first English edition, 1769.)

Radine, Lawrence B. 1983. "Pangolins and Advocates: Vulnerability and Self-Protection in a Mental Patients' Rights Agency." In *The Anthropology of Medicine.* L. Romanucci-Ross, D. Moerman, and L. Tancredi, eds. New York: Praeger 366–87.

Reich, Walter, 1986. "Diagnostic Ethics: The Uses and Limits of Psychiatric Explanation." In *Ethical Issues in Epidemiologic Research.* L. Tancredi, ed. New Brunswick, N.J.: Rutgers University Press, 37–69.

Rollins, N. 1972. *Child Psychiatry in the Soviet Union*. Cambridge, Mass.: Harvard University Press.

Romanucci-Ross, Lola, and Laurence Tancredi. 1986. "Psychiatry, the Law, and Cultural Determinants of Behavior." *International Journal of Law and Psychiatry* 9(3):265–93.

Sanders, M., F. White, and C. Bloor. 1977. "Cardiovascular Responses of Dogs and Pigs Exposed to Similar Physiological Stress." *Comparative Physiology and Biochemistry* 58(A):365–70.

Schlick, M. 1925. *Allgemeine Erkenntnislehre*. 2nd ed. Berlin: Springer.

Selzer, Richard. 1976. *Mortal Lessons: Notes on the Art of Surgery*. New York: Simon and Schuster.

Shapiro, A. K. 1968. "The Placebo Response." In *Modern Perspectives in World Psychiatry*. J. G. Howells, ed. Edinburgh: Oliver and Boyd.

Snellen, H. A. 1984. *History of Cardiology*. Rotterdam: Donker Academic Publications.

Spiegelberg, H. 1960. *The Phenomenological Movement*. The Hague: Mouton.

Tancredi, Laurence. 1983. "Psychiatry and Social Control." In *The Anthropology of Medicine*. L. Romanucci-Ross, D. Moerman, and L. Tancredi, eds. New York: Praeger, 284–97.

Tomoike, H., D. Franklin, W. Scott Kemper, S. W. McKown, and John Ross, Jr. 1981. "Functional Evaluation of Coronary Collateral Development in Conscious Dogs." *American Journal of Physiology: Heart Circulation Physiology* 241: H519–24.

Wilder, Raymond. 1952. *Introduction to the Foundation of Mathematics*, New York: Wiley, 256–61.

Williams, Bernard. 1967. René Descartes. *The Encyclopedia of Philosophy*. Vol. 2. Paul Edwards, ed. New York: Macmillan, 344–54.

World Health Organization. 1973. *Report of the International Pilot Study of Schizophrenia*. Vol. 1. Geneva: WHO.

Wright, P., and A. Treacher. 1982. *The Problem of Medical Knowledge: Examining the Social Construction of Medicine*. Edinburgh: Edinburgh University Press.

19

"Medical Anthropology": Convergence of Mind and Experience in the Anthropological Imagination

LOLA ROMANUCCI-ROSS, DANIEL E. MOERMAN, AND LAURENCE R. TANCREDI

There is an uneasy fit of the biomedical into anthropological discourse. Medical discourse also finds integrating "the cultural" problematic. It often seems very difficult to translate things from one domain to the other; the organization, style, and sense of what is important differ between the two fields.

Works that claim to be biocultural anthropology seem usually to be mainly "bio" with a few inserts of the cultural here and there. The primary reason for this, we think, is that the "bio" aspect is the more quantifiable part, and thus appears more scientific, more manageable, less subject to challenge in an argument. Such quatified material is reified as data.

In the older anthropological tradition we had, in contrast, a more apparently intuitive ethnographic method, tribal studies and peasant studies. Subsequently we became somewhat more statistical, then we became ethnoscolars, and have since become interpretative. From this tradition in anthropology, how can we carry out an anthropology of biology or medicine and in that exercise emerge with a genuine appreciation of biomedical systems and, as well, learn the possible levels of integration of biomedical phenomena with cultural phenomena? A medical event is both biological *and* cultural, and since investigators are usually aligned with one aspect or the other of such an event, the simultaneity of the two aspects needs to be acknowledged. Integrating facts from the two realms of knowing has not been, and will not be, accomplished easily while we search for cause and effect. In this chapter we will first discuss the stance of an exponent of the biocultural approach as currently conceived. This will be followed by a consideration of rhetoric and intentionality in the physical sciences; we will then focus on what can be gleaned from some current research frontiers in the medical sciences to find a resolution to the biocultural dilemma.

TANGLED HYPOTHESES

We give an example that typifies the intellectual style in biocultural studies: Melvin Konner wrote a book called *The Tangled Wing* (1982) that presumably was meant to bridge the gap between the biological and the cultural. But note the subtitle: *Biological Constraints on the Human Spirit.* While he might have chosen to focus on culture as a device by which people can be liberated from biological constraints, he chose the reverse. The critical reader should be alerted.

Consider Konner's approach to one study he analyzes to illustrate bioanthropology. In a paper published in a well-known medical journal, the investigators described three intermarrying rural villages in the Dominican Republic (Imperato-McGinley et al. 1979). Over four generations, 19 persons appeared at birth to be female and were so raised. At puberty, they failed to develop breasts, male testes in the abdominal cavity descended, voices deepened, and the male genitalia appeared. At this point "physically and psychologically they became men." They were described by the researchers as genetically male with one X and one Y chromosome but lacking a single enzyme of the male sex hormone, 5-alpha-reductase:

The most extraordinary thing is that they became completely and securely men of their culture in every sense of the word. After twelve or more years of rearing as girls, with all the psychological influences encouraging that gender role in a rather sexist society, they are able to transform themselves into an almost typical example of the masculine gender. Of course they did not make the transformation with ease; some had years of psychological anguish. But they made it. (Konner 1982: 124–25)

The researchers reasoned that the testosterone circulating during the course of growth in these *machi-hembras* (male-females) had a masculinizing effect on the brain, an effect that "appears to contribute substantially to the formation of male gender identity when combined with the transforming effect of the further testosterone surge at puberty. . . . The effect of testosterone predominates, overriding the effect of rearing as girls" (Imperato-McGinley et al. 1979:1236).

Konner accepts this explanation without question. In fact, he places the author of this article in the company of his collection of distinguished "tough-minded" female researchers who devoted themselves "with great courage" (Konner 1982:106) to the question of whether sex differences in behavior have a basis that is in part biological. (We are not aware of any previous inquiry that has put such an assertion, thus stated, in doubt.) But he concludes, "After sexism is wholly stripped away . . . after differences in training have gone the way of the whalebone corset, there will still be something different, something that is grounded in biology . . . because men are more violent . . . that is merely a statement of plain observable fact" (Konner 1982:107).

Yet Konner appears to hold in highest esteem the sex-difference studies of Margaret Mead. Such studies made culture the salient (but not the exclusive) determinant of behavior (e.g., Mead 1962). He also appears to know that knowledge of the gender of the newborn is the first and most important question asked by its parents, so that they will "know how to act" toward the child—and, we might add, know how to *elicit the behavior* that the family and society need and want (Konner 1982:144).

A culture provides the conscious models for sex role behaviors, and one learns not only one's role but the complementary sex role as well. Both role descriptors are ascribed by society and internalized by the individual, and are responsive to external signs and signals. The culture of origin of the *machi-hembras* does indeed feature powerful disincentives to continuing female development along with the presence of male organs, a cultural rather than a biological constraint. We contend that the bioanthropologists should not rush to judgment in attributing the sudden assumption of masculinity to "a rush of testosterone."

Konner's delightful (if at times less than meticulously reasoned) book presents us with many studies that find biological bases for feelings of rage, fear, joy, lust, and love. Problematic with his approach, however, is the usual bioanthropological argument in which facts and creeds from the biological and social sciences are juxtaposed, but the mechanisms connecting them are not the demonstrable casual loops found in well-controlled prospective studies, which require controlling both cultural and biological differences simultaneously. Rather, we are confronted with myriad tropes in free association. Such casual approaches to complex problems have kept us, and will keep us, dangling from a pendulum that swings from cultural and psychosocial explanations to anatomical and physiological explanations, an exercise well exemplified by the history of psychiatry that we might try to avoid.

It takes sufficient sensitivity to the details of any culture to recognize that one learns not only one's own role but also and simultaneously the roles which contrast with it. In other words, while you are learning how to act, how to speak, how to dress, how to walk and talk, you are confronted with contrasting sets of how not to act, speak, dress, walk, and talk. The opposite role model is as important as the apposite one. Romanucci-Ross was struck with this in Italian fieldwork when she noted the relationship between the saints, who literally starved and wasted away, and the believers in these saints, who died from heart attacks, overeating for decades on long pilgrimages to shrines. Some of the saints had relinquished youthful lives of gluttony and carnality to achieve their sanctified states. No one thinks it necessary to introduce a hormone to explain the change from debauchery to abstinence, from indulgence to mutilation, from dominance to obedience.

Nowhere is this reversion to biology in the name of science more rampant then in the decades of studies on male-female differences in intelligence and other kinds of performance, although accounts of racial differences might be close in the movement toward old paradigms of causality. We do not assert that physiology has no influence on behavior or that cultural explanations are inevitably complete. Rather, we note that with reckless regularity biocultural explanations heavily emphasize the biological while tossing in a few statements to the effect that culture is also important, usually in the least relevant manner.

A BLACK HOLE HAS NO HAIR

We tend to think that the cultural part of biocultural anthropology is text and rhetorical, and that it relies heavily on the usage of tropes. This is taken by some as criticism. But we suggest that bioscience, indeed any science, has *always* used tropes and that *rhetoric* has always played a central role in science, even in the most technical treatises. We give many examples from the biological sciences. (See chapter 18 in this volume.) As is inevitably the case, however, the speakers do not recognize their own metaphors as being such; one of the most powerful aspects of culture is that it appears to its bearers as "natural."

Consider an example from the work of a renowned leader of the most physical of the physical sciences. [Stephen Hawking's interesting book *A Brief History of Time* (1988) was on the *New York Times* best-seller list for years.] Whether all those who have purchased a copy have read it is not clear; but if they have, they have been exposed to a wonderfully compelling, persuasive rhetorical and metaphorical argument. Here, for example, are the kernels of a series of sentences taken from the central chapter, "Black Holes." We leave out the substance of the argument, retaining only the rhetorical devices used to create what the author puts forth as logical linkages; the italics are added.

On this assumption ... Michell wrote. ... Michell *suggested*. ... [P]erhaps [Laplace] *decided* that it [black holes] was a *crazy* idea. ... How would it [a certain kind of star] *know* that it had to lose weight? ... Eddington was *shocked*. ... he *refused* to believe. ... Eddington thought it was simply not possible. ... Einstein ... *claimed*. ... The hostility of other scientists ... persuaded Chandrasekhar to abandon. ... This scenario is not entirely realistic. ... However, we *believe*. ... there *must* be a singularity. ... There are some solutions of the equations ... in which it is possible for ... [e.g., solutions are chosen, not proven]. There was, however, a different interpretation of [a certain] result ... *advocated* by [other scientists]. ... They *argued*. ... [Certain] calculations *supported* this view ... [while supposedly others supported another]. It was *conjectured* that . . . a black hole must settle down. . . . "A black hole has no hair." The "no hair" theorem . . . greatly restricts the possible types of black holes. . . . A black hole seems to be the only really *natural* explanation of the observations. (Hawking 1988:81–94)

Much could be made of the above in analysis but we confine ourselves to two emergent points in the reasoning. One, that theorems constrain nature (with which we completely agree); and two, that these analytical constructions (black holes)—inventions (fabulations, fabrications) of Hawking and his colleagues—are aspects of "nature," with which we also agree, insofar as we are prepared to argue that nature is a cultural invention.

ON BIOMEDICINE AND CAUSALITY

Physics is not without its interpretative slants and concomitant ambiguities of natural phenomena, as we have seen with some of Hawking's perceptions, but nowhere in science is the issue of causation regarding influences on natural events more problematic than in biomedicine. This can be well illustrated in the two areas of biomedicine currently representing the cutting edge of research: genetics and the neurosciences. Many geneticists would argue that the nature-nurture issue is near resolution (Wilson 1975; Paul 1988). The discovery and elucidation at this time of over four thousand diseases of genetic origin would appear to fuel the proposition that genes and biochemistry determine our destiny, parallel to Konner's interpretation of the *machi-hembras*. However, belief that genetics is the sole determinant of individual development ignores two critical factors affecting the manifestation of a genetic trait: *gene penetrance* and *gene expressivity*.

Penetrance refers to the presence of a gene that is causally related to the development of, for example, a disease; it does not mean that every individual carrying that gene will eventually develop that disease. To use Huntington's chorea as an example, it is argued that everyone who has that particular autosomal dominant gene will develop the disease—if he or she lives long enough (Chandler et al. 1960). The vast majority will develop the disease in their forties or fifties. A small tail effect will represent those who might develop the symptoms of Huntington's chorea at ten or eleven years of age or at sixty or sixty-five years of age (Farrer et al. 1984). However, Huntington's chorea appears to be 100 percent penetrating. On the other hand, many autosomal dominant conditions are penetrating in a varying percentage of cases, occasionally skipping generation(s), and may have a wide variety of expressions (Conneally 1984). For instance, neurofibromatosis (Von Recklinghausen's disease) may feature mild conditions identified only by the presence of café-au-lait spots; it may cause seriously deforming conditions involving the presence of fibromatous skin tumors, meningiomas,

acoustic neuroma, mental retardation, scoliosis, optic neuroma, and hypogly-
cemia (Crowe et al. 1956; Nicolls 1969; Riccardi 1981).

Why, if genetics is determinative of the individual, don't 100 percent of
those with the gene develop the condition? One explanation appears to be
that cofactors are essential to bring a condition into being. Such cofactors
include the presence of other genes creating biochemical substances, and
cultural or environmental factors interacting with genetic or biochemical determinants that either result in the penetration of the gene or impede its
development. The dynamics of penetrance, seen frequently with autosomal-
dominant conditions such as neurofibromatosis, has by no means been thoroughly understood. Schools of thought embrace various notions, of which
cofactors, genetic or cultural-environmental, tip the balance. Penetrance and
expressivity, discussed below, may more clearly explain the instancing of a
disease such as schizophrenia, which is considered not an autosomal-
dominant condition but a multigenetically caused condition in which environmental and cultural factors are strongly involved in causality. In
schizophrenia we find a concordance (of approximately 60%) among mono-
zygotic twins, giving support to the argument of the powerful effects of
environmental and cultural factors (Connor and Ferguson-Smith 1987).

The second critical factor is expressivity. Let us consider an individual
with the gene for a particular condition that has penetrated, that is, the
individual develops symptoms and signs associated with the genetic disease
(Holtzman 1989:233–35). We have seen here that the range of the ways in
which these symptoms manifest themselves is wide. Some individuals with
genetic conditions, such as Charcot-Marie-Tooth disease, may have minimal
symptoms and be nearly normal despite the presence of the autosomal-
dominant gene (McKusick 1986:no. 11820). Others may inherit the gene
and manifest severe disability consistent with the typical characterization of
a particular disease.

Differences in expressivity, despite the similarity of the genetic component, may reflect the presence or absence of genetic cofactors but in some
instances have been shown to be due to cultural or environmental differences. An excellent example of this is phenylketonuria (PKU), a genetically
autosomal-dominant condition with varying penetrance. However, even
where this condition occurs and an individual is susceptible to the symptomatology of PKU, habits of nutrition can affect its expressivity in a major
way. For example, in a culture relatively devoid of phenylalanine in the diet,
the expressivity of PKU would be markedly diminished in intensity. Ordinarily an individual with PKU would be severely retarded. However, when
the diet is modified very early, the retardation can be significantly attenuated. Cultural factors that influence diet and nutrition will directly influence
whether this disease will be manifested in its most severe form. It is con-
ceivable that an individual born with PKU in a culture in which the diet is

modified as a matter of (cultural) course would be seen as simply a minor deviation from the norm.

One might argue that this example does not directly address the thesis of those who argue that genetic or biohumoral agents determine such basic elements as personality, behavior, and personal identity. But does the inheriting of a genetic condition labeled "disease" really differ from gender identity? It is a genetically transmissible condition that affects biology and behavior, just as traits of "maleness" and "femaleness" affect biology and behavior? In part, we designate something as a disease if it has symptoms and disabilities that are incompatible with cultural values of normalcy. The designation of "disease" is very fluid, particularly with regard to behavioral and psychological conditions. Even in the case of physical conditions, what is considered a disease differs in various cultures on the basis of the percentage of individuals who possess the condition and the impact of that condition on other, potentially more serious disabilities (Nelkin and Tancredi 1989).

For example, in parts of Africa the sickle cell gene reaches substantial frequencies. The homozygous condition for this gene results in sickle cell anemia, a genetic disease that is nearly always fatal. However, it has been shown that heterozygous individuals—said to have the sickle cell trait—are less susceptible to malaria, which is endemic in the areas where the gene occurs (Livingstone 1958). The biogenetic condition leading to sickle cell trait therefore is pervasive and associated with a benefit thus rendering it unlikely to be classified as a disease; it is seen as merely a variant of the normal condition. Indeed, it is easy to show that if, in such a situation, one somehow eliminated the sickle cell gene from the population, thus eliminating mortality from sickle cell anemia, the overall mortality rate would actually increase due to malaria in unprotected individuals.

Biomedical notions of causality in the neurosciences are also problematic. In recent years research on the brain has been considered one of the major frontiers of biomedical explanation of the human condition (National Institute of Mental Health 1988). Consequently the brain is rapidly being targeted as the most exciting area of biomedical investigation. Developments such as the use of complex imaging technologies—positron emission tomography (PET), single photo emission tomography (SPECT), magnetoencephalography (SQUID), and computerized electroencephalography (CEEG and BEAM), to name a few—are major advances over earlier imaging technologies in that they provide for direct evaluation of brain function in normal living humans (Volkow and Tancredi 1991).

Such technologies have reinforced observations about brain function that had been, even in the recent past, highly inferential and based on clinical observation alone. With the use of positron emission tomography, for example, it is now possible to measure the brain's utilization of glucose, a substance necessary for cellular function, and thereby to determine which areas of the brain are activated under well-defined circumstances. Through the use of this technology, principles of brain function, such as brain organization, human variability, and openness and plasticity, can be examined directly from a biochemical and biophysiological perspective. Of these principles the most important, from the standpoint of examining the interaction of nature and nurture, is that of plasticity and openness.

"Plasticity" refers to the capacity of the brain to alter itself by virtue of external stimuli. Obviously this is most conspicuously seen through the process of learning, which essentially produces a "different" individual. External stimuli result in activation and stimulation of segments of the brain that create transformations not only of neurochemical characteristics but also of structural characteristics (Kolers 1979; Rose 1981). In addition to the activity of learning, other processes are responsible for brain remodeling. These include intervention through the use of pharmacological agents (Duncan et al. 1989), endocrinological alterations (Nottebohm 1989), a range of external insults (Cotman and Nieto-Sampedro 1985), and stress (Inoue et al. 1985). In relating external stimuli to internal response, the brain must be thought of as an open system. For although in some respects the brain is limited by its physical boundaries, in terms of its ability to transform and to be transformed it extends into both the world within and the world without; it influences the external world but at the same time incorporates features of that world in an integrative biological fashion (Gomez-Mont and Volkow 1982).

Clinical syndromes can be identified that demonstrate defects in the ability of the individual to interact with the environment. In the Kline-Levine syndrome of hypersomnia and hyperphagia (Lichtenberg 1982:344–45), a person loses the capacity to integrate the external environment effectively (Volkow and Tancredi 1991). In some variations of the syndrome, behaviors may be triggered by the external environment and dominate internal needs and desires. Such behaviors are frequently automated routines in the brain; a person may eat whenever food is placed in front of him, for example, even though he consumed a full meal only 15 minutes earlier; the mere presence of the food activates intention and behavior. Similarly, someone with this syndrome may, when placed in a bedroom, fall asleep immediately. Here again, the environment influences and in some respects controls behavior.

A similar syndrome (but in reverse, as it were) indicates a severe obsessive-compulsive disorder in which the internal environment elicits behaviors frequently dissonant with the external environment. An obsession becomes so compelling that it obfuscates the integrative function which normally would balance external stimuli with internal needs to inform individual action. In both of these illustrations, that of the Klein-Levine syndrome and that of the obsessive-compulsive disorder, conscious personal needs and desires give way to external or internal environmental influences (Zohar and Insel 1987).

Positron emission tomography studies have frequently documented abnormal function of the caudate and orbital frontal cortex of these patients (Baxter et al. 1987). They are in agreement with studies involving animals that have shown repetitive compulsive behavior when the caudate nuclei or orbital frontal cortex is destroyed (Kolb 1977). It has been postulated that a circuit exists involving the orbital frontal cortex, the ventral palladium, the caudate nucleus, and the medical thalamic nucleus that serves a major role in the pathogenesis of obsessive-compulsive disease (Volkow and Tancredi 1991; Modell et al. 1989).

Both clinical studies and position emission tomography studies indicate that brain remodeling involves a complex interplay of biological and cultural factors. Furthermore, it is important to note that there have been demonstrations, both clinical and biochemical, to suggest quite convincingly that externally or internally derived stimuli can bring about remodeling of the brain not only on a neurochemical level but also in terms of structural change (Volkow and Tancredi 1991). To this process we must add the fact of human variability indicating structural and functional differences in the brains of individuals; we are left with a complex calculus.

Because of this complex circuitry, much needs to be done to show causative linkages between specific external stimuli, be they learning or the introduction of pharmacological agents, and specific structural and neurochemical changes of the brain. Fortunately, we now have biochemical and biophysiological evidence to support inferential observations from clinical studies that the outside world *does* have an impact on shaping the brain of the individual. Social and cultural factors, coupled with the capacity of the brain to integrate information and to *intend* certain activities, create a direct interactive pattern. We have, in the studies alluded to above, a scientific basis to discredit simplistic studies that imply that sex differentiation, for example, is purely biochemical and biophysiological. The openness and plasticity of the brain do not dismiss the role of the biochemical and the biophysiological as mediating processes, but suggest instead that all the outside world, including the sociocultural, has a direct impact on biophysiological structure and function.

TOWARD A NEW LEVEL OF DISCOURSE

What should be questioned, then, is the finality and authority that many of our colleagues grant to science, to biology, to nature, as we puzzle things out. We assert that, insofar as we have any sense of them, these are things that we—anthropologists, biologists, physicians, physicists—construct in much the same manner as we construct anything else—hand axes, bridges, poems, equations, rituals—as concepts/objects that "hang together," "make sense," "seem right," and generally "fit."

Moreover, we challenge the notion endemic to much biological anthropology and biomedical research that we are observing a mechanical "other" through the two-way glass, as emic observers of the etic, whether the other be a pansy, a savage, or a thought, a disease, an illness, or a gene. "The notion that a numerical result should depend on the relation of an object to observer is in the spirit of physics in this century and is even an exemplary illustration of it" (Mandelbrot 1977:26). The observer in this view may be correct, but perhaps not completely. For we are now confronted with a tangle of wide arcs of causality in negotiating "facts" about the physical world, with more emicity in the process and with a growing recognition of both trends (see Bohr 1958; see also Feynman et al. 1966).

In the biological and medical sciences, as well as in the social sciences, we find objects of the same order studying classes of objects of which they are members, simultaneously subject to self and object to others. And, as indicated in examples above, in such sciences we test theories based on complementary and converging results that come from disparate methods of investigation. Negotiating facts and truths in such problem areas as we describe above may not be too different from negotiating "correct" ethnographic description in anthropology (for discussion of negotiating ethnography, see Geertz 1973; Habermas 1984; Romanucci-Ross 1985).

NEW DIRECTIONS

The debate as to whether culture or biology is the salient vector of behavior appears to continue unabated. We have given enough examples to indicate that it is not this illusory dichotomy which should now be problematic. In Western medical culture, however, we are historically accustomed to dualistic thought; even in our popular culture we speak of the "horns of a dilemma" (two dual symbols in this phrase, one a referent to an iconic sign, one linguistic). But it is possible to escape the paradigm entirely, and for our purposes it is necessary to learn to interpret properly the epistemological fallout of our new technologies and the possible interpretations of our studies of culture and events.

The newer technologies will give us the information (certainly not the values) to help us confront the chaos; we have alluded to several areas that provide opportunities for thinking on the frontier. In addition, again in the illustrations in this chapter, we can begin to understand that the manner in which we think about biological and physical data is not just a cultural act; the "hard data" themselves are, if you will, contaminated with, or constructed of, cultural inputs. All of this resolves itself into a question of where we situate our subjectivity.

Bourdieu asserts that we need a unified science of practice, and that such a science must describe those laws of transformation which govern the changing of different kinds of capital into symbolic capital (Bourdieu 1977: 117). He refers to economic structures, of course, but we borrow his metaphor, finding it appropriate to view information from various disciplines as capital. Different systems of information translated into "symbolic capital" can lead us to better appreciate the relationship between things or objects, and those persons (agents) shaped by their culture. We shape and define the nature of those knowledge domains which we revere as reality and therefore, with our consent, they rule the imagination. We have alluded to an example in the rhetorical devices of physicists to exemplify what is characteristic of many established scientific disciplines—an intention-based semantics. The reader is driven to ascribe meaning, but the road to meaning is carefully guided by the intent of the scientist-authors, an intent to convert the reader to a belief system. This is done through a subtle shift from words conveying thoughts to words presumably conveying things: "facts," causes, relationships (Grice 1989). Nor do we think that anthropology as a discipline is free of intentional works and pronouncements. Many anthropologists have thought of culture as the ultimate explanation, which raises the interesting question of where one could stand outside of it or find a lever long enough to arrange cultural words into meaningful constellations that are also dependable maps.

Medical anthropology has indeed enriched both anthropology and medicine, and will undoubtedly continue to do so. It is also a promising area for research in those knowledge domains composing the field; these are the domains that can be restructured into a new semantic field, a new grammar for avoiding the old paradigms of either/or. We need not look to biology or culture for the unique, "real," and exclusive cause for any of the phenomena we study. Biological events *are* biocultural; cultural events are also biological. Biological events and cultural events are equally and simultaneously biocultural. The materials we need to reach a new level of discourse are in our grasp; we have only to abandon outmoded approaches/disciplines to achieve an enlightening beginning for a new science.

REFERENCES

Baxter, L. R., M. E. Phelps, J. B. Mazziotta, B. H. Guze, J. M. Schwartz, and C. E. Selin. 1987. "Local Cerebral Glucose Metabolic Rates in Obsessive-Compulsive Disorder: A Comparison with Rates in Unipolar Depression and in Normal Controls." *Archives of General Psychiatry* 44:211–18.

Bohr, N. 1958. *Atomic Physics and Human Knowledge.* New York: John Wiley and Sons.

Bourdieu, Pierre. 1977. *Outline of a Theory of Practice.* Cambridge: Cambridge University Press.

Chandler, J. H., T. E. Reed, and R. N. Dejong. 1960. "Huntington's Chorea in Michigan." *Neurology* 10:148–53.

Conneally, P. M. 1984. "Huntington Disease: Genetics and Epidemiology." *American Journal of Human Genetics* 36:506–29.

Connor, J. F., and M. A. Ferguson-Smith. 1987. *Essential Medical Genetics*, 2nd ed. St. Louis, Mo.: Blackball Scientific Publications.

Cotman, C. W., and M. Nieto-Sampedro. 1985. "Progress in Facilitating the Recovery of Function after Central Nervous System Trauma." In *Hope for a New Neurology*. F. Nottebohm, ed. New York: New York Academy of Sciences, 83–204.

Crowe, F. W., W. J. Schull, and J. V. Neel. 1956. *A Clinical Pathological and Genetic Study of Multiple Neurofibromatosis*. Springfield, Ill.: Charles C. Thomas.

Duncan, G. E., I. A. Paul, K. R. Powell, J. B. Fassberg, W. E. Stumpf, and G. R. Breese. 1989. "Neuroanatomically Selective Down-Regulation of Beta Adrenergic Receptors by Chronic Imipramine Treatment." *Journal of Pharmacology and Experimental Therapeutics* 248:470–77.

Farrer, L. A., P. M. Conneally, and P. Yu. 1984. "The Natural History of Huntington Disease: Possible Role of 'Aging Genes.'" *Am J Med Genet* 18:115–23.

Fausto-Sterling, Anne. 1985. *Myths of Gender*. New York: Basic Books.

Feynman, R. F., R. B. Leighton, and M. Sands. 1966. *The Feynman Lectures on Physics*. Reading, Mass.: Addison-Wesley.

Freeman, Derek. 1983. *Margaret Mead and Samoa. The Making and Unmaking of an Anthropologic Myth*. Cambridge, Mass.: Harvard University Press.

Geertz, C. 1973. *The Interpretation of Cultures*. New York: Basic Books.

Gomez-Mont, F. A., and N. D. Volkow. 1982. "The Relevance of Systems Thinking for Psychiatry." In *General Systems Theory and the Psychological Sciences*. W. Gray, J. Fidler and J. Batttista, eds. Seaside, Calif.: Intersystems Publications, 91–102.

Grice, Paul. 1989. *Studies in the Way of Words*. Cambridge, Mass.: Harvard University Press.

Habermas, J. 1984. *The Theory of Communicative Action*. Trans. Thomas McCarity. London: Heinemann.

Hawking, Stephen W. 1988. *A Brief History of Time: From the Big Bang to Black Holes*. New York: Bantam.

Holtzman, N. A. 1989. *Proceed with Caution*. Baltimore, Md.: Johns Hopkins University Press.

Imperato-McGinley, J., R. E. Peterson, T. Gautier, and E. Sturlo. 1979. "Androgens and the Evolution of the Male Gender-Identity Among Male Pseudohermaphodites with 50-Reductase Deficiency." *New England Journal of Medicine* 300(22):1233–37.

Inoue, O., G. Akimoto, K. Hashimoto, and T. Yamasaki. 1985. "Alterations in Biodistribution of ^{3}H Ro 15–1788 in Mice by Acute Stress: Possible Changes in *in Vivo* Binding Availability of Brain Benzodiazepine Receptors." *International Journal of Nuclear Medicine and Biology* 12:369–74.

Kolb, B. 1977. "Studies on the Candate-Putamen and the Dorsomedial Thalamic Nucleus of the Rat: Implications for Mammalian Frontal Lobe Functions." *Physiological Behavior* 18:234–44.

Kolers, P. A. 1979. "A Pattern-Analyzing Basis of Recognition." In *Levels of Processing in Human Memory*. L. S. Cermak and F. I. M. Craik, eds. Hillsdale, N.J.: Lawrence Erlbaum.

Konner, Melvin. 1982. *The Tangled Wing: Biological Constraints on the Human Spirit*. New York: Holt, Rinehart and Winston.

Lichtenberg, R. 1982. *The Psychiatrist's Guide to Diseases of the Nervous System*. New York: John Wiley and Sons.

Livingstone, Frank B. 1958. "Anthropological Implications of Sickle Cell Distribution in West Africa." *American Anthropologist* 60:533–62.

McKusick, V. A. 1986. *Mendelian Inheritance in Man*. 7th edition. Baltimore, Md. and London: Johns Hopkins University Press.

Mandelbrot, Benoit. 1977. *The Fractal Geometry of Nature*. New York: Freeman.

Mead, Margaret. 1962. *Sex and Temperament in Three Primitive Societies*. New York: Mentor Books. (First published in 1935.)

Modell, J. G., J. M. Mountz, G. Curtis, and J. F. Gieden. 1989. "Neurophysiologic Dysfunction in Basal Ganglia/Limbic Striatal and Thalamocortical Circuits as a Pathogenetic Mechanism of Obsessive-Compulsive Disorder." *Journal of Neuropsychiatry* 1:27–36.

National Institute of Mental Health. 1988. *Approaching The Twenty-first Century: Opportunities for NIMH Neurosciences Research. Report to Congress on the Decade of the Brain*. Washington, D.C.: U.S. Department of Health and Human Services.

Nelkin, D., and L. Tancredi. 1989. *Dangerous Diagnostics: The Social Power of Biological Information*. New York: Basic Books.

Nicolls, E. M. 1969. "Somatic Variation and Multiple Neurofibromatosis." *Human Heredity* 19:473–79.

Nottebohm, F. 1989. "Testosterone Triggers Growth of Brain Vocal Control Nuclei in Adult Female Canaries." *Brain Research* 189:429–36.

Paul, Diane. 1988. "Eugenic Origins of Clinical Genetics." (Mimeodraft.) Boston: University of Massachusetts, Boston.

Riccardi, V. M. 1981. "Von Recklinghausen Neurofibromatosis." *New England Journal of Medicine* 305:1617–26.

Romanucci-Ross, Lola. 1983. "Apollo Alone and Adrift in Samoa: Early Mead Reconsidered." *Reviews in Anthropology* 10(3):85–92.

———. 1985. *Mead's Other Manus: Phenomenology of the Encounter*. South Hadley, Mass.: Bergin & Garvey.

Rose, S. P. 1981. "What Should a Biochemistry of Learning and Memory Be About?" *Neuroscience* 6:811–21.

Volkow, N. D., and L. Tancredi. 1991. "Biological Correlates of Mental Activity Studied with PET." *American Journal of Psychiatry* 148:439–43.

Wilson, E. O. 1975. *Sociobiology*. Cambridge, Mass.: Belknap Press.

Zohar, J., and T. R. Insel. 1987. "Obsessive-Compulsive Disorder: Psychological Approaches to Diagnosis, Treatment and Pathophysiology." *Biological Psychiatry* 22:667–87.

INDEX

About the Editors and Contributors

BARRY BOGIN is Professor of Anthropology at the University of Michigan, Dearborn.

LIBBET CRANDON-MALAMUD was, at the time of her untimely death, Associate Professor of Anthropology at the University of Arkansas.

JOEL E. DIMSDALE is Professor of Psychiatry at the University of California, San Diego, School of Medicine, and the Veteran's Administration Hospital in La Jolla, California. He is Editor-in-Chief of *Psychosomatic Medicine.*

NINA L. ETKIN is Professor of Anthropology at the University of Hawaii, Honolulu. She has conducted ethnological field research in Nigeria, Hawaii, and Indonesia, combining inquiry in ethnomedicine, diet and health, pharmaceuticals, and the pharmacology of foods and medicinal plants. She is Editor-in-Chief of the journal *Reviews in Anthropology.*

MICHAEL HEINRICH is anthropologist as well as biologist and Assistant Professor ("Hochschulassistent") at the Institute for Pharmaceutical Biology (School of Chemistry and Pharmacy) at the Albert-Ludwigs-University of Freiburg, Germany.

CLARA SUE KIDWELL is Professor of Native American Studies at the University of Oklahoma in Norman, Oklahoma.

ROBERT KUGELMANN is Professor of Psychology at the University of Dallas, Irving, Texas.

DANIEL E. MOERMAN is William E. Stirton Professor of Anthropology at the University of Michigan, Dearborn, and the author of the definitive work on the medicinal use of plants by Native Americans, *Medicinal Plants of Native America* (1986).

BERNARDO NG is Clinical Assistant Professor in the Department of Psychiatry at the University of California, San Diego, School of Medicine in La Jolla, California.

ALLEN F. ROBERTS is Professor of Sociology at the University of Iowa.

JENS D. ROLLNIK is in the Department of Medicine Psychology at Ruhr University of Bochum, Germany.

LOLA ROMANUCCI-ROSS is Professor of Family and Preventive Medicine at the University of California, San Diego, School of Medicine in La Jolla, California. She is also on the faculty of the Department of Anthropology at UCSD. She has done anthropological fieldwork in the South Pacific, Mexico, Italy, and among American Indian tribes. Among her books are *Conflict, Violence, and Morality in a Mexican Village*; *Mead's Other Manus*; *Phenomenology of the Encounter*; *One Hundred Towers, an Italian Odyssey of Cultural Survival*; and *Ethnic Identity, Creation, Conflict, Accommodation*.

PAUL J. ROSS is Adjunct Instructor in the Department of Anthropology at the University of Hawaii, and a member of the Oncology Staff at The Queens Medical Center, Honolulu. His present inquiries focus on applications in transcultural nursing.

HARVEY SHAPIRO is Professor of Anesthesiology at the University of California, San Diego, School of Medicine in La Jolla, California.

LAURENCE R. TANCREDI is Clinical Professor in the Department of Psychiatry, New York University School of Medicine, and a Research Associate at Brookhaven National Laboratories. He is author of numerous books and articles on Forensic Psychiatry, medical ethics, and the relationships between law and medicine. He practices psychiatry in New York City.

LINDA M. VAN BLERKOM is Professor of Anthropology at Drew University in Madison, New Jersey.

ISBN 0-89789-490-1

HARDCOVER BAR CODE